ADOLESCENT MEDICINE: STATE OF THE ART REVIEWS

Metabolic Challenges to Adolescent Health

GUEST EDITORS

Victor C. Strasburger, MD
Susan M. Coupey, MD

December 2008 • Volume 19 • Number 3

THE AMERICAN ACADEMY OF PEDIATRICS®

ADOLESCENT MEDICINE:
STATE OF THE ART REVIEWS
December 2008
Editor: Diane E. Lundquist
Marketing Manager: Marirose Russo
Production Manager: Shannan Martin

Volume 19, Number 3
ISBN 978-1-58110-289-5
ISSN 1934-4287
MA0435
SUB1006

Adolescent Medicine: State of the Art Reviews is published three times per year by the American Academy of Pediatrics, 141 Northwest Point Blvd, Elk Grove Village, IL 60007-1098. Periodicals postage paid at Arlington Heights, IL.

POSTMASTER: Send address changes to American Academy of Pediatrics, Department of Marketing and Publications, Attn: AM:STARs, 141 Northwest Point Blvd, Elk Grove Village, IL 60007-1098.

Subscriptions: Subscriptions to *Adolescent Medicine: State of the Art Reviews* (AM:STARs) are provided to members of the American Academy of Pediatrics' Section on Adolescent Health as part of annual section membership dues. All others, please contact the AAP Customer Service Center at 866/843-2271 (7:00 am–5:30 pm Central Time, Monday–Friday) for pricing and information.

Adolescent Medicine: State of the Art Reviews

Official Journal of the American Academy of Pediatrics
Section on Adolescent Health

EDITORS-IN-CHIEF

VICTOR C. STRASBURGER, MD, FAAP, Professor of Pediatrics, Division of Adolescent Medicine, University of New Mexico, School of Medicine, Albuquerque, New Mexico

DONALD E. GREYDANUS, MD, FAAP, Professor of Pediatrics, Michigan State University; and Pediatrics Program Director, Kalamazoo Center for Medical Studies, Kalamazoo, Michigan

GUEST EDITORS

VICTOR C. STRASBURGER, MD, FAAP, Professor of Pediatrics, Division of Adolescent Medicine, University of New Mexico, School of Medicine, Albuquerque, New Mexico

SUSAN M. COUPEY, MD, Professor of Pediatrics and Chief, Adolescent Medicine, Albert Einstein College of Medicine, Children's Hospital at Montefiore, Bronx, New York

CONTRIBUTORS

LEE A. BRICKER, MD, Department of Internal Medicine, Michigan State University/Kalamazoo Center for Medical Studies, Kalamazoo, Michigan

MONIQUE COLLIER, MD, Division of Adolescent Medicine, Departments of Pediatrics, Children's Hospital at Montefiore, Albert Einstein College of Medicine, Bronx, New York

MARTIN B. DRAZNIN, MD, FAAP, Departments of Pediatrics and Human Development, Michigan State University College of Human Medicine, East Lansing, Michigan; Pediatric Endocrinology Subspecialty Clinics, Michigan State University Kalamazoo Center for Medical Studies, Kalamazoo, Michigan

SHIRA FELDMAN, MPH, RD, Division of Epidemiology and Community Health, School of Public Health, University of Minnesota, Minneapolis, Minnesota

COLLEEN FREEH FLATTUM, MS, RD, Division of Epidemiology and Community Health, School of Public Health, University of Minnesota, Minneapolis, Minnesota

DONALD E. GREYDANUS, MD, FAAP, Departments of Pediatrics, Michigan State University/Kalamazoo Center for Medical Studies, Kalamazoo, Michigan

ZEEV HAREL, MD, Division of Adolescent Medicine/Hasbro Children's Hospital/ Rhode Island Hospital, Providence, Rhode Island; Department of Pediatrics, Warren Alpert Medical School of Brown University, Providence, Rhode Island

MARJORIE J. HOGAN, MD, Department of Pediatrics, University of Minnesota, Minneapolis, Minnesota; Department of Pediatrics, Hennepin County Medical Center, Minneapolis, Minnesota

MARC S. JACOBSON, MD, Department of Pediatrics and Epidemiology, Albert Einstein College of Medicine, Great Neck, New York

BRIAN P. JENSSEN, BA, University of Rochester School of Medicine and Dentistry, Rochester, New York

AMY B. JORDAN, PhD, Annenberg Public Policy Center, University of Pennsylvania, Philadelphia, Pennsylvania

UNAB I. KHAN, MD, Division of Adolescent Medicine, Departments of Pediatrics and Family and Social Medicine, Children's Hospital at Montefiore, Albert Einstein College of Medicine, Bronx, New York

EMILY K. KRAMER-GOLINKOFF, BA, Marketing Communications, University of Pennsylvania Health System, Philadelphia, Pennsylvania

NICOLE LARSON, PhD, MPH, RD, Division of Epidemiology and Community Health, School of Public Health, University of Minnesota, Minneapolis, Minnesota

PAMELA J. MURRAY, MD, MHP, Department of Pediatrics, Children's Hospital of Pittsburgh and University of Pittsburgh School of Medicine, Pittsburgh, Pennsylvania

DIANNE NEUMARK-SZTAINER, PhD, MPH, RD, Division of Epidemiology and Community Health, School of Public Health, University of Minnesota, Minneapolis, Minnesota

REBECKA PEEBLES, MD, FAAP, Division of Adolescent Medicine, Department of Pediatrics, Stanford University School of Medicine

CHRISTINE A. PETRICH, MEd, Division of Epidemiology and Community Health, School of Public Health, University of Minnesota, Minneapolis, Minnesota

ERIC SIGEL, MD, Department of Pediatrics, University of Colorado Denver Health Science Center, Children's Hospital, Aurora, Colorado

MARY STORY, PhD, RD, Division of Epidemiology and Community Health School of Public Health, University of Minnesota, Minneapolis, Minnesota

VICTOR C. STRASBURGER, MD, FAAP, Departments of Pediatrics and Family and Community Medicine and Division of Adolescent Medicine, Department of Pediatrics, University of New Mexico School of Medicine, Albuquerque, New Mexico

METABOLIC CHALLENGES TO ADOLESCENT HEALTH

CONTENTS

Preface

Metabolic Challenges to Adolescent Health

The problem of metabolic disorders in adolescence has recently exploded onto the scene with the epidemic of childhood and adolescent obesity. Many of us "vintage" pediatricians and adolescent specialists have never had to deal with type 2 diabetes or metabolic syndrome until recently. Adolescence is a time of rapid growth, but sometimes it is not rapid enough to out-distance the accumulation of total body fat from a variety of different sources. Do the media cause obesity? Are there programs that have been successful in dealing with overweight and obese adolescents? Can we safely offer the option of bariatric surgery to severely obese teenagers? At the same time, constant progress is being made with more "traditional" problems such as eating disorders and bone growth. What can the practitioner do in his or her own office with these significant metabolic problems? The authors of this issue of *AM:STARs* seek to provide the answers to at least some of these vexing questions.

This issue represents the last issue with Dr Susan Coupey as a guest editor and as a member of the editorial board. Similarly, Dr Manny Schydlower is also retiring from the editorial board after this issue. *AM:STARs* is now in its 19th year of publication. Drs Coupey and Schydlower have been with us from the beginning, and they have been invaluable to both Don Greydanus and I as co–editors-in-chief. Their cheerful counsel and willingness to volunteer are deeply appreciated. We will miss them dearly.

Victor C. Strasburger, MD
Chief, Division of Adolescent Medicine
University of New Mexico School of Medicine
Albuquerque, New Mexico

 ISSN 1934-4287

Adolesc Med 19 (2008) 357–379

The Adolescent Obesity Epidemic: Why, How Long, and What to Do About It

Nicole Larson, PhD, MPH, RD*, Mary Story, PhD, RD

Division of Epidemiology and Community Health, School of Public Health, University of Minnesota, 1300 South Second Street, Suite 300, Minneapolis, MN 55454, USA

The epidemic of obesity among adolescents is a serious public health concern bearing great health and economic consequences.[1] Obese adolescents are at increased risk for several adverse health outcomes and are ~3 times more expensive for the health care system than the average young person.[2] Consequently, increases in the prevalence of obesity have been associated with dramatic increases in US health care costs.[3] Metabolic and physiologic abnormalities associated with obesity in adolescence (eg, hypertension, dyslipidemias, orthopedic problems, type 2 diabetes) tend to track into adulthood along with the condition of obesity itself.[4–6] One in 8 obese adolescents will remain obese as an adult. If the epidemic of obesity is not stemmed or reversed, it may result in a decrease in life expectancy for the first time in 200 years.[7]

The public health response to obesity needs to be informed by current knowledge of what groups are at greatest risk and modifiable contributing factors. In this literature review we address (1) trends and identified disparities in the prevalence of adolescent obesity, (2) behavioral and environmental factors that contribute to the development of obesity, and (3) what efforts are needed to reduce obesity.

NATIONAL TRENDS IN ADOLESCENT OBESITY

A striking worldwide increase in the prevalence of obesity occurred among young people during the latter part of the 20th century. Among adolescents in the United States, the prevalence of obesity tripled between 1966 and 1999 (from 4.6% to 15.5%).[8] During this same period, obese adolescents as a group became heavier. The average extent by which adolescents exceeded the BMI (weight/height^2 [kg/m^2]) threshold for obesity more than doubled.[9] National surveillance data for the years 1999–2006 indicate that the prevalence of obesity has not significantly increased in recent years; however, rates of overweight (85th per-

*Corresponding author.
E-mail address: larsonn@umn.edu (N. Larson).

 ISSN 1934-4287

centile $<$ BMI $<$ 95th percentile) and obesity (BMI $\geq$ 95th percentile) have remained high.[10] Current estimates indicate that one third of adolescents aged 12 to 19 years are either overweight (16.5%) or obese (17.6%).[10]

GROUPS AT HIGH RISK FOR OBESITY

Increases in the prevalence of obesity have occurred among adolescents of all socioeconomic, racial, and ethnic groups, but notable disparities exist. There is considerable evidence that low parental education increases risk for obesity.[11] For example, a study that primarily used parental education to determine socioeconomic status in 4746 Minnesota adolescents found large differences in obesity rates across socioeconomic groups. The results showed that 33% of girls and 36% of boys in families of low socioeconomic status were either overweight or obese compared with 21% of girls and 28% of boys in families of high socioeconomic status.[12] Other determinants of socioeconomic status, such as parental income and occupation, may also have an impact but are less consistently related to risk for obesity in youth.[11] National surveillance data for youth aged 15 to 17 years indicate that obesity rates are greater among adolescents from poor families (23%) than adolescents from nonpoor families (14%).[13] Similar income disparities were observed in male and female adolescents of non-Hispanic white race, but no income disparities were found among adolescents of non-Hispanic black race or youth aged 12 to 14 years.

Socioeconomic disparities in obesity differ across racial and ethnic groups and do not fully explain noted racial and ethnic disparities in rates of obesity.[14] National surveillance data indicate that rates of overweight and obesity are greater among non-Hispanic black and Mexican American youth when compared with rates among non-Hispanic white youth (12 to 19 years).[10] The prevalence of overweight or obesity is 44% in non-Hispanic black girls and 37% in Mexican American girls compared with just below 32% in non-Hispanic white girls. Among boys, the prevalence of overweight or obesity is similar in non-Hispanic white (34%) and non-Hispanic black (32%) adolescents but notably higher in Mexican American (40%) adolescents. There are limited data on obesity rates in American Indian and Asian/Pacific Islander youth; however, the data suggest that the burden of obesity is also great among these groups. For example, a study that measured youth on 12 reservations in North Dakota, South Dakota, Nebraska, and Iowa revealed that >37% of American Indian boys and >40% of American Indian females girls aged 12 to 17 years were either overweight or obese.[15]

In addition to the considerable disparities across socioeconomic, racial, and ethnic groups, there are regional differences in the prevalence of obesity. Rates of overweight and obesity are increased among youth residing in rural areas and southern US states. The 2003 National Survey of Children's Health showed that youth (aged 5–18 years) residing in rural areas had 25% higher odds of being overweight or obese compared with youth living in metropolitan areas, independent of race and household income.[16] Data from this survey also showed the prevalence of obesity to be much greater in the east southcentral (19%) and west southcentral (18%) regions of the United States than in the mountain region (11%).[17] After statistical adjustment for regional differences in race, ethnicity, household poverty, and physical activity behaviors, youth (aged 10–17 years) living in east southcentral and west southcentral regions had 46% and 52% higher odds, respectively, of being obese compared with youth living in the mountain region.

FACTORS CONTRIBUTING TO OBESITY IN ADOLESCENTS

A wide range of behavioral, environmental, and genetic factors contribute to the development of obesity in adolescents (see Fig 1). Obesity develops when there is a regular imbalance between the amount of energy consumed as food and beverages and the energy expended to support normal growth and development, metabolism, and physical activity.[1] However, the balance between energy intake and energy expenditure is not simple; many factors influence what and how much youth eat and how much and what types of physical activity they do. Behavioral factors that have been identified as important targets for population-based and

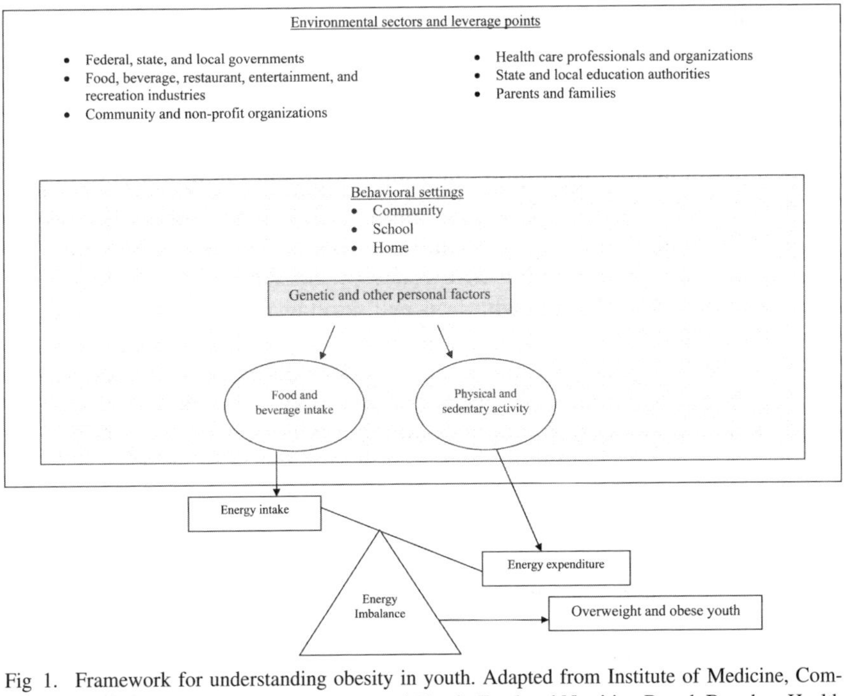

Fig 1. Framework for understanding obesity in youth. Adapted from Institute of Medicine, Committee on Prevention of Obesity in Children and Youth, Food and Nutrition Board, Board on Health Promotion and Disease Prevention. *Preventing Childhood Obesity: Health in the Balance*. Washington, DC: National Academies Press; 2005.

primary care interventions are highlighted here along with influencing factors in the eating and activity environments of youth.[1,18–20]

Sugar-Sweetened Beverage Consumption

National survey data show that sugar-sweetened beverages provide 13% of adolescents' total energy intake and are the single leading source of added sugars in the diets of male and female adolescents.[21,22] The majority of calories from sugar-sweetened beverages are consumed in the home. Adolescents have reported that the purchase source of most sugar-sweetened beverage calories is a store (69%); however, 18% are obtained from restaurants, and ~5% are obtained from vending machines or school cafeterias.[22] Evidence from observational and experimental research indicates that youth do not completely compensate for the energy they consume in sugar-sweetened beverages.[23] As a result, regular consumption of sugar-sweetened beverages may lead to increases in total energy intake and weight gain. Research suggests that interventions designed to reduce intakes of sugar-sweetened beverages could help to prevent excess weight gain in adolescents. Environmental influences on consumption, including parental norms for soft-drink consumption and the availability of beverages at home, school, and restaurants, should be addressed as part of interventions.[24,25]

Fruit and Vegetable Consumption

Fewer than 1% of boys and only 1.5% of girls aged 14 to 18 years consume the recommended amount of fruits (1.5–2.5 cups) and vegetables (2–4 cups) per day, which is based on individual energy needs.[26] Eating more fruits and vegetables could help youth to reduce their energy intake and avoid excess weight gain, because these foods are high in fiber and tend to have a low energy density (kcal/g). Because of their composition, fruits and vegetables are filling and can help to displace more energy-dense foods in the diet.[27] The evidence base directly linking weight status with fruit and vegetable consumption in youth is not strong; however, increasing consumption of these foods may also benefit overall nutritional health and reduce risk for future chronic disease. Research in adolescents has found that several factors in their home, school, and neighborhood environments are related to consumption.[28–33] For example, when a pilot study lowered prices on fresh fruits and vegetables by 50% in 2 high school cafeterias, sales of fruit were found to increase fourfold, and sales of baby carrots doubled.[28] Other research suggests that young people eat more fruits and vegetables if they observe their parents eating these foods and live in a neighborhood with ready supermarket access and limited access to convenience stores.[29–33]

Eating at Fast-Food Restaurants

Although youth consume the majority of their total energy intakes at home, national nutrition surveys have indicated that 50% of adolescents eat something from a fast-food restaurant on any given day.[34,35] Adolescents report eating at a fast-food restaurant an average of 2 days/week and have higher intakes of total energy on days when fast food is consumed.[35–37] Because fast-food menu items are typically energy dense and offered in large portion sizes, eating frequently at fast-food restaurants may lead to a positive energy balance and excess weight gain over time.[38–40] Several cross-sectional and prospective observational studies have found that frequency of eating at fast-food restaurants is a risk factor for obesity and increased weight gain over time.[36,41–43] Fast foods are frequently promoted to adolescents and are widely available in environments where youth spend time. Adolescents view an average of 4 advertisements for fast foods on television every day and may also be exposed to fast-food marketing when they go to school.[44] Brand-name fast foods (eg, Pizza Hut, Taco Bell, Subway) are sold in 19% of middle schools and 23% of high schools.[45] In addition, other research has indicated that fast-food restaurants tend to cluster in school neighborhoods; nationwide, 37% of secondary schools are within walking distance of at least 1 fast-food restaurant.[46–48] These findings suggest that efforts to reduce obesity in adolescents should address food marketing and neighborhood access to fast foods.

Food and Beverage Portion Sizes

Average portion sizes for most foods and beverages consumed in fast-food restaurants and at home have increased since the 1970s, concurrently with population increases in the prevalence of obesity.[38,49] For example, salty snacks consumed by the US population aged 2 years and older increased in size from an average of 1.0 to 1.6 oz (from 552 to 941 kJ [132–225 kcal]) between 1977 and 1996.[49] Few studies have examined the influence of portion sizes on obesity in adolescents; however, at least 1 study has observed a positive relationship between meal portion size and age-specific BMI percentile.[50] In addition, there is strong evidence that youth tend to eat less when they are served an age-appropriate portion or allowed to self-select their own portion.[51,52] Research suggests that eating environments should optimally provide a variety of nutrient-dense foods and allow youth to decide how much they will eat by serving themselves.

Physical Activity

The majority of adolescents in the United States have physical activity levels that are lower than recommended. For example, the 2007 Youth Risk Behavior Surveillance System survey of high school students revealed that only 44% of boys and 26% of girls met the guideline to accumulate at least 60 minutes of physical activity ≥5 days/week.[53] The expenditure of energy in regular physical activity can help young people to balance their energy intakes. There is strong evidence that daily moderate-to-vigorous physical activity can help overweight and obese youth to reduce their weight.[19] Although there is not consistent evidence to support a relationship between physical activity and reduced risk of excess weight gain among youth at a healthy weight, maintaining an active lifestyle benefits several aspects of health.[19] As young people accumulate physical activity throughout the day in active transportation (eg, biking to the store), free play (eg, swimming at the beach), structured activity (eg, competing in organized sports), and work-related activities (eg, mopping the floor, mowing the lawn), overall activity levels may be influenced by multiple layers of the environment. Environmental characteristics that have been found to be positively associated with physical activity among adolescents include the number of exercise aids (eg, fitness equipment) in their home,[54,55] parent and peer support for physical activity,[56,57] school campus size,[58] and the number of recreational facilities and other destinations of interest within walking distance from home.[55,59,60]

Recreational Screen Time

In contrast to current recommendations to limit recreational screen time to no more than 1 or 2 hours/day,[61] youth have reported report high levels of media exposure. A nationally representative survey found that, on average, adolescents aged 11 to 14 years spend 4.5 hours and adolescents aged 15 to 18 years spend 3.5 hours daily with screen media (see Fig 2). In addition, youth have reported spending >1 hour/day using a computer for recreation (ie, playing video games, surfing the Internet).[62] Several observational studies have revealed a relationship between screen time and increased rates of obesity and metabolic syndrome in youth, and intervention studies have further demonstrated that reducing screen time helps to prevent excess weight gain.[63–67] Recreational screen time may contribute to energy imbalance and the development of obesity by (1) consuming time that might otherwise be spent burning energy in physical activity, (2)

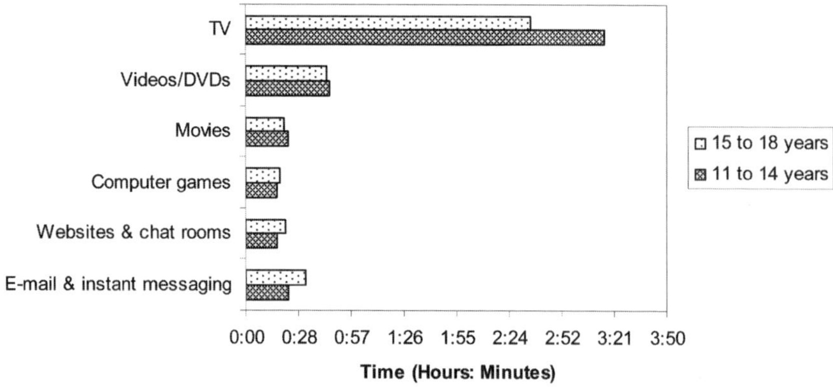

Fig 2. Average daily screen time among adolescents aged 11 to 14 and 15 to 18 years. Source: Roberts D, Foehr U, Rideout V. Generation M: Media in the lives of 8–18 year-olds. Available at: www.kff.org/entmedia/entmedia030905pkg.cfm.

decreasing resting metabolic rate during screen time, (3) increasing snacking during screen time, and (4) promoting the consumption of energy-dense foods and beverages.[1] Adolescents (aged 13–17 years) view ~17 food or beverage advertisements on television each day, which amounts to an average of 40 hours over 1 year.[44] Advertisements for energy-dense products such as candy, snack foods, sugary cereals, and fast foods are viewed most often.[44,68,69] Other research in adolescents suggests that several characteristics in the home environment may influence screen time. Adolescents have been found to spend more time with screen media if they have a television in their bedroom or have pay television, there are few household rules regarding screen time, and their parents have high levels of media exposure.[63,70–72]

EFFORTS NEEDED TO REDUCE OBESITY

Reducing adolescent obesity has been identified as a national public health priority by the Institute of Medicine (IOM) and numerous other expert groups.[1,73,74] Interventions designed to establish healthy eating and physical activity behaviors are needed to treat and prevent obesity; however, research has indicated that it is unlikely that such efforts will be sufficient to reverse population increases in obesity. The public health response to obesity should be broad-based, emphasize prevention, and target corrective changes in the eating and activity environments of youth. Although much remains to be learned about the efficacy of various environmental and policy interventions, such efforts have the potential to greatly impact obesity in the population and reduce inequities. Future efforts to reduce obesity should be informed by ongoing efforts across the nation and the research-based recommendations of expert groups. The IOM has developed an action plan that includes recommendations for each level of government, industries, local communities, health care professionals and organizations, schools, and families.[1,75] Recommendations of particular relevance to adolescents are listed in Table 1, and selected examples of ongoing efforts to reduce obesity are reviewed briefly below.

Federal, State, and Local Governments

On the federal level, despite increased attention to the obesity epidemic and the introduction of several bills designed to address contributing factors, few bills have been passed.[76] Recent examples of federal legislation that address obesity in youth include the 2008 Farm Bill and the 2004 Child Nutrition and the WIC (Special Supplemental Nutrition Program for Women, Infants, and Children) Reauthorization Act. The 2008 Farm Bill allocates funding for demonstration projects to address obesity in low-income communities and provides for a nationwide expansion of the Fresh Fruit and Vegetable Program.[77,78] By 2012 the expansion of this program will provide for the school-based distribution of free fresh fruits and vegetables to 3 million low-income youth in all 50 states.[77] The 2004 Child Nutrition and WIC Reauthorization Act also addresses supports

Table 1
Summary of selected recommendations for promoting healthful eating behaviors and regular physical activity

Federal government	Program and research efforts designed to prevent and reduce obesity in high-risk youth populations should be provided expanded funding.
	Federal nutrition-assistance programs and agricultural policies should be assessed and modified as needed to ensure that they promote healthy behaviors for all youth.
	Pilot projects designed to promote healthful dietary intake and physical activity should be developed and evaluated within the nutrition-assistance programs.
State and local governments	Coordinated leadership, funding, and policy development should support obesity-prevention efforts in youth, particularly those focused on high-risk populations.
	Public health agencies and community coalitions should be provided support for collaborative efforts to promote and evaluate obesity-prevention interventions.
	Comprehensive plans, capital-improvement programs, zoning guidelines, and subdivision ordinances should be revised to increase the availability and accessibility of opportunities for physical activity (ie, recreational facilities, parks, playgrounds, sidewalks, bike paths) in new and existing areas.
	The street, sidewalk, and street-crossing safety of routes to school should be improved, and schools should be built within walking and bicycling distance of the neighborhoods they serve.
Industry	Products, packaging, and marketing strategies that help youth and families make healthful choices in terms of energy density, nutrient density, and serving sizes should be developed by food and beverage industries.
	A greater number and variety of healthful food options should be made available in restaurants, along with information on the calorie and nutritional content of products at the point of purchase.
	Products and opportunities that promote regular physical activity and reduce sedentary behaviors should be developed by leisure, entertainment, and recreation industries.
	Rigorous standards for food and beverage marketing to youth should be established and enforced in collaboration with government, scientific, public health, and consumer groups.
Community and nonprofit organizations	The availability of opportunities for physical activity and healthful eating should be measured.
	Programs that address social, economic, and environmental barriers to healthy eating and physical activity should be provided expanded support.
	New and existing programs that promote healthful eating behaviors and regular physical activity in youth populations should be developed, evaluated, and supported over the long-term.
	Access to supermarkets, farmers' markets, and community gardens should be expanded to support healthful food options.

(Continued)

Table 1
(Continued)

Health care professionals and organizations	BMI should be routinely tracked, and relevant evidence-based counseling should be provided to youth and their families.
	Evidence-based clinical guidance and programs should be disseminated to providers by their respective professional organizations.
	Obesity-prevention knowledge and skills should be required as part of training programs for health care providers.
Schools and state and local education authorities	Nutritional standards should ensure that all food and beverage items sold or served in schools are healthful.
	Meals served or sold in schools should be in compliance with the Dietary Guidelines for Americans.
	Youth should participate in a minimum of 30 min of moderate-to-vigorous physical activity during the school day.
	Opportunities for physical activity should be expanded through physical education classes; sports programs and physical activity clubs; use of school recreation facilities outside of school hours; and walking- and biking-to-school programs.
	Health curricula should be enhanced to devote adequate attention to the development of lifestyle behaviors that promote energy balance (ie, improving eating habits, increasing regular physical activity, reducing sedentary behaviors).
	School policies should ensure that facilities are advertising-free to the greatest possible extent.
	Annual assessments of each student's weight, height, and gender- and age-specific BMI percentile should be performed and provided to parents.
	Policies and practices relevant to nutrition and physical activity should be reviewed periodically, and the implementation of policies should be monitored.
Parents and families	Healthful food and beverage options should be available at home and served at meals.
	Youth should be provided with guidance in making healthful decisions regarding the types of foods and beverages to consume, how often, and in what portion size.
	Regular physical activity should be encouraged and supported.
	Television viewing and recreational screen time should be limited to <2 h/d.
	Caregivers should model healthful eating and physical activity behaviors for their children.

Adapted from Institute of Medicine, Committee on Prevention of Obesity in Children and Youth, Food and Nutrition Board, Board on Health Promotion and Disease Prevention. *Preventing Childhood Obesity: Health in the Balance*. Washington, DC: National Academies Press; 2005. Dietary Guidelines for Americans from US Department of Agriculture. Dietary guidelines for Americans 2005. Available at: www.health.gov/dietaryguidelines. Accessed June 9, 2008.

for eating and physical activity at school but emphasizes local control over universal standards. Schools participating in federal child nutrition programs are required to have a wellness policy that addresses nutritional guidelines for all foods available on campus and goals for physical activity.[79] However, the law does not require that wellness policies be made more restrictive than limited federal regulations. In addition, many school wellness policies are not being implemented as planned.[80] Research conducted to identify obesity policy options that would be politically feasible and likely to have a significant public health impact might be used to guide the next steps of policy makers and opinion leaders (see Table 2).[76] It is evident from this research that much work is needed to change public opinion and build a solid scientific foundation for higher-impact policies such as bans and mandates to increase their political feasibility.

Much attention has also been focused on the obesity epidemic at the state and local levels of government. In recent years several states have enacted legislation to promote healthy eating and physical activity.[81] Selected examples of legislation introduced in 2007 are highlighted in Table 3. The work of policy makers across the country to address obesity in youth have led to[81]:

- the creation of a task force or the launching of a pilot project in 25 states;
- new legislation to increase farm-to-school programs or improve the nutritional quality of school breakfasts, lunches, à la carte selections, or vending machine offerings in 16 states;
- new legislation to promote farmers' markets in 7 states;
- support for policies to strengthen physical education classes or physical activity programs at school in 16 states; and
- new legislation concerning student BMI measures and/or physical fitness assessments in 11 states.

Although much work is still needed, ongoing policy work is helping to shape healthier futures and may inspire legislative action across the country.

Table 2
Youth obesity policies identified as politically feasible and likely to have a significant public health impact

- Allocating funds for research on prevention and cost-effective interventions
- Aligning federal nutrition-assistance programs with obesity-prevention efforts
- Providing free or subsidized fruits and vegetables at school lunch
- Allocating funds for public-service advertising campaigns regarding portion sizes and the dangers of obesity
- Allocating funds to assess the impact of interventions
- Mandating or encouraging reduced-fat (1% or skim) milk in schools
- Allocating transportation funding for the promotion of physical activity (eg, establishing and maintaining bike and walking paths)
- Establishing federal standards for portion sizes in school cafeterias
- Promoting media literacy among youth
- Applying federal school lunch standards to à la carte options
- Funding indoor activity centers, especially in low-income neighborhoods

Source: Brescoll V, Kersh R, Brownell K. *Ann Am Acad Pol Soc Sci.* 2008;615(1):178–194.

Table 3
Selected examples of state action to promote nutrition, increase physical activity, and prevent obesity in youth

Type of Policy	Sample Legislation
Task forces, commissions, and study groups	Arkansas: Duties of the Healthy Advisory Committee were amended to include examining the progress of the Coordinated School Health Program and making recommendations to the Department of Health and Education and the Division of Health.
	Delaware: A statewide Health Advisory Council was established to provide advice to the Department of Education on current and future physical education and physical activity programs in public schools. In addition, the new council will report on fitness levels and obesity in youth.
Initiatives and pilot programs	Minnesota: Mini grants were established to test school wellness policies that target youth who are at high risk for obesity in school districts that have a high percentage of free and reduced-price lunch recipients.
	New York: Collaborative programs were established involving the YMCA and Alliance of Boys & Girls Club to promote better nutrition and physical activity policies in after-school settings.
	Rhode Island: An initiative was established to restructure school environments to promote healthy nutrition and physical activity and create safe routes to schools in low-income communities.
Food, snack, and beverage taxes	Louisiana: Schools participating in the National School Lunch and Breakfast programs were exempted from having a sales or use tax imposed on them.
	Rhode Island: Farmers were given a 5% income tax credit for the cost of farm products grown or produced in the state and sold to local education agencies.
Farmers' markets	Kentucky: The Kentucky Farmers' Market Nutrition Program was created to provide services including the provision of fresh, locally grown produce to low-income citizens and school food programs.
	Utah: The opportunity for counties and municipalities was established to operate a farmers' market on a county- or municipality-owned property to promote economic development and indemnify a food producer participating in the farmers' market.
Pedestrian and recreational safety	California: The Safe Routes to School construction program was established to be administered by the California Department of Transportation.
	Hawaii: A percentage of federally eligible moneys from the state highway fund was earmarked to establish multiuse paths, bicycle paths, and bicycle lanes and to install signage and safety devices along bikeways.

(*Continued*)

Table 3
(Continued)

Type of Policy	Sample Legislation
School breakfast and lunch	Oregon: Minimum nutrition standards were established for all food and beverage items sold in public schools to students in kindergarten through grade 12.
	Pennsylvania: The Department of Education was directed to establish a School Nutrition Incentive Program. The program will provide a supplemental school lunch and breakfast reimbursement to any school in a local education agency that adopts and implements nutritional guidelines for foods and beverages.
	Oklahoma: Schools and farms were linked through the creation of a farm-to-school program within the Department of Agriculture, Food, and Forestry. The goal of the program is to provide schools with fresh farm products in meals and snacks and help students develop healthy eating habits.
Physical education in schools	Arizona: A pilot program was established to require students in grades 1–12 to participate in physical education class for at least 150 min/wk. At least 50% of the physical education time must be devoted to moderate-to-vigorous exercise.
	Mississippi: Minimum requirements for students in kindergarten through grade 8 were established and include at least 150 min/wk of physical activity–based instruction and 45 min/wk of health education; minimum requirements were also established for grades 9–12 of 1 semester of physical education or physical activity for high school graduation.
	Washington: An outdoor education and recreation program was established to provide a large number of underserved students with opportunities to directly experience nature.
BMI and fitness testing in schools	Maine: The requirement to confidentially assess and report either BMI or height and weight was established for all students in kindergarten and grades 1, 3, 5, 7, and 9 in public and private schools.
	Florida: The requirement for school health service programs was established to test students' physical fitness levels and encourage the evaluation of students' BMI in grades 1, 3, 6, and 9.

Adapted from the Robert Wood Johnson Foundation. Balance: a report on state action to promote nutrition, increase physical activity and prevent obesity. Available at: www.healthyeatingresearch.org/uploads/balance122007Final.pdf.

Industry

The food, beverage, restaurant, entertainment, and recreation industries have begun to make changes in response to the growing concerns of consumers and public-interest groups around obesity.[75] The food, beverage, and restaurant industries have taken some positive steps to make their products healthier, provide smaller portion sizes, label and promote healthy options, and provide nutrition information to young consumers and families.[82–84] Although 13 food and beverage companies have pledged to limit the marketing of unhealthy food to children, most companies have not addressed marketing directed to youth over the age of 12 years.[83] The entertainment and recreation industries have responded in a similar fashion by sponsoring community-based obesity-prevention initiatives and developing computer games that promote healthy eating and physical activity.[75] For example, in 2006 Nintendo introduced the Wii, a game console that features a wireless controller with the ability to detect motion. Software sold with the Wii provides youth with the options of playing baseball, golf, tennis, boxing, or bowling games. Research conducted to evaluate the new technology has shown that playing the Wii simulated sport games uses less energy than playing the actual sports but uses significantly more energy than playing sedentary computer games.[85]

Although the actions of industry to date suggest that future advances could greatly strengthen efforts by the public health community to reduce obesity, much work remains to be done to create an environment that is fully supportive of healthful food and beverage choices and an active lifestyle. One growing area of concern is the use of new interactive digital media by food and beverage companies to reach and promote their products to adolescents. The current “marketing ecosystem” includes a number of digital platforms from online games to cell phones to three-dimensional virtual worlds. Behavioral targeting and “social media marketing” have grown dramatically because companies can now reach young people through Web sites such as MySpace and Facebook.[86] These new marketing practices target adolescents with unprecedented reach and sophistication and warrant close scrutiny to ensure that they promote the health of youth rather than undermine it.[86]

Community and Nonprofit Organizations

Although there is great variation in the extent to which communities across the nation are engaged in efforts to reduce obesity and limited outcome data exist, there are many encouraging examples of actions and initiatives on which future obesity intervention efforts may be built.[75] For example, the PedNet Coalition in Missouri is working to restore a network of nature trails and pedestrian walkways between schools, residential areas, shopping districts, and parks. The Pennsylvania Fresh Food Financing Initiative is providing financial support to improve the availability of supermarkets and grocery stores in communities with limited resources. A federal program, BodyWorks, provides materials to communities for teaching healthful nutrition and physical activity behaviors to young adolescent girls and their families.[87] The expanding program has been able to reach >700 families nationwide across communities that hire instructors and secure facilities for the counseling sessions.

There are also a growing number of philanthropies involved in funding efforts to improve the health of communities across the nation. The Healthy Eating/Active Living (HEAL) Convergence Partnership is a joint effort by the California

Endowment, Kaiser Permanente, Nemours Health and Prevention Services, the Robert Wood Johnson Foundation (RWJF) and the W. K. Kellogg Foundation.[88] The Centers for Disease Control and Prevention (CDC) serves as a technical advisor. The HEAL Convergence Partnership shares information, pools resources, and coordinates strategy. In 2007, the RWJF committed $500 million to reversing the obesity epidemic among youth by improving coordination between leaders, researchers, and activists; supporting research; putting research into action in schools and communities; and advocating for change. The RWJF developed a 5-steps framework (see Table 4) to help guide communities and policy makers in their efforts to increase physical activity and healthy eating and reduce obesity among youth.[88] Past and ongoing efforts in communities to reduce obesity, such as the examples mentioned here, have also led to the identification of key strategies (see Table 5) and stakeholders (eg, community youth organizations, faith-based groups, policy makers) to involve in the design of future programs and initiatives.[75] Evaluation data and the broad dissemination of successful programs are needed to advance community-level efforts around the country.

Health Care Professionals and Organizations

Health care professionals have taken many steps to address adolescent obesity in primary care practice and in the communities they serve.[75] As experts in healthy weight management, health care professionals are taking active roles in advocating for policies to prevent and reduce obesity. For example, recent efforts to

Table 4
Five-steps framework for increasing physical activity and healthy eating in youth

1. Provide healthier foods to students at school.
   All foods served and sold in schools should meet or exceed US Department of Agriculture guidelines, and schools should limit access to high-calorie snacks and drinks, whether sold in cafeterias, vending machines or school stores, given as rewards, or sold as fund-raisers.
2. Improve the availability of healthy foods at home.
   To ensure that all families have access to affordable, nutritious food, efforts and incentives are needed to bring new food sources, such as supermarkets and farmers' markets, to underserved communities.
3. Increase the frequency, intensity, and duration of physical activity at school.
   Increasing the amount of time that children spend in physical education and improving the quality of delivered physical education can help to prevent obesity; schools and communities should look for innovative ways to increase physical activity before, during, and after the school day.
4. Improve access to safe places where youth can play.
   Creating parks, athletic fields, and other places to play is crucial, but that is only half the battle; those places need to be accessible, safe, and well maintained.
5. Limit screen time.
   Youth who spend less time in front of a television, DVD player, or video game screen are less likely to be obese.

Source: Lavizzo-Mourey R. RWJF childhood obesity update: 2008. Available at: www.rwjf.org/files/research/rlm2008cobupdate.pdf.

Table 5
Key strategies for community-based efforts to reduce adolescent obesity

- Developing committed and sustained leadership
- Building community coalitions with well-defined goals
- Building on cultural assets
- Identifying sufficient resources
- Addressing community safety
- Engaging community-group members
- Supporting efforts that can produce multiple social and health benefits

Adapted from Institute of Medicine, Committee on Progress in Preventing Childhood Obesity. *Progress in Preventing Childhood Obesity: How Do We Measure Up?* Washington, DC: National Academies Press; 2007.

introduce legislation (the Child Nutrition Promotion and School Lunch Protection Act of 2006) that would update the nutrition standards for foods and beverages sold in schools have been supported by numerous professional organizations including the American Dietetic Association, the National Association of School Nurses, the American Public Health Association, and the American Academy of Pediatrics (AAP).[89] Individual providers and their professional organizations have further been active in the implementation of obesity prevention programs. Professional organizations such as the AAP have developed evidence-based guidelines, positions, training programs, and tool kits for providers.[19,20,90] The AAP guidelines provide physicians with a protocol for counseling youth about their weight in primary care (see Table 6), counseling strategies, a set of recommended behaviors for healthy weight management (see Table 7), and several suggestions for getting involved in community obesity-prevention efforts. Continued efforts to train health care professionals in the use of effective strategies for primary care prevention and promote their increased involvement in advocacy efforts will be a critical part of the ongoing work to reduce obesity.

Schools and State and Local Education Authorities

There has been much variation in efforts to address obesity in schools across the nation.[75] Several schools have taken steps to improve supports for healthful eating and physical activity, and national survey data indicate recent improvements. However, much work is still needed to ensure that all students have access to healthy food and beverage options and opportunities to be physically active (see Figs 3 and 4).[45,91] A number of action steps can be taken in schools to influence students' health behavior and create an environment that is conducive to healthy eating and physical activity. The CDC has identified 10 key strategies that schools can implement to improve student nutrition and increase physical activity (see Table 8).[92]

Federal guidelines currently require that reimbursable school breakfast and lunch programs meet nutrition standards and prohibit the sale of certain foods and

Table 6
Pediatric obesity-prevention protocol for primary care

Step 1: Assess
- a. Explain and conduct assessments of
  - weight, height, and BMI percentile;
  - dietary intake (fruit, vegetables, sweetened beverages, and fast food);
  - activity (screen time, moderate-to-vigorous activity); and
  - eating behaviors (breakfast, portion sizes, family meals)
- b. Provide and elicit feedback on BMI and behaviors found to be inside the optimal range and outside the optimal range

Step 2: Set agenda
- a. Explore interest in changing behaviors not in the optimal range
- b. Agree on target behaviors with the patient and caregiver

Step 3: Assess motivation and confidence
- a. In regard to interest in changing weight status or behaviors, assess
  - willingness;
  - the perceived importance; and
  - confidence in having success
- b. Probe the patient regarding ratings of willingness, perceived importance, and confidence to explore the advantages and disadvantages of changing

Step 4: Summarize and probe possible changes
- a. Summarize the advantages and disadvantages of change
- b. Query about possible next steps
- c. Offer ideas for getting started in making a change as needed
- d. Summarize the change plan
- e. Provide positive feedback

Step 5: Schedule follow-up visit
- a. If a change plan is made, agree on a follow-up appointment within a specified number of weeks or months
- b. If no change plan is made, agree to revisit the topic within a specific number of weeks or months

Adapted from Davis M, Gance-Cleveland B, Hassink S, Johnson R, Paradis G, Resnicow K. *Pediatrics.* 2007;120(suppl 4):S229–S253.

beverages that have minimal nutritional value (soft drinks, water ices, chewing gum, and certain candies) in foodservice areas during meal periods. As reviewed earlier, schools are also required to have a wellness policy that addresses nutritional guidelines for all foods available on campus and opportunities for physical activity; however, the legislation does not require that wellness policies be made more restrictive than federal guidelines.[79] To address this gap, the National Alliance for Nutrition and Physical Activity has developed model school-wellness policies, and the IOM has developed science-based nutrition standards for foods sold outside the federal school-meal program (competitive foods).[93,94] It has further been suggested that the redesign of school spaces (physical fitness grounds, cafeterias, etc) might provide opportunities for promoting nutrition and physical activity.[95] Future research is needed to evaluate school-wellness policies, guide spatial designs, and illuminate other promising opportunities.

Table 7
Recommended behaviors that physicians and allied health care providers should provide counsel on for youth whose BMI is between the 5th and 84th percentiles

- Limit consumption of sugar-sweetened beverages.
- Consume recommended quantities of fruits and vegetables.
- Limit television and other screen time by allotting no more than 2 h/d.
- Remove television and computer screens from primary sleeping areas.
- Eat breakfast daily.
- Limit eating at restaurants.
- Have frequent family meals in which parents and youth eat together.
- Limit portion sizes.

Adapted from Davis M, Gance-Cleveland B, Hassink S, Johnson R, Paradis G, Resnicow K. *Pediatrics*. 2007;120(suppl 4):S229–S253.

Parents and Families

The development of best-practice recommendations for the parents and families of adolescents has been hindered by a lack of efficacy and effectiveness data.[75] Parents and other household caregivers may influence the eating and physical activity behaviors of youth as role models and change agents in the home. However, few family-based obesity interventions have been tested to determine the efficacy of various strategies in adolescents aged 13 years and older. Much research is needed to make progress in improving the home eating and activity environments of youth. Until efficacy data are available, family-based interventions for adolescents should focus on improving the behaviors of adult role models and rely on the best available evidence from observational studies and interventions tested in young children. National survey data indicate that the majority of US adults are not modeling healthy behaviors. For example, 3 of every 4 adults do not consume adequate amounts of fruits and vegetables, and ~1 of every 4 adults report doing no physical activities in the past month.[96] Available evidence from research in families strongly suggests that parents and

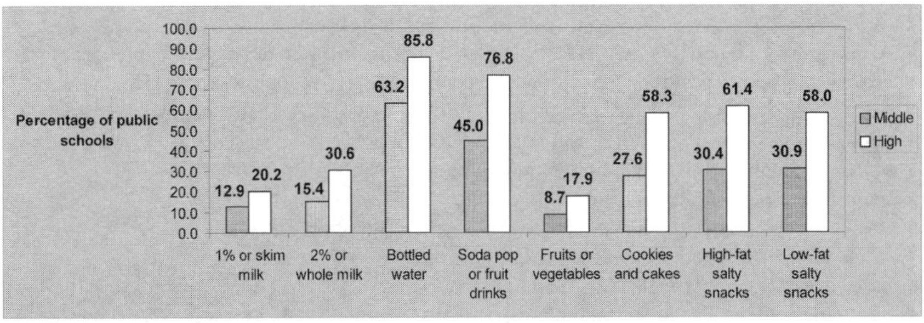

Fig 3. Percentage of US public secondary schools in which students could purchase foods and beverages from vending machines or in a school store, canteen, or snack bar. Source: O'Toole T, Anderson S, Miller C, Guthrie J. *J Sch Health*. 2007;77(8):500–521.

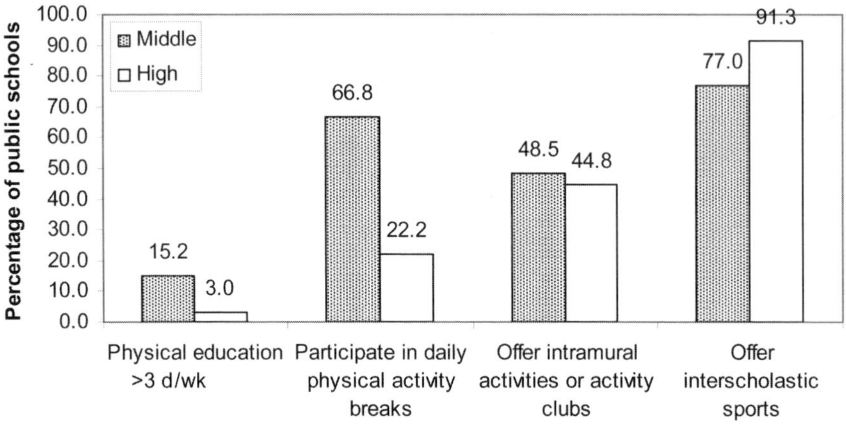

Fig 4. Percentage of US public secondary schools that offer opportunities for physical activity. Source: Lee SM, Burgeson CR, Fulton JE, Spain CG. *J Sch Health.* 2007;77(8):435–463.

families should engage in supportive communication with their adolescents around behaviors rather than weight status; make healthy food options readily available at home; limit the availability of high-calorie, low-nutrition foods at home; be active together; and model healthy weight behaviors and attitudes.[97]

CONCLUSIONS

Much effort has been invested in the public health response to adolescent obesity; however, there is still a great need for additional research, behavioral interventions, and corrective changes in the eating and activity environments of youth. The future investment of resources for research and involvement of professionals with the diverse skills necessary to positively influence environmental and policy action will be critical for preventing the staggering health and economic consequences of obesity.

Table 8
Key strategies for schools to improve the nutrition and physical activity of students

- Address physical activity and nutrition through a coordinated school health program approach.
- Designate a school health coordinator and maintain an active school health council.
- Assess the school's health policies and programs and develop a plan for improvement.
- Strengthen the school's nutrition and physical activity policies.
- Implement a high-quality health-promotion program for school staff.
- Implement a high-quality course of study in health education.
- Implement a high-quality course of study in physical education.
- Increase opportunities for students to engage in physical activity.
- Implement a quality school meals program.
- Ensure that students have appealing, healthy choices in foods and beverages offered outside of the school-meals program.

Source: Wechsler H, McKenna M, Lee S, Dietz W. *State Educ Stand.* 2004;5(2):4–12.

REFERENCES

1. Institute of Medicine, Committee on Prevention of Obesity in Children and Youth, Food and Nutrition Board, Board on Health Promotion and Disease Prevention. *Preventing Childhood Obesity: Health in the Balance*. Washington, DC: National Academies Press; 2005
2. Thomson Medstat. Childhood obesity: costs, treatment patterns, disparities in care, and prevalent medical conditions. Available at: www.medstat.com/pdfs/childhood_obesity.pdf. Accessed June 8, 2008
3. Wang G, Dietz W. Economic burden of obesity in youths aged 6 to 17 years: 1979–1999 [published correction appears in *Pediatrics*. 2002;109(6):1195]. *Pediatrics*. 2002;109(5). Available at: www.pediatrics.org/cgi/content/full/109/5/e81
4. Wang LY, Chyen D, Lee S, Lowry R. The association between body mass index in adolescence and obesity in adulthood. *J Adolesc Health*. 2008;42(5):512–518
5. Whitaker R, Wright J, Pepe M, Seidel K, Dietz W. Predicting obesity in young adulthood from childhood and parental obesity. *N Engl J Med*. 1997;337(13):869–873
6. Freedman DS, Khan LK, Serdula MK, Dietz WH, Srinivasan SR, Berenson GS. The relation of childhood BMI to adult adiposity: the Bogalusa Heart Study. *Pediatrics*. 2005;115(1):22–27
7. Olshansky SJ, Pasaro DJ, Hershow RC, et al. A potential decline in life expectancy in the United States in the 21st century. *N Engl J Med*. 2005;352(11):1138–1145
8. Ogden CL, Flegal KM, Carroll MD, Johnson CL. Prevalence and trends in overweight among U.S. children and adolescents, 1999–2000. *JAMA*. 2002;288(14):1728–1733
9. Jolliffe D. Extent of overweight among U.S. children and adolescents from 1971 to 2000. *Int J Obes Relat Metab Disord*. 2004;28(1):4–9
10. Ogden CL, Carroll MD, Flegal KM. High body mass index for age among US children and adolescents, 2003–2006. *JAMA*. 2008;299(20):2401–2405
11. Shrewsbury V, Wardle J. Socioeconomic status and adiposity in childhood: a systematic review of cross-sectional studies 1990–2005. *Obesity (Silver Spring)*. 2008;16(2):275–284
12. Neumark-Sztainer D, Story M, Hannan PJ, Croll J. Overweight status and eating patterns among adolescents: where do youths stand in comparison with the *Healthy People 2010* objectives? *Am J Public Health*. 2002;92(5):844–851
13. Miech RA, Kumanyika S, Stettler N, Link B, Phelan J, Chang V. Trends in the association of poverty with overweight among US adolescents, 1971–2004. *JAMA*. 2006;295(20):2385–2393
14. Gordon-Larsen P, Adair LS, Popkin BM. The relationship of ethnicity, socioeconomic factors, and overweight in US adolescents. *Obes Res*. 2003;11(1):121–129
15. Zephier E, Himes JH, Story M, Zhou X. Increasing prevalences of overweight and obesity in Northern plains American Indian children. *Arch Pediatr Adolesc Med*. 2006;160(1):34–39
16. Singh GK, Kogan MD, van Dyck PC. A multilevel analysis of state and regional disparities in childhood and adolescent obesity in the United States. *J Community Health*. 2008;33(2):90–102
17. Lutfiyya MN, Lipsky MS, Wisdom-Behounek J, Inpanbutr-Martinkus M. Is rural residency a risk factor for overweight and obesity for U.S. children? *Obesity (Silver Spring)*. 2007;15(9):2348–2356
18. Sherry B. Food behaviors and other strategies to prevent and treat pediatric overweight. *Int J Obes (Lond)*. 2005;29(suppl 2):S116–S126
19. Davis M, Gance-Cleveland B, Hassink S, Johnson R, Paradis G, Resnicow K. Recommendations for prevention of childhood obesity. *Pediatrics*. 2007;120(suppl 4):S229–S253
20. Kohn M, Rees J, Brill S, et al. Preventing and treating adolescent obesity: a position paper of the Society for Adolescent Medicine. *J Adolesc Health*. 2006;38(6):784–787
21. Murphy M, Douglass J, Latulippe M, Barr S, Johnson R, Frye C. Beverages as a source of energy and nutrients in diets of children and adolescents [abstract]. *FASEB J*. 2005;19(4 suppl S pt 1):A434
22. Wang Y, Bleich S, Gortmaker S. Increasing caloric contribution from sugar-sweetened beverages and 100% fruit juices among US children and adolescents, 1988–2004. *Pediatrics*. 2008;121(6). Available at: www.pediatrics.org/cgi/content/full/121/6/e1604

23. Vartanian L, Schwartz M, Brownell K. Effects of soft drink consumption on nutrition and health: a systematic review and meta-analysis. *Am J Public Health.* 2007;97(4):667–675
24. Grimm G, Harnack L, Story M. Factors associated with soft drink consumption in school-aged children. *J Am Diet Assoc.* 2004;104(8):1244–1249
25. Wiecha JL, Finkelstein D, Troped PJ, Fragala M, Peterson KE. School vending machine use and fast-food restaurant use are associated with sweetened beverage intake in youth. *J Am Diet Assoc.* 2006;106(10):1624–1630
26. Guenther P, Dodd K, Reedy J, Krebs-Smith S. Most Americans eat much less than recommended amounts of fruits and vegetables. *J Am Diet Assoc.* 2006;106(9):1371–1379
27. Newby P. Are dietary intakes and eating behaviors related to childhood obesity? A comprehensive review of the evidence. *J Law Med Ethics.* 2007;35(1):35–60
28. French SA, Story M, Jeffery RW, et al. Pricing strategy to promote fruit and vegetable purchase in high school cafeterias. *J Am Diet Assoc.* 1997;97(9):1008–1010
29. Young EM, Fors SW, Hayes DM. Associations between perceived parental behaviors and middle school student fruit and vegetable consumption. *J Nutr Educ Behav.* 2004;36(1):2–8
30. Hanson NI, Neumark-Sztainer D, Eisenberg ME, Story M, Wall M. Associations between parental report of the home food environment and adolescent intakes of fruits, vegetables and dairy foods. *Public Health Nutr.* 2005;8(1):77–85
31. Timperio A, Ball K, Roberts R, Campbell K, Andrianopoulos N, Crawford D. Children's fruit and vegetable intake: associations with the neighborhood food environment. *Prev Med.* 2008; 46(4):331–335
32. Jago R, Baranowski T, Baranowski J, Cullen K, Thompson D. Distance to food stores and adolescent male fruit and vegetable consumption: mediation effects. *Int J Behav Nutr Phys Act.* 2007;4:35
33. Rose D, Richards R. Food store access and household fruit and vegetable use among participants in the US Food Stamp Program. *Public Health Nutr.* 2004;7(8):1081–1088
34. Nielsen SJ, Siega-Riz AM, Popkin BM. Trends in food locations and sources among adolescents and young adults. *Prev Med.* 2002;35(2):107–113
35. Paeratakul S, Ferdinand D, Champagne C, Ryan D, Bray G. Fast-food consumption among U.S. adults and children: dietary and nutrient intake profile. *J Am Diet Assoc.* 2003;103(10):1332–1338
36. Niemeier H, Raynor H, Lloyd-Richardson E, Rogers M, Wing R. Fast food consumption and breakfast skipping: predictors of weight gain from adolescence to adulthood in a nationally representative sample. *J Adolesc Health.* 2006;39(6):842–849
37. Ebbeling CB, Sinclair KB, Pereira MA, Garcia-Lago E, Feldman HA, Ludwig DS. Compensation for energy intake from fast food among overweight and lean adolescents. *JAMA.* 2004; 291(23):2828–2833
38. Young LR, Nestle M. The contribution of expanding portion sizes to the US obesity epidemic. *Am J Public Health.* 2002;92(2):246–249
39. Diliberti N, Bordi PL, Conklin MT, Roe LS, Rolls BJ. Increased portion size leads to increased energy intake in a restaurant meal. *Obes Res.* 2004;12(3):562–568
40. Prentice AM, Jebb SA. Fast foods, energy density and obesity: a possible mechanistic link. *Obes Rev.* 2003;4(4):187–194
41. French S, Story M, Neumark-Sztainer D, Fulkerson J, Hannan P. Fast food restaurant use among adolescents: associations with nutrient intake, food choices and behavioral and psychosocial variables. *Int J Obes Relat Metab Disord.* 2001;25(12):1823–1833
42. Thompson O, Ballew C, Resnicow K, et al. Food purchased away from home as a predictor of change in BMI *z*-score among girls. *Int J Obes Relat Metab Disord.* 2004;28(2):282–289
43. Taveras E, Berkey C, Rifas-Shiman S, et al. Association of consumption of fried food away from home with body mass index and diet quality in older children and adolescents. *Pediatrics.* 2005;116(4). Available at: www.pediatrics.org/cgi/content/full/116/4/e518
44. Gantz W, Schwartz N, Angelini J, Rideout V. Food for thought: television food advertising to children in the United States. Available at: www.kff.org/entmedia/entmedia032807pkg.cfm. Accessed June 14, 2008

45. O'Toole T, Anderson S, Miller C, Guthrie J. Nutrition services and foods and beverages available at school: results from the School Health Policies and Programs Study 2006. *J Sch Health.* 2007;77(8):500–521
46. Kipke M, Iverson E, Moore D, et al. Food and park environments: neighborhood-level risks for childhood obesity in East Los Angeles. *J Adolesc Health.* 2007;40(4):325–333
47. Austin S, Melly S, Sanchez B, Patel A, Buka S, Gortmaker S. Clustering of fast-food restaurants around schools: a novel application of spatial statistics to the study of food environments. *Am J Public Health.* 2005;95(9):1575–1581
48. Zenk S, Powell L. US secondary schools and food outlets. *Health Place.* 2008;14(2):336–346
49. Nielsen SJ, Popkin BM. Patterns and trends in food portion sizes, 1977–1998. *JAMA.* 2003; 289(4):450–453. Available at: http://jama.ama-assn.org/cgi/content/full/289/4/450. Accessed August 8, 2008
50. Huang T, Howarth N, Lin B, Roberts S, McCrory M. Energy intake and meal portions: associations with BMI percentile in US children. *Obes Res.* 2004;12(11):1875–1885
51. Orlet Fisher J, Rolls B, Birch L. Children's bite size and intake of an entrée are greater with large portions than with age-appropriate or self-selected portions. *Am J Clin Nutr.* 2003;77(5):1164–1170
52. Fisher J. Effects of age on children's intake of large and self-selected food portions. *Obesity.* 2007;15(2):403–412
53. Eaton DK, Kann L, Kinchen S, et al. Youth Risk Behavior Surveillance: United States, 2007. *MMWR Surveill Summ.* 2008;57(4):1–131. Available at: www.cdc.gov/HealthyYouth/yrbs/pdf/yrbss07_mmwr.pdf. Accessed July 1, 2008
54. Kerr J, Norman G, Sallis J, Patrick K. Exercise AIDS, neighborhood safety, and physical activity in adolescents and parents. *Med Sci Sports Exerc.* 2008;40(7):1244–1248
55. Evenson K, Birnbaum A, Bedimo-Rung A, et al. Girls' perception of physical environmental factors and transportation: reliability and association with physical activity and active transport to school. *Int J Behav Nutr Phys Act.* 2006;3:28
56. Price S, McDivitt J, Weber D, Wolff L, Massett H, Fulton J. Correlates of weight-bearing physical activity among adolescent girls: results from a national survey of girls and their parents. *J Phys Act Health.* 2008;5(1):132–145
57. Trost S, Sallis J, Pate R, Freedson P, Taylor W, Dowda M. Evaluating a model of parental influence on youth physical activity. *Am J Prev Med.* 2003;25(4):277–282
58. Cradock A, Melly S, Allen J, Morris J, Gortmaker S. Characteristics of school campuses and physical activity among youth. *Am J Prev Med.* 2007;33(2):106–113
59. Pate R, Colabianchi N, Porter D, Almeida M, Lobelo F, Dowda M. Physical activity and neighborhood resources in high school girls. *Am J Prev Med.* 2008;34(5):413–419
60. Kligerman M, Sallis J, Ryan S, Frank L, Nader P. Association of neighborhood design and recreation environment variables with physical activity and body mass index in adolescents. *Am J Health Promot.* 2007;21(4):274–277
61. American Academy of Pediatrics, Committee on Public Education. Children, adolescents, and television. *Pediatrics.* 2001;107(2):423–426
62. Roberts D, Foehr U, Rideout V. Generation M: Media in the lives of 8–18 year-olds. Available at: www.kff.org/entmedia/entmedia030905pkg.cfm. Accessed June 14, 2008
63. Delmas C, Platat C, Schweitzer B, Wagner A, Oujaa M, Simon C. Association between television in bedroom and adiposity throughout adolescence. *Obesity.* 2007;15(10):2495–2503
64. Mark A, Janssen I. Relationship between screen time and metabolic syndrome in adolescents. *J Public Health (Oxf).* 2008;30(2):153–160
65. Must A, Bandini L, Tyler D, Phillips S, Naumova E, Dietz W. Activity, inactivity, and screen time in relation to weight and fatness over adolescence in girls. *Obesity.* 2007;15(7):1774–1781
66. Boone J, Gordon-Larsen P, Adair L, Popkin B. Screen time and physical activity during adolescence: longitudinal effects on obesity in young adulthood. *Int J Behav Nutr Phys Act.* 2007;4:26
67. Gortmaker SL, Peterson K, Wiecha J, et al. Reducing obesity via a school-based interdisciplinary intervention among youth: Planet Health. *Arch Pediatr Adolesc Med.* 1999;153(4):409–418

68. Powell L, Szczypka G, Chaloupka F. Exposure to food advertising on television among US children. *Arch Pediatr Adolesc Med.* 2007;161(6):553–560
69. Powell L, Szczypka G, Chaloupka F. Adolescent exposure to food advertising on television. *Am J Prev Med.* 2007;33(4 suppl):S251–S256
70. Barradas D, Fulton J, Blanck H, Huhman M. Parental influences on youth television viewing. *J Pediatr.* 2007;151(4):369–373, 373e.1–373e.4
71. Barr-Anderson D, van den Berg P, Neumark-Sztainer D, Story M. Characteristics associated with older adolescents who have a television in their bedrooms. *Pediatrics.* 2008;121(4):718–724
72. Hardy L, Baur L, Garnett S, et al. Family and home correlates of television viewing in 12–13 year old adolescents: the Nepean Study. *Int J Behav Nutr Phys Act.* 2006;3:24
73. Barlow S; Expert Committee. Expert committee recommendations regarding the prevention, assessment, and treatment of child and adolescent overweight and obesity: Summary report. *Pediatrics.* 2007;120(suppl 4):S164–S192
74. Kumanyika SK, Obarzanek E, Stettler N, et al. Population-based prevention of obesity: the need for comprehensive promotion of healthful eating, physical activity, and energy balance: a scientific statement from American Heart Association Council on Epidemiology and Prevention, Interdisciplinary Committee for Prevention. *Circulation.* 2008;118(4):428–464
75. Institute of Medicine, Committee on Progress in Preventing Childhood Obesity, Food and Nutrition Board. *Progress in Preventing Childhood Obesity.* Washington, DC: National Academies Press; 2007
76. Brescoll V, Kersh R, Brownell K. Assessing the feasibility and impact of federal childhood obesity policies. *Ann Am Acad Pol Soc Sci.* 2008;615(1):178–194
77. Rosenbaum D; Center on Budget and Policy Priorities. Farm bill contains significant domestic nutrition improvements. Available at: www.cbpp.org/5-8-08fa.htm. Accessed July 15, 2008
78. House Committee on Agriculture. 2008 Farm Bill Nutrition Title: promoting health and fighting hunger in the United States. Available at: http://agriculture.house.gov/inside/Legislation/110/FB/Conf/Title_IV_fs.pdf. Accessed July 12, 2008
79. Food Research and Action Center. Local school wellness policies. Available at: www.frac.org/html/federal_food_programs/programs/school_wellness.html. Accessed July 16, 2008
80. School Nutrition Association, School Nutrition Foundation. From cupcakes to carrots: local wellness policies one year later. Available at: www.schoolnutrition.org/uploadedFiles_old/ASFSA/newsroom/pressreleases/From_Cupcakes_to_Carrots.pdf. Accessed June 19, 2008
81. Robert Wood Johnson Foundation. Balance: a report on state action to promote nutrition, increase physical activity and prevent obesity. Available at: www.healthyeatingresearch.org/uploads/balance122007Final.pdf. Accessed July 3, 2008
82. Grocery Manufacturers of America. Industry report on health and wellness. Available at: www.gmabrands.com/publications/docs/hwreport.pdf. Accessed June 27, 2006
83. Better Business Bureau. Children's food and beverage advertising initiative. Available at: http://us.bbb.org/WWWRoot/SitePage.aspx?site=113&id=dba51fbb-9317-4f88-9bcb-3942d7336e87. Accessed June 28, 2008
84. Langlois A, Crossley R. The proof of the pudding: benchmarking ten of the world's largest food companies' response to obesity and related health concerns. Available at: http://whattoeatbook.com/wp-content/uploads/2008/04/proof-of-the-pudding-final.pdf. Accessed 9, 2008
85. Graves L, Stratton G, Ridgers N, Cable N. Comparison of energy expenditure in adolescents when playing new generation and sedentary computer games: cross sectional study. *BMJ.* 2007;335(7633):1282–1284
86. Chester J, Montgomery K. *Interactive Food and Beverage Marketing: Targeting Children and Youth in the Digital Age.* Berkeley, CA: Berkeley Media Studies Group; 2007. Available at: www.digitalads.org Accessed June 14, 2008
87. Office on Women's Health, US Department of Health and Human Services. BodyWorks: a toolkit for healthy girls and strong women. Available at: www.womenshealth.gov/bodyworks. Accessed July 18, 2008
88. Lavizzo-Mourey R. RWJF childhood obesity update: 2008. Available at: www.rwjf.org/files/research/rlm2008cobupdate.pdf. Accessed July 24, 2008

89. Center for Science in the Public Interest. Improve school foods. Available at: www.schoolfoods.org. Accessed July 18, 2008
90. American Dietetic Association. Position of the American Dietetic Association: individual-, family-, school-, and community-based interventions for pediatric overweight. *J Am Diet Assoc.* 2006;106(6):925–945
91. Finkelstein D, Hill E, Whitaker R. School food environments and policies in US public schools. *Pediatrics.* 2008;122(1). Available at: www.pediatrics.org/cgi/content/full/122/1/e251
92. Wechsler H, McKenna M, Lee S, Dietz W. The role of schools in preventing childhood obesity. *State Educ Stand.* 2004;5(2):4–12
93. Institute of Medicine, Committee on Nutrition Standards for Foods in Schools. *Nutrition Standards for Foods in Schools: Leading the Way Toward Healthier Youth.* Washington, DC: National Academies Press; 2007. Available at: www.iom.edu/Object.File/Master/42/505/Food%20in%20Schools.pdf. Accessed July 15, 2008
94. National Alliance for Nutrition and Activity. Model local school wellness policies. Available at: www.schoolwellnesspolicies.org/WellnessPolicies.html. Accessed July 16, 2008
95. Gorman N, Lackney J, Rollings K, Huang T. Designer schools: the role of school space and architecture in obesity prevention. *Obesity.* 2007;15(11):2521–2530
96. Centers for Disease Control and Prevention, National Center for Chronic Disease Prevention and Health Promotion. Behavioral Risk Factor Surveillance System survey data, 2007. Available at: http://apps.nccd.cdc.gov/brfss/index.asp. Accessed July 19, 2008
97. Neumark-Sztainer D. *"I'm, Like, SO Fat!": Helping Your Teen Make Healthy Choices about Eating and Exercise in a Weight-Obsessed World.* New York, NY: Guilford Press; 2005

Adolesc Med 19 (2008) 380–405

Adolescent Obesity: Etiology, Office Evaluation, and Treatment

Rebecka Peebles, MD, FAAP*

Division of Adolescent Medicine, Department of Pediatrics, Stanford University School of Medicine, 1174 Castro Street, Suite 250A, Mountain View, CA 94040, USA

Overweight and obesity are now commonly encountered clinical diagnoses for adolescents and have emerged as a serious threat to public health. Of US children aged 2 to 19 years in 2003–2006, 11.3% were above the 97th percentile for BMI, and 31.9% were at or above the 85th percentile for BMI, and these rates have been fairly stable since 1999.[1,2] Multiple studies have shown black and Hispanic children to be disproportionately affected.[1–4] With costs mounting for obesity-associated treatment and sequelae, these rates have dramatic implications for our health care economy.[5]

Obesity carries multiple extraphysical risks as well. Overweight is associated with fewer years of school completion and household poverty in women, independent of baseline socioeconomic status and aptitude-test scores.[6] Pediatric obesity is often associated with significantly lower health-related quality of life (equal to those of children diagnosed with cancer) compared with normal-weight peers.[7–9]

Finally, adolescent obesity predicts overweight in adulthood,[10,11] in addition to weight-related medical complications during childhood and later in life.[10] Multiple studies have documented the increased risk of mortality for adults associated with poor diet, physical inactivity, and an excessive BMI.[12,13] Overweight and obesity in adulthood are associated with diabetes, high blood pressure, high cholesterol levels, asthma, arthritis, and poor health status.[14]

DEFINITION OF OVERWEIGHT IN ADOLESCENCE

BMI, or body weight in kilograms divided by height in meters squared and then plotted against age and gender-specific percentiles, is the measure of choice for defining childhood weight norms. Adolescents younger than 20 are

*Corresponding author.
E-mail address: rpeebles@stanford.edu (R. Peebles).

 ISSN 1934-4287

defined as "obese" if their BMI exceeds the 95th percentile for age and as "overweight" if their BMI exceeds the 85th percentile for age[15–18] (see www.cdc.gov/nccdphp/dnpa/bmi/bmi-for-age.htm). Often, BMI at the 95th percentile is said to represent "obesity," leading to some inconsistencies from one report to another. BMI measurements have some inherent limitations in that they are not a direct measure of adiposity, and as such, some patients with a high BMI may not have excess adiposity but, rather, a high degree of lean body mass. However, BMI measurements have correlated reasonably well with adiposity in numerous studies across different ethnic groups.[15]

Other measures of adiposity have been studied, including skinfold-thickness measurements by calipers, electrical impedance techniques, waist circumference, dual-energy radiograph absorptiometry (DEXA), densitometry, and MRI. However, although these have some utility in describing visceral fat and body composition beyond a measure of BMI, few of them have pediatric norms, and some are expensive and not accessible on a widespread basis; for these reasons, they are not used routinely for adolescents.

ETIOLOGIES

It is generally agreed that the etiologies of obesity in the adolescent years are usually multifactorial and are frequently exogenous. However, there are other biological factors to be considered, some of which are described below.

Prenatal and Early Childhood Growth Influences

Certain growth periods of childhood are especially influential on future weight. The prenatal period is now understood as a critical growth period, with prenatal deprivation, gestational diabetes, and high birth weights correlating positively with rates of obesity later in life.[19] In addition, early onset of "adiposity rebound" (defined as the age at which adiposity reaches a postinfancy low point and then increases) is inversely associated with BMI and positively correlated with impaired glucose tolerance later in life.[20,21] Puberty is also a particularly dynamic time of growth and body-composition changes, and early menarche has also been shown to increase the risk of later developing obesity and metabolic syndrome.[22,23]

Exogenous Influences

Excessive food intake is a focal contributor to the development and maintenance of obesity. Fast food, prepackaged foods, fewer fruits and vegetables, and added sugars are all frequently consumed by today's youth and are key contributors to weight gain.[24,25] Diets containing foods with a high glycemic index (Table 1), or propensity to cause a rise in blood glucose level after a

Table 1
Common dietary interventions to combat obesity in adolescents

Diet/Diet Change	Description	Studies/Evidence Base
Increased dairy consumption	Increased intake of milk, yogurt, and other dairy products	The Coronary Artery Risk Development in Young Adults (CARDIA) study: increased dairy consumption was strongly and inversely associated with obesity, glucose intolerance, hypertension, and hyperlipidemia; risk of developing metabolic syndrome involving these conditions was 72% lower among those in the highest dairy consumption category[30]
Low-fat diet	20%–30% of daily caloric intake from dietary fats; often use US Department of Agriculture food pyramid as a guide; new emphasis also targets reducing trans fats	Low-fat diet including additional supplementation with plant sterols, soy proteins, and extra fiber led to impressive reductions in serum LDL and total cholesterol levels[120]
Increased fiber	Increase fiber intake to >20 g/d	Increased fiber intake is inversely associated to BMI, inflammatory markers, and insulin levels; fiber intake is often low in adolescents, and it is a helpful target for change[121,122]
Moderate-fat diet	~35% of daily calories are derived from fat	Allows capitalization of health benefits of omega-3 fatty acids; similar weight loss is achieved to those on low-fat regimens but with improved metabolic parameters[123–126]
Traffic Light/Stop Light diet	Categorizes foods as green (may have unlimited quantities), yellow (limited but good nutrient density), and red (try to minimize intake, higher in fat and refined sugars)	Multiple studies in children and adolescents have shown feasibility of approach; enhanced by significant parental component[96,127]
Low-carbohydrate diet	Restrict carbohydrate grams; often advocate initial extreme restriction followed by longer phase during which some carbohydrates are added back to diet in moderation	Adolescents on low-carbohydrate regimens in some trials have lost more weight and lowered insulin levels more than those on low-fat diets[128,129]; a recent study of adults showed more long-term weight loss for those on the Atkins diet, a low-carbohydrate approach[130]
Low-GI diet	The GI ranks carbohydrate-containing foods according to their ability to produce fluctuations in blood glucose levels; this dietary approach emphasizes foods that produce only small fluctuations or have a low GI	Multiple studies of low-to-moderate GI diets have shown that they may be helpful in achieving meaningful weight loss,[26,92] improving insulin profiles over time,[27] and prolonging satiety[28]

(*Continued*)

Table 1
(Continued)

Diet/Diet Change	Description	Studies/Evidence Base
PSMF	Generally reserved for adolescents suffering from severe obesity and often initiated when inpatient; requires close medical monitoring, daily supplements, adequate water intake, and frequent measurement of electrolyte levels to be safe; the diet typically allows for 2520–3780 kJ/d (600–900 cal/d), with 1.5–2.5 g of protein per kilogram per day, with intakes of carbohydrate (20–40 g/d) and fat very restricted; these diets are usually not used for periods >12 wk; described complications of the PSMF include cholelithiasis, hyperuricemia, orthostatic hypotension, halitosis, and diarrhea	Because of high dropout rates for this regimen, studies have been difficult to interpret[92,104]; 1 study showed greater weight loss at 10 wk in children taking the PSMF, but at 1 y the weight loss was not significantly different from that of controls on a standard low-calorie diet[131]
Intuitive eating	A nondiet approach to weight regulation that has no forbidden foods or specific dietary constraints but instead emphasizes eating only when hungry and stopping when comfortably satisfied; identified saboteurs of intuitive eating are eating when distracted, upset, or on the move; this approach does not emphasize weight loss but instead focuses on healthful eating and acceptance of a natural shape; it is often combined with a movement component in practice	Adult women taking a nondiet approach showed less weight loss than controls on a traditional weight-loss program but showed similar metabolic changes; in long-term follow-up, dieters had regained the weight they had lost initially and had not maintained behavior changes, whereas nondiet participants had maintained both weight and lifestyle changes[132,133]

GI indicates glycemic index; PSMF, protein-sparing modified fast.

meal, have been shown to increase food intake and are associated with higher insulin and glucose levels in obese adolescent boys.[26–28] Finally, dairy foods also have a protective influence on body weight. The intake of calcium from dairy foods correlates negatively with 2-year changes in total body weight and body fat in young women, even when exercise level and energy intake are taken into account,[29] and is also associated with reduced insulin resistance.[30]

Suboptimal Physical Activity

Of US high school students, 65.3% did not meet recommended levels of physical activity in 2007, and 24.9% did not participate in even 1 day/week of ≥60 minutes of physical activity.[31] Girls were less likely than boys to show adequate physical activity rates, and other studies have shown both ethnic disparities in activity levels and differences between immigrant and native children.[32] Physical activity has been directly linked to overweight status in overweight early adolescents; in fact, when multiple diet, sedentary, and activity behaviors were studied, the only factor shown to be predictive of a higher BMI in adolescent boys was decreased physical activity.[33]

Sedentary Behaviors

Patterns of inactivity and an unhealthy lifestyle are often established in adolescence.[34] Twenty-five percent of children's waking hours are spent watching television or playing video games, which is concerning because increased television time has been correlated with increased BMI and the development of type 2 diabetes.[35–37] In addition, television constitutes a predominant source of media influence on food choices and obesity. Even brief exposures to televised food commercials have been found to influence preschool-aged children's food preferences. It is possible that limiting exposure to food advertisements from the media would positively affect body composition in children.[38]

Genetics

Some genetic syndromes, such as Prader-Willi, Turner, and Lawrence-Moon-Biedl syndromes, are known to lead to obesity. Of note is that these disorders are generally accompanied by poor linear growth relative to an excessive body weight and that mental deficiency and hypogonadism are frequent features. Other genetic loci have been identified in recent years as strongly associated with obesity, such as one that encodes for the melanocortin 4 receptor. Alterations in this receptor have been shown to lead to binge-eating and obesity phenotypes.[39,40]

Family Risk Factors

A prospective study of 150 children from birth to 9.5 years of age found the strongest risk factor for childhood obesity to be parent overweight, which was mediated by child temperament.[41] After the age of 7 years, children with 2 overweight parents had consistently elevated BMIs, compared with children with either no overweight parents or 1 overweight parent.[42] Parental obesity also more than doubles the risk of adult obesity among both obese and nonobese children younger than 10 years of age.[43] Finally, family meal patterns can also influence these outcomes; family meals together are positively associated with improved dietary quality in adolescent children.[44]

Data have also suggested that disordered eating patterns can emerge during early childhood, possibly as a result of parental characteristics. Research has shown that the risk for emergence of inhibited eating, secretive eating, overeating, and vomiting increases annually through age. Maternal body dissatisfaction, internalization of the thin ideal, dieting, bulimic symptoms, and maternal and paternal body mass prospectively predicted the emergence of childhood eating disturbances.[45] These disordered eating patterns could potentially progress to a dysregulated pattern of binge eating and obesity in adolescence.

Psychological Factors

Disordered eating behaviors, especially binge-eating episodes, have been shown to be associated with greater weight gain.[46] Depressed adolescents are likely to have a higher BMI in adult life than would adolescents who are free of depression.[47] Ironically, attempts at concerning weight-control behaviors such as dietary restraint, self-labeled dieting, exercise for weight-control purposes, and appetite-suppressant/laxative use predict an increased risk for obesity onset in female adolescents.[48]

Hormonal/Physiological Factors

A few hormones are well-documented contributors to the pathogenesis of obesity. Insulin resistance has been shown to increase weight gain, and fasting plasma insulin levels are significantly greater in obese adolescents than in lean controls.[49] Disturbances in pathways of insulin-mediated lipolysis also play a role in the origin of obesity and in type 2 diabetes mellitus.[50] Leptin is secreted from adipocytes and helps to moderate food intake and energy expenditure, and circulating levels correlate with body fat and BMI.[51] Leptin actively increases during the peripubertal years, even before the appearance of other pubertal hormones, and is thought to interplay with pubertal initiation. Boys have lower leptin levels than girls, and decreases in boys coincide with rises in testosterone levels during puberty.[52] Finally, ghrelin is a gastric hormone with adipogenic properties, and increased levels are thought to contribute to hyperphagia. It has been shown to modulate pituitary hormones.[53]

Other hormones that are often considered to be important to the development and maintenance of obesity are corticotropin-releasing hormone (CRH), arginine vasopressin, melanocyte-stimulating hormone, glucocorticoids, neuropeptide Y (NPY), and the catecholamines, norepinephrine and epinephrine. Most of these help to promote weight gain, and may increase visceral abdominal fat stores,[54] as well as adverse metabolic changes.

COMORBIDITIES

Common obesity-related comorbidities are described in Table 2, with details following on the most well-described conditions below. Most of these are connected by a common thread of decreased insulin sensitivity; hyperlipidemia, hypertension, obstructive sleep apnea (OSA), polycystic ovarian syndrome (PCOS), nonalcoholic steatohepatitis (NASH), elevated inflammatory markers, and type 2 diabetes all have been strongly linked to insulin resistance.[55]

Hyperlipidemia and Cardiovascular Risk

Hyperlipidemia is commonly diagnosed in overweight adolescents. Studies have shown the occurrence of atherosclerotic lesions in the vasculature by late adolescence. They have also shown that hyperlipidemia is a common causal factor in the development of these lesions. The National Cholesterol Education Program guidelines suggest that all overweight adolescents undergo testing with a fasting lipid profile. Low-density lipoprotein (LDL) cholesterol levels of <110 mg/dL are considered acceptable, and levels of >130 mg/dL are considered elevated. LDL cholesterol levels of 110 to 130 mg/dL are considered borderline and necessitate repeat measurement in 1 year. Abnormal lipid profiles should prompt testing for other components of the metabolic syndrome, such as insulin resistance and hypertension. The finding of elevated LDL cholesterol values should trigger an individualized treatment plan, including dietary advice.[56] Statins should be considered for adolescents >10 years of age with LDL levels of >190 or >160 mg/dL with at least 2 other risk factors for premature coronary artery disease, and patients should be followed closely with regular laboratory work if these are initiated.[57] In addition, physical activity, omega-3 fatty acids, and dietary fiber have all been shown to have beneficial effects on lipoprotein profiles.[57]

Increases in BMI correlate with markers of elevated cardiovascular risk[58,59] and increased left ventricular size and relative wall thickness, all considered risk factors for future cardiovascular disease.[60] Obese pediatric subjects have higher levels of hemostatic and inflammatory markers, possibly putting children with this profile at greater risk for future cardiovascular disease.[61,62]

Hypertension

Obese adolescents commonly present with hypertension. Risk factors such as a positive family history of hypertension, an ethnic predisposition to hypertensive disease, and insulin resistance all make high blood pressure more likely. BMI is positively correlated with elevations in blood pressure, and weight loss can dramatically improve hypertension.[63]

Table 2
Common Comorbidities

Illness	Testing	Abnormal Levels	Treatment
Cardiac			
Hyperlipidemia	Fasting lipid profile	LDL >130–160 mg/dL, dependent on risk factors; HDL <40 mg/dL; cholesterol >180–200 mg/dL; triglycerides >150–200 mg/dL	Diet change (fewer saturated fats; omega 3 fatty acids may be helpful); exercise; pharmacotherapy can be considered if LDL level is >190 mg/dL
Hypertension	Blood pressure reading with appropriately sized cuff on 3 separate occasions	Systolic and/or diastolic blood pressure at >95th percentile for age and gender; prehypertension: >85th percentile	Prehypertension: dietary change, weight loss, and physical activity; grade I (95th–99th percentile): add pharmacotherapy if symptomatic; grade II (>99th percentile): pharmacotherapy should be considered
Metabolic syndrome (Adult Treatment Panel III)	Presence of ≥3 of the abnormal levels listed	Abdominal obesity, high triglyceride level, low HDL level, high blood pressure, high fasting glucose level	Treat individual components
Endocrine			
Diabetes type 2	Screen adolescents every 2 y if at risk of overweight (BMI >85th percentile) and 2 of the following: family history in first- or second-degree relatives; race/ethnicity; and associated conditions (acanthosis, PCOS hypertension, dyslipidemia)	Impaired fasting glucose level: 100–125 mg/dL; diabetes: fasting glucose >126 mg/dL; random glucose >200 mg/dL; 2-h oral glucose-tolerance test level >200 mg/dL	Dietary change; weight management; physical activity; metformin; bariatric surgery may be indicated for patients who have not improved with conventional therapy
PCOS	Consider testing if menstrual irregularity and some sign of androgen excess (acne, extra hair growth in unwanted areas, overweight, and/or abnormal blood values)	Androgen excess by laboratory tests or physical examination in the absence of other causes	Physical activity; metformin

(*Continued*)

Table 2
(Continued)

Illness	Testing	Abnormal Levels	Treatment
Pulmonary			
OSA	Polysomnogram (sleep study)	Abnormal sleep study results	Weight management; physical activity; continuous positive airway pressure; bariatric surgery may be indicated if severe
Restrictive lung disease and obesity hypoventilation syndrome	Lung function testing; polysomnogram	Restrictive lung function, build-up of carbon dioxide in the blood, excessive sleepiness, signs of heart failure over time	Weight management
Asthma	History, examination, lung function testing	Obstructive lung function	Physical activity; optimize asthma management; weight management; physical activity
Gastrointestinal			
NAFLD	Laboratory tests, ultrasound	Elevated liver function	Weight management, address insulin resistance; vitamin E sometimes helpful
Reflux or heartburn	Liver biopsy; history and physical; tests often unnecessary	Abnormal ultrasound or liver biopsy; nonspecific	Proton-pump inhibitors; weight management; dietary changes
Gallstones	Examination, ultrasound	Periodic abdominal pain, gallstones seen on ultrasound	Weight management, dietary changes, surgery, or lithotripsy sometimes necessary
Orthopedic			
Blount disease	Radiographs, physical examination, MRI when necessary; more common in black populations	Tibial bowing, chronic pain, abnormal radiologic tests	Surgical: tibial osteotomy; nonsurgical: weight management
Slipped capital femoral epiphysis	Radiographs, physical examination, MRI when necessary	Abnormal radiograph results; limp can be present; pain at hip, knee, or ankle; can be acute or subacute	Emergent surgery
Knee, back, and hip disease	Radiographs, physical examination, MRI when necessary		Weight management; nonsteroidal antiinflammatory medication; weight management; surgery occasionally necessary
Neurologic: IIH	Comprehensive eye examination, visual fields testing, lumbar puncture, MRI may be indicated	Persistent headaches, papilledema; blind spots in vision; elevated spinal fluid pressure	Weight management; ventricular shunts if severe; bariatric surgery

(*Continued*)

Table 2
(Continued)

Illness	Testing	Abnormal Levels	Treatment
Genitourinary			
Stress incontinence	History	Incontinence while laughing, coughing, or sneezing	Weight management
Gout	History, examination, uric acid level	Joint inflammation, high uric acid level in the blood	Dietary change; weight management; pharmacotherapy
Skin and blood vessels			
Infections	Physical examination	Red skin with an odor, especially in skinfolds and creases, under the breasts, beneath the abdomen, in leg skinfolds; fungal infections of the nails; poor wound healing resulting from poor circulation in the extremities	Improved hygiene in intertriginous regions; antifungal powders/creams; caution with steroid creams; culture if uncertain organism
Varicose veins	Physical examination	Dark purple veins on the lower legs	Laser therapy
Deep venous thrombosis	Physical examination, ultrasound	Clot seen on ultrasound; pain in calf	Support stockings; anticoagulation; emergent evaluation

HDL indicates high-density lipoprotein.

Type 2 Diabetes/Glucose Intolerance

Type 2 diabetes (non–insulin-dependent diabetes mellitus) accounts for nearly half of all reported diabetes cases in children and adolescents.[64] Impaired glucose tolerance is even more common in obese youth. Additional risk factors include a positive family history of type 2 diabetes, increased body and abdominal fat, insulin resistance, ethnicity (with greater risk in black, Hispanic, and Native American children), and earlier onset of puberty. These risk factors seem to be cumulative in their interactions and may be even more problematic during early adolescence, with changes in body-fat stores and hormonal signaling.[65]

Metabolic Syndrome

The metabolic syndrome is a clustering of metabolic risk factors, described as involving increased risk for premature cardiovascular disease and other comorbidities of insulin resistance. The factors include abdominal obesity, decreased high-density lipoprotein levels, elevated triglyceride levels, insulin resistance or diabetes, and elevated blood pressure, and having ≥3 criteria present qualifies patients for the diagnosis of metabolic syndrome. The metabolic syndrome seems to be quite prevalent in obese children.[66] However, there are different existing definitions of these criteria published, and no age-specific guidelines for diagnosis have been agreed on for adolescents. Most specialists adapt these guidelines for pediatric patients, but there is some controversy as to the diagnostic utility of this risk cluster.[67–69]

PCOS and Menstrual Irregularities

PCOS is diagnosed in women with a history of menstrual irregularity (usually oligomenorrhea or amenorrhea) in a setting of hyperandrogenism, either biochemical or clinical. Common clinical signs of hyperandrogenism are acne, hirsutism, or overweight, and only 1 of these signs needs to be present for the diagnosis of PCOS; it is even possible for none to be present if laboratory work shows increased androgen activity in the absence of other pathology. Other conditions of hyperandrogenism must be considered, such as late-onset congenital adrenal hyperplasia and ovarian or adrenal tumors, particularly when a patient shows virilization, and should be ruled out by either physical examination or laboratory findings before presuming that PCOS is present.

The name "PCOS" is a misnomer, because many patients with the condition do not have polycystic ovaries on ultrasound, and many young women with multiple cysts on their ovaries do not have PCOS. Ovarian cysts can be a normative finding in pubertal girls. Approximately 50% to 75% of women with PCOS are obese, most of whom are characterized by visceral abdominal obesity. Obesity may play a causative role in the development of PCOS in susceptible individuals. It certainly seems to contribute to the insulin resistance experienced by many women with PCOS.[70–72]

Sleep Apnea

OSA is also growing more and more common in obese adolescents and is significantly associated with future cardiovascular disease.[73,74] Current recommendations state that all children should be screened for snoring and that those who snore should be tested by polysomnography to determine if they have OSA.[73,75]

Nonalcoholic Steatohepatitis/Nonalcoholic Fatty Liver Disease

Nonalcoholic fatty liver disease (NAFLD) is commonly seen in association with obesity, diabetes, insulin resistance, hypertension, and hypertriglyceridemia. Most patients are asymptomatic and usually present with mild elevations in aminotransferase levels. The natural history of NAFLD is not clearly defined, but it can progress to cirrhosis and end-stage liver disease. Insulin resistance seems to play a key role, leading to altered glucose and lipid metabolism, culminating in hepatic steatosis. This then can progress to NASH or cirrhosis through mechanisms that are not yet well elucidated.[76–78] It is as yet unknown how common this disorder is in obese children and adolescents.

Gastroesophageal Reflux Disease

Gastroesophageal reflux disease is found frequently in obese populations and improves after weight loss. It should be considered and treated whenever an overweight adolescent complains of chronic epigastric pain after meals.[79]

Gall Bladder Disease

Nearly 50% of cases of cholecystitis are associated with obesity, although ironically, weight loss can also be complicated by cholelithiasis. Patients should be screened for abdominal pain, and this condition should be considered, particularly if coupled with a family history of gall bladder disease.[10]

Orthopedic Complications

Overweight children are at increased risk for a number of weight-related orthopedic complications. Chronic excess weight can lead to a bowing of the tibia and femur, causing an overgrowth on the medial aspect of the proximal tibial metaphysis called Blount disease; it is seen more commonly in both obese and nonobese black adolescents. Slipped capital femoral epiphysis can also result from excess weight and is considered an orthopedic emergency. Finally, many overweight patients have degenerative disease of the spine, leading to discomfort and decreased mobility as a result of excess pressure on the lower spine from their body mass.[10]

Idiopathic Intracranial Hypertension (Pseudotumor Cerebri)

Idiopathic intracranial hypertension (IIH) is a rarer condition in adolescents, although up to 59% of children and 91% of late adolescents with IIH are also obese.[80,81] It is characterized by increased intracranial pressure (ICP) in the absence of other intracranial pathology. Patients will typically complain of headaches and sometimes can experience severe visual impairment or blindness. Papilledema is often found during a physical examination. To diagnose IIH, the following criteria must be present: symptoms of increased ICP, a normal neurologic examination and mental status, normal brain-imaging results, evidence of increased ICP on examination and by lumbar puncture opening pressure, normal cerebrospinal fluid findings, and no identifiable cause of increased ICP. These criteria, also called the Dandy criteria, must be met to diagnose IIH. Once diagnosed, IIH requires prompt treatment with weight reduction, which is paramount to reduce the risk of further complications.[82]

Psychiatric Conditions

Overweight children and adolescents seem to be at risk of disordered eating, most commonly overeating and binge-eating disorder but also bulimia nervosa and night eating syndrome.[83–86] Overweight adolescents tend to experience more psychosocial distress than their nonoverweight peers.[87] BMI is positively associated with depressive symptoms in preadolescent girls, mediated by overweight concerns, but not in boys.[88] Other studies have demonstrated increased victimization and bullying behaviors with increased BMI.[89]

Overeating seems to be quite common in young people, with 17.3% of girls and 7.8% of boys reporting such behavior. Youth who overeat are more likely to be overweight or obese, to have dieted in the past year, to be trying to lose weight currently, and to report that weight and shape are very important to their overall feelings about themselves. Youth who binge eat have lower satisfaction with their body, lower self-esteem, and higher measures of depressive mood than those who report either subclinical or no binge eating. In 1 study, 28.6% of girls and 27.8% of boys who met criteria for binge-eating syndrome reported that they had attempted suicide.[90]

There are other life issues that obese individuals contend with daily and that impact their quality of life that are not well quantified by current research. These include, for example, difficulty fitting into airline seats, finding clothes that are stylish and also fit, facing discrimination in the workplace, and being exposed to contempt or criticism at times from our society in general, as well as from noncompassionate friends, family members, spouses, and children. These day-to-day issues are often quite prominent for adolescents with obesity, more so than the comorbidities that we are used to evaluating in an office visit, and it is important to consider them during a complete assessment.

EVALUATION

The first step in evaluating an adolescent suspected to be overweight is to calculate and plot the BMI for age and gender. If the BMI is ≥85th percentile with complications caused by obesity or is ≥95th percentile with or without complications, an evaluation and possible treatment plan should be initiated.[91]

Nutrition Assessment

Obtaining a full dietary history during the evaluation is important. A registered dietician, if available, can help with calorie counts and recommended treatment plans. However, assessing the frequency of sugared-drink and juice and convenience-food and fast-food consumption and the content of school lunches should be completed regardless of the dietician's availability.[92] Food diaries should be interpreted with caution, because self-reporting of food intake has known limitations.[93] Indirect calorimetry can be a helpful adjunct to determining resting energy-expenditure levels, especially for patients whose food reports do not match their clinical presentation.[94] Practitioners should remember to ask about risky eating behaviors (such as purging or diet-pill usage, binge eating, and night eating) and need not worry that this will increase such behaviors in children and adolescents.[95]

History and Physical Examination

If an adolescent is determined by BMI to be overweight, a thorough medical and nutritional assessment should be undertaken. Clinicians should examine and screen clinically for signs of rare exogenous causes of obesity. However, these are rarely seen and can often be ruled out on physical examination. If there is no delay in linear growth, an endocrinologic cause is unlikely. If no developmental delay and no dysmorphisms are present, genetic conditions are unlikely. It is recognized that parents and patients often seek a medical cause. Frequently, reassurance must be given that no further workup is necessary but that screening for comorbidities and treatment should be initiated without delay.

The American Academy of Pediatrics Expert Committee on Obesity in Children and Adolescents recommends screening by physical examination or laboratory test for hypertension, hyperlipidemia, orthopedic difficulties, OSA, gall bladder disease, and insulin resistance.[18] In addition, pseudotumor cerebri should be screened for by asking about headaches or vision loss and conducting a fundoscopic examination. PCOS should be considered in adolescent girls with obesity, because the condition is extremely common in this population and can increase future diabetes and lipid risk levels. Many people with obesity are diagnosed with asthma when their breathing difficulties are caused more by thoracic restriction from their increased BMI and undertraining. Therefore, it is important to elicit a history of breathing difficulties, along with a family history of asthma and allergies. Before starting chronic long-term antiinflammatory agents, a full round of pulmonary function tests should be considered. Screening for binge-eating and purging behaviors, along with body-image dysmorphisms and dietary supplement usage, is also wise, because these issues frequently coexist with difficulties in regulating weight.

Severe obesity can, at times, be difficult to manage in the primary care setting. Although each practitioner develops his or her own comfort level in this management, referrals to a subspecialist may be appropriate, particularly if the teenager has a significant comorbidity. American Academy of Pediatrics guidelines for further referral to a pediatric obesity specialist include pseudotumor cerebri, sleep disorders, orthopedic problems, morbid or severe obesity, or obesity in children <2 years of age.[91]

TREATMENT

General Considerations

Educating adolescents about healthy eating behaviors, the importance of physical activity, and sound nutritional practices is paramount to both the prevention and treatment of obesity in this age group. Sometimes, weight maintenance is the soundest course rather than initiating an aggressive weight-loss plan. If patients are likely to undergo additional linear growth, weight maintenance may be indicated. In addition, if they have already undergone multiple periods of weight cycling, with significant losses and regains and subsequent decreases in self-efficacy, it may be more empowering and productive in the long run to first focus on weight maintenance. However, when clinically severe comorbidities are present that impact quality of life, medically supervised weight loss is recommended. An important part of the assessment is to what degree both patients and family members are committed to engaging in treatment. Most successful long-term weight-treatment programs for adolescents include some family component. Helping with appropriate teaching of parenting skills and family support is a foundation of any weight-maintenance or weight-loss program for adolescents.[91,96] Finally, provider patience is important as well, because sometimes providers can feel frustrated at the time it takes for true lifestyle change to onset and take hold.

Frequent sessions, longer treatment, and the inclusion of individualized counseling with the group sessions have all been shown to be helpful components of behavioral change in young people with obesity. Cognitive behavior therapy is an emerging approach that also shows some promise.[97] Regardless of behavioral treatment approaches, clear and simple diets, physical activity programs, emphasis on reduction of sedentary behaviors, teaching skills for high-risk situations, and relapse prevention are important components of a well-structured pediatric weight program.[98]

Physical Activity

Physical activity has protective health effects at all weight ranges[99] and is sometimes even more predictive of cardiac risk factors and coronary artery disease than BMI.[100,101] Youth with poor fitness levels and high adiposity have higher levels of hemostatic markers, which may increase their risk of future cardiovascular disease.[61] Most weight-loss experts advocate a combination of aerobic and strength exercises, combined with behavioral modifications and calorie reduction, for optimal results in weight reduction.[34,97] A referral to physical therapy can be helpful in establishing such a program, particularly for adolescents whose obesity has imposed mobility constraints.

Decreasing Sedentary Behaviors

Media usage is more prominent now than ever. Identifying sedentary behaviors, particularly in the form of "screen time" (television, video game, or computer viewing) is as helpful as increasing physical activity in the adolescent population.[102] School-based interventions to reduce television, videotape, and video game usage in third- and fourth-graders have shown statistically significant decreases in BMI, in triceps skinfold thickness, waist circumference, and waist/hip ratio in the intervention group as compared with controls. These studies highlight the importance of reducing sedentary behaviors to achieve effective weight control in the pediatric population.[35]

Nutrition

No weight program can be successful without some ordered approach to improved nutrition. The most commonly used nutritional interventions and philosophies are reviewed in Table 1. Liquid diets have not been well studied in adolescents and, therefore, are not reviewed. It is important to remember that very few studies have assessed long-term efficacy in weight loss with any dietary intervention in adolescents, and most long-term studies in adults have not documented sustained weight loss at 1- or 5-year follow-ups. Thus, our emphasis on dietary modification is important and common sense in origin but should not be the sole emphasis when treating obese adolescents.

Pharmacotherapy

Few weight-loss medications have been studied in adolescents, and usually such medications are only indicated for severe obesity that has not responded to other measures.[91] To date, no studies have been conducted to examine these medications in a long-term, randomized, double-blind, placebo-controlled trial and compare them with a program that involves diet, exercise, and behavior modification. Thus, the findings in children and adolescents of certain currently used weight-loss medications (detailed in Table 3) should be interpreted with caution, because studies are limited and the medications carry risk.[103,104] Over-the-counter diet pills, which are abundant and highly available and marketed to obese adolescents, are, nonetheless, very poorly studied and should be discouraged.

Weight-Loss Surgery

The most common weight-loss procedure performed in adolescents is Roux-en-Y gastric bypass (RYGB). Adjustable gastric banding (AGB), currently only US Food and Drug Administration–approved for adults, has been performed in research trials for adolescents, and the results published to date are promising. The RYGB is the procedure most commonly performed and accepted. It is both restrictive, by creating a small (1-oz) gastric pouch, and malabsorptive, in that

Table 3
Pharmacotherapy in adolescent obesity

Medication	Mechanism of Action	Evidence/Studies
Sibutramine	Inhibitor of norepinephrine, serotonin, and dopamine uptake; adverse effects: mild hypertension and tachycardia, but can also include dry mouth, headache, insomnia, and constipation; should not be administered in conjunction with monoamine oxidase inhibitors or other serotonin-reuptake inhibitors[103,104]	Decreased weight in adults in randomized, double-blind, placebo-controlled study[134]; trials involving adolescents have shown that sibutramine-treated groups lose significantly more weight, report less hunger, and have improved metabolic profiles than placebo group or behavior-change groups[135–137]
Orlistat	Gastrointestinal lipase inhibitor; adverse effects: decreased levels of fat-soluble vitamins, flatulence, fecal incontinence, and steatorrhea[103,104]	Showed significant weight loss in a randomized, controlled trial in adolescents when compared with dietary and behavioral intervention[138]
Metformin	Inhibits hepatic glucose production and intestinal glucose absorption; increases insulin sensitivity; adverse effects: nausea, flatulence, bloating, and diarrhea; black-box warning for lactic acidosis, a rare complication that is fatal in 50% of cases, and affects primarily patients with renal insufficiency, decreased perfusion, cardiac or pulmonary insufficiency, and liver disease; the use of metformin is contraindicated in those with these conditions[103,104]	A randomized, placebo-controlled trial of obese adolescents with hyperinsulinemia showed significant decreases in BMI and favorable metabolic changes in the treated group compared with the placebo group[139,140]
Octreotide	Suppresses pancreatic insulin secretion; must be injected and can cause pain at the injection site; adverse effects: gallstones, diarrhea, abdominal pain, nausea, cardiac abnormalities, vitamin B_{12} deficiency, hypothyroidism, suppression of growth hormone secretion, and type 1 diabetes	Studied in children with hypothalamic obesity after intracranial therapy for cancer with good results, but not in other pediatric populations; still requires more study before increased use[103,104]

this pouch then drains via a narrow passageway to the middle part of the small intestine, the jejunum, and thereby bypasses the duodenum. AGB entails placing an adjustable band around the upper portion of the stomach to create a smaller gastric pouch and, thus, is a restrictive procedure. Criteria for bariatric surgery in the pediatric population are listed in Table 4. Contraindications to surgery include a medically correctable cause of obesity, recent history of substance abuse, any con-

Table 4
Criteria for bariatric surgery in adolescents[105]

BMI ≥ 40 and at least 1 of the following
- Diabetes mellitus type 2
- Sleep apnea
- Pseudotumor cerebri

or

BMI ≥50 with less-serious comorbidities
- Hypertension
- Dyslipidemia
- NASH
- Venous stasis
- Impaired activities of daily living
- Intertriginous infection
- Stress incontinence
- Gastroesophageal reflux disease
- Weight-related arthropathies
- Weight-related arthropathies
- Obesity-related psychosocial disease

Additional criteria
- Skeletal maturation
- Girls, ≥13 y old
- Boys, ≥15 y old
- Psychiatric evaluation that shows no contraindication and cognitive maturity to make decisions and comply with recommendations
- Good social support system
- Participation in at least 6 mo of organized attempts at weight management or other good demonstration of an ability to comply with medical recommendations over time

New in-press surgical criteria modify BMI cutoffs to ≥35 with comorbidities (and include severe NASH) and ≥40 in adolescents with other comorbidities.[141]

dition that would impair adherence to postoperative dietary or medication regimens, current lactation or pregnancy, or planned pregnancy within 2 years after the surgery. Potential postoperative complications can include intestinal leakage, strictures, small-bowel obstruction, infection, cholelithiasis, nutritional deficiencies, thromboembolism, and even death.[105–107]

New guidelines are in press that revise previous recommendations of when weight-loss surgery might be considered for treatment of severe refractory obesity in the pediatric population, because this procedure is being performed increasingly.[105,106] Both published and in-press guidelines are listed in Table 4. Gastric-bypass surgery has been shown to be curative for diabetes mellitus in some adult and adolescent subjects[108] and dramatically improves sleep apnea and pseudotumor cerebri. Results published from studies in adolescents have been promising, with case series showing weight reductions in excess of 30 kg and a cohort-controlled multicenter study comparing laparoscopic RYGB to 1 year in a pediatric behavioral treatment program showing BMI changes in the intervention group from 56.5 to 35.8 kg/m^2, with significant resolution of comorbidities, as compared with no significant change in BMI in the comparison group with a family-based behavioral intervention.[109,110] Long-term studies have been too small to adequately assess longitudinal success and risks, but they have shown few unanticipated complications in the initial postoperative periods.[111,112]

Hazards of Weight Loss

Rapid and profound weight loss is associated with dangers of its own. When obese subjects are placed on very low calorie diets, they experience a loss of myocardial muscle mass. Ventricular tachyarrhythmias, prolongation of the QT interval, syncope, and sudden death are known complications of such regimens.[113–115] It is clearly important not to casually endorse a regimen that is dangerously low in calories or causes extremely rapid weight loss.

Studies that have examined the risk of developing eating disorders after efforts at weight loss have shown that girls who have great concern about their weight are more likely to develop eating disorders.[116,117] Much has been published on dieting in adolescents ultimately leading to weight gain and unhealthy weight-control practices over time.[118] Few studies have examined the risk of developing disordered eating after participation in organized programs aimed at weight loss. However, a school-based obesity-prevention program showed significantly decreased rates of disordered eating in the intervention group compared with controls.[119] Therefore, it may be that reaching preadolescents and younger children with obesity prevention rather than treatment is key to the combined efforts of reducing obesity and eating disorders.

CONCLUSIONS

Obesity and its complications are commonly found in adolescent populations. BMI for age is the measure of choice for defining obesity in pediatric patients. Thorough evaluations should screen for all related comorbidities, because they are becoming more common. Therapy rests on behavior change, increased activity, decreased sedentary activities, and diet modifications. However, in extreme cases, pharmacotherapy, even bariatric surgery, may be considered in the therapeutic plan. Continuing advocacy on the part of both patients and health care providers will be instrumental in providing much-needed education and support to be able to adequately care for this population.

REFERENCES

1. Ogden CL, Carroll MD, Flegal KM. High body mass index for age among US children and adolescents, 2003–2006. *JAMA*. 2008;299(20):2401–2405
2. Ogden CL, Carroll MD, Curtin LR, McDowell MA, Tabak CJ, Flegal KM. Prevalence of overweight and obesity in the United States, 1999–2004. *JAMA*. 2006;295(13):1549–1555
3. Dietz WH. Overweight in childhood and adolescence. *N Engl J Med*. 2004;350(9):855–857

4. Ahn MK, Juon HS, Gittelsohn J. Association of race/ethnicity, socioeconomic status, acculturation, and environmental factors with risk of overweight among adolescents in California, 2003. *Prev Chronic Dis.* 2008;5(3):A75
5. Wang G, Dietz WH. Economic burden of obesity in youths aged 6 to 17 years: 1979–1999 [published correction appears in *Pediatrics.* 2002;109(6):1195]. *Pediatrics.* 2002;109(5). Available at: www.pediatrics.org/cgi/content/full/109/5/e81
6. Gortmaker SL, Must A, Perrin JM, Sobol AM, Dietz WH. Social and economic consequences of overweight in adolescence and young adulthood. *N Engl J Med.* 1993;329(14):1008–1012
7. Schwimmer JB, Burwinkle TM, Varni JW. Health-related quality of life of severely obese children and adolescents. *JAMA.* 2003;289(14):1813–1819
8. Modi AC, Loux TJ, Bell SK, Harmon CM, Inge TH, Zeller MH. Weight-specific health-related quality of life in adolescents with extreme obesity. *Obesity (Silver Spring).* 2008;16(10):2266–2271
9. de Beer M, Hofsteenge GH, Koot HM, Hirasing RA, Delemarre-van de Waal HA, Gemke RJ. Health-related-quality-of-life in obese adolescents is decreased and inversely related to BMI. *Acta Paediatr.* 2007;96(5):710–714
10. Dietz WH. Health consequences of obesity in youth: childhood predictors of adult disease. *Pediatrics.* 1998;101(3 pt 2):518–525
11. Wang LY, Chyen D, Lee S, Lowry R. The association between body mass index in adolescence and obesity in adulthood. *J Adolesc Health.* 2008;42(5):512–518
12. Calle EE, Thun MJ, Petrelli JM, Rodriguez C, Heath CW Jr. Body mass index and mortality in a prospective cohort of U.S. Adults. *N Engl J Med.* 1999;341(15):1097–1105
13. Mokdad AH, Marks JS, Stroup DF, Gerberding JL. Actual causes of death in the United States, 2000. *JAMA.* 2004;291(10):1238–1245
14. Mokdad AH, Ford ES, Bowman BA, et al. Prevalence of obesity, diabetes, and obesity-related health risk factors, 2001. *JAMA.* 2003;289(1):76–79
15. Dietz WH, Robinson TN. Use of the body mass index (BMI) as a measure of overweight in children and adolescents. *J Pediatr.* 1998;132(2):191–193
16. Krebs NF, Jacobson MS; American Academy of Pediatrics, Committee on Nutrition. Prevention of pediatric overweight and obesity. *Pediatrics.* 2003;112(2):424–430
17. Hammer LD, Kraemer HC, Wilson DM, Ritter PL, Dornbusch SM. Standardized percentile curves of body-mass index for children and adolescents. *Am J Dis Child.* 1991;145(3):259–263
18. Barlow SE; Expert Committee. Expert committee recommendations regarding the prevention, assessment, and treatment of child and adolescent overweight and obesity: summary report. *Pediatrics.* 2007;120(suppl):S164–S192
19. Whitaker RC, Dietz WH. Role of the prenatal environment in the development of obesity. *J Pediatr.* 1998;132(5):768–776
20. Skinner JD, Bounds W, Carruth BR, Morris M, Ziegler P. Predictors of children's body mass index: a longitudinal study of diet and growth in children aged 2–8 years. *Int J Obes Relat Metab Disord.* 2004;28(4):476–482
21. Bhargava SK, Sachdev HS, Fall CHD, et al. Relation of serial changes in childhood body-mass index to impaired glucose tolerance in young adulthood. *N Engl J Med.* 2004;350(9):865–875
22. Freedman DS, Khan LK, Serdula MK, Dietz WH, Srinivasan SR, Berenson GS. The relation of menarcheal age to obesity in childhood and adulthood: the Bogalusa heart study. *BMC Pediatr.* 2003;3:3
23. Frontini M, Srinivasan SR, Berenson GS. Longitudinal changes in risk variables underlying metabolic syndrome X from childhood to young adulthood in female subjects with a history of early menarche: the Bogalusa Heart Study. *Int J Obes Relat Metab Disord.* 2003;27(11):1398–1404
24. Bowman SA, Gortmaker SL, Ebbeling CB, Pereira MA, Ludwig DS. Effects of fast-food consumption on energy intake and diet quality among children in a national household survey. *Pediatrics.* 2004;113(1 pt 1):112–118

25. Ebbeling CB, Sinclair KB, Pereira MA, Garcia-Lago E, Feldman HA, Ludwig DS. Compensation for energy intake from fast food among overweight and lean adolescents. *JAMA.* 2004;291(23):2828–2833
26. Ludwig DS. Dietary glycemic index and the regulation of body weight. *Lipids.* 2003;38(2): 117–121
27. Ebbeling CB, Leidig MM, Sinclair KB, Hangen JP, Ludwig DS. A reduced-glycemic load diet in the treatment of adolescent obesity. *Arch Pediatr Adolesc Med.* 2003;157(8):773–779
28. Ball SD, Keller KR, Moyer-Mileur LJ, Ding YW, Donaldson D, Jackson WD. Prolongation of satiety after low versus moderately high glycemic index meals in obese adolescents. *Pediatrics.* 2003;111(3):488–494
29. Lin YC, Lyle RM, McCabe LD, McCabe GP, Weaver CM, Teegarden D. Dairy calcium is related to changes in body composition during a two-year exercise intervention in young women. *J Am Coll Nutr.* 2000;19(6):754–760
30. Pereira MA, Jacobs DR Jr, Van Horn L, Slattery ML, Kartashov AI, Ludwig DS. Dairy consumption, obesity, and the insulin resistance syndrome in young adults: the CARDIA Study. *JAMA.* 2002;287(16):2081–2089
31. Eaton DK, Kann L, Kinchen S, et al. Youth risk behavior surveillance: United States, 2007. *MMWR Surveill Summ.* 2008;57(4):1–131
32. Singh GK, Yu SM, Siahpush M, Kogan MD. High levels of physical inactivity and sedentary behaviors among US immigrant children and adolescents. *Arch Pediatr Adolesc Med.* 2008; 162(8):756–763
33. Patrick K, Norman GJ, Calfas KJ, et al. Diet, physical activity, and sedentary behaviors as risk factors for overweight in adolescence. *Arch Pediatr Adolesc Med.* 2004;158(4):385–390
34. Amisola RVB, Jacobson M. Physical activity, exercise, and sedentary activity: relationship to the causes and treatment of obesity. *Adolesc Med.* 2003;14(1):23–35
35. Robinson TN. Reducing children's television viewing to prevent obesity: a randomized controlled trial. *JAMA.* 1999;282(16):1561–1567
36. Robinson TN, Hammer LD, Killen JD, et al. Does television viewing increase obesity and reduce physical activity? Cross-sectional and longitudinal analyses among adolescent girls. *Pediatrics.* 1993;91(2):273–280
37. Robinson TN, Killen JD, Kraemer HC, et al. Dance and reducing television viewing to prevent weight gain in African-American girls: the Stanford GEMS pilot study. *Ethn Dis.* 2003;13(1 suppl 1):S65–S77
38. Borzekowski DL, Robinson TN. The 30-second effect: an experiment revealing the impact of television commercials on food preferences of preschoolers. *J Am Diet Assoc.* 2001;101(1): 42–46
39. Farooqi IS, Keogh JM, Yeo GS, Lank EJ, Cheetham T, O'Rahilly S. Clinical spectrum of obesity and mutations in the melanocortin 4 receptor gene. *N Engl J Med.* 2003;348(12):1085–1095
40. Branson R, Potoczna N, Kral JG, Lentes KU, Hoehe MR, Horber FF. Binge eating as a major phenotype of melanocortin 4 receptor gene mutations. *N Engl J Med.* 2003;348(12):1096–1103
41. Agras WS, Hammer LD, McNicholas F, Kraemer HC. Risk factors for childhood overweight: a prospective study from birth to 9.5 years. *J Pediatr.* 2004;145(1):20–25
42. Safer DL, Agras WS, Bryson S, Hammer LD. Early body mass index and other anthropometric relationships between parents and children. *Int J Obes (Lond).* 2001;25(10):1532–1536
43. Whitaker RC, Wright JA, Pepe MS, Seidel KD, Dietz WH. Predicting obesity in young adulthood from childhood and parental obesity. *N Engl J Med.* 1997;337(13):869–873
44. Larson NI, Neumark-Sztainer D, Hannan PJ, Story M. Family meals during adolescence are associated with higher diet quality and healthful meal patterns during young adulthood. *J Am Diet Assoc.* 2007;107(9):1502–1510
45. Stice E, Agras WS, Hammer LD. Risk factors for the emergence of childhood eating disturbances: a five-year prospective study. *Int J Eat Disord.* 1999;25(4):375–387
46. Morgan CM, Yanovski SZ, Nguyen TT, et al. Loss of control over eating, adiposity, and psychopathology in overweight children. *Int J Eat Disord.* 2002;31(4):430–441

47. Stunkard AJ, Faith MS, Allison KC. Depression and obesity. *Biol Psychiatry.* 2003;54(3):330–337
48. Stice E, Cameron RP, Killen JD, Hayward C, Taylor CB. Naturalistic weight-reduction efforts prospectively predict growth in relative weight and onset of obesity among female adolescents. *J Consult Clin Psychol.* 1999;67(6):967–974
49. Attia N, Tamborlane WV, Heptulla R, et al. The metabolic syndrome and insulin-like growth factor I regulation in adolescent obesity. *J Clin Endocrinol Metab.* 1998;83(5):1467–1471
50. Blaak E. Fatty acid metabolism in obesity and type 2 diabetes mellitus. *Proc Nutr Soc.* 2003;62(3):753–760
51. Moran O, Phillip M. Leptin: obesity, diabetes and other peripheral effects: a review. *Pediatr Diabetes.* 2003;4(2):101–109
52. Garcia-Mayor RV, Andrade MA, Rios M, Lage M, Dieguez C, Casanueva FF. Serum leptin levels in normal children: relationship to age, gender, body mass index, pituitary-gonadal hormones, and pubertal stage. *J Clin Endocrinol Metab.* 1997;82(9):2849–2855
53. Pagotto U, Gambineri A, Vicennati V, Heiman ML, Tschöp M, Pasquali R. Plasma ghrelin, obesity, and the polycystic ovary syndrome: correlation with insulin resistance and androgen levels. *J Clin Endocrinol Metab.* 2002;87(12):5625–5629
54. Cavagnini F, Croci M, Putignano P, Petroni ML, Invitti C. Glucocorticoids and neuroendocrine function. *Int J Obes Relat Metab Disord.* 2000;24(suppl 2):S77–S79
55. Reaven G. Insulin resistance, type 2 diabetes mellitus, and cardiovascular disease: the end of the beginning. *Circulation.* 2005;112(20):3030–3032
56. Belay B, Belamarich P, Racine AD. Pediatric precursors of adult atherosclerosis. *Pediatr Rev.* 2004;25(1):4–16
57. McCrindle BW, Urbina EM, Dennison BA, et al. Drug therapy of high-risk lipid abnormalities in children and adolescents: a scientific statement from the American Heart Association, Atherosclerosis, Hypertension, and Obesity in Youth Committee, Council of Cardiovascular Disease in the Young, with the Council on Cardiovascular Nursing. *Circulation.* 2007;115(14): 1948–1967
58. Freedman DS, Khan LK, Dietz WH, Srinivasan SR, Berenson GS. Relationship of childhood obesity to coronary heart disease risk factors in adulthood: the Bogalusa Heart Study. *Pediatrics.* 2001;108(3):712–718
59. Freedman DS, Dietz WH, Srinivasan SR, Berenson GS. The relation of overweight to cardiovascular risk factors among children and adolescents: the Bogalusa Heart Study. *Pediatrics.* 1999;103(6 pt 1):1175–1182
60. Humphries MC, Gutin B, Barbeau P, Vemulapalli S, Allison J, Owens S. Relations of adiposity and effects of training on the left ventricle in obese youths. *Med Sci Sports Exerc.* 2002;34(9): 1428–1435
61. Barbeau P, Litaker MS, Woods KF, et al. Hemostatic and inflammatory markers in obese youths: effects of exercise and adiposity. *J Pediatr.* 2002;141(3):415–420
62. Hackam DG, Anand SS. Emerging risk factors for atherosclerotic vascular disease: a critical review of the evidence. *JAMA.* 2003;290(7):932–940
63. Sorof J, Daniels S. Obesity hypertension in children: a problem of epidemic proportions. *Hypertension.* 2002;40(4):441–447
64. Rowell HA, Evans BJ, Quarry-Horn JL, Kerrigan JR. Type 2 diabetes mellitus in adolescents. *Adolesc Med.* 2002;13(1):1–12, v
65. Goran MI, Ball GD, Cruz ML. Obesity and risk of type 2 diabetes and cardiovascular disease in children and adolescents. *J Clin Endocrinol Metab.* 2003;88(4):1417–1427
66. Weiss R, Dziura J, Burgert TS, et al. Obesity and the metabolic syndrome in children and adolescents. *N Engl J Med.* 2004;350(23):2362–2374
67. Goodman E. Metabolic syndrome and the mismeasure of risk. *J Adolesc Health.* 2008;42(6): 538–540
68. Love-Osborne KA, Nadeau KJ, Sheeder J, Fenton LZ, Zeitler P. Presence of the metabolic syndrome in obese adolescents predicts impaired glucose tolerance and nonalcoholic fatty liver disease. *J Adolesc Health.* 2008;42(6):543–548

69. Grundy SM, Brewer HB Jr, Cleeman JI, Smith SC, Lenfant C. Definition of metabolic syndrome: report of the National Heart, Lung, and Blood Institute/American Heart Association Conference on Scientific Issues Related to Definition. *Circulation.* 2004;109(3):433–438
70. Gordon CM. Menstrual disorders in adolescents: excess androgens and the polycystic ovary syndrome. *Pediatr Clin North Am.* 1999;46(3):519–543
71. Franks S. Polycystic ovary syndrome. *N Engl J Med.* 1995;333(13):853–861
72. Gambineri A, Pelusi C, Vicennati V, Pagotto U, Pasquali R. Obesity and the polycystic ovary syndrome. *Int J Obes Relat Metab Disord.* 2002;26(7):883–896
73. American Academy of Pediatrics, Section on Pediatric Pulmonology, Subcommittee on Obstructive Sleep Apnea Syndrome. Clinical practice guideline: diagnosis and management of childhood obstructive sleep apnea syndrome. *Pediatrics.* 2002;109(4):704–712
74. Shamsuzzaman ASM, Gersh BJ, Somers VK. Obstructive sleep apnea: implications for cardiac and vascular disease. *JAMA.* 2003;290(14):1906–1914
75. Matiz A, Roman EA. In brief: apnea. *Pediatr Rev.* 2003;24(1):32–34
76. American Gastroenterological Association medical position statement: nonalcoholic fatty liver disease. *Gastroenterology.* 2002;123(5):1702–1704
77. Harrison SA, Di Bisceglie AM. Advances in the understanding and treatment of nonalcoholic fatty liver disease. *Drugs.* 2003;63(22):2379–2394
78. Beymer C, Kowdley KV, Larson A, Edmonson P, Dellinger EP, Flum DR. Prevalence and predictors of asymptomatic liver disease in patients undergoing gastric bypass surgery. *Arch Surg.* 2003;138(11):1240–1244
79. Suter M, Dorta G, Giusti V, Calmes JM. Gastro-esophageal reflux and esophageal motility disorders in morbidly obese patients. *Obes Surg.* 2004;14(7):959–966
80. Kesler A, Fattal-Valevski A. Idiopathic intracranial hypertension in the pediatric population. *J Child Neurol.* 2002;17(10):745–748
81. Balcer LH, Liu GT, Forman S, et al. Idiopathic intracranial hypertension: relation of age and obesity in children. *Neurology.* 1999;52(4):870–872
82. Binder DK, Horton JC, Lawton MT, McDermott MW. Idiopathic intracranial hypertension. *Neurosurgery.* 2004;54(3):538–552; discussion 551–552
83. Colles SL, Dixon JB, O'Brien PE. Night eating syndrome and nocturnal snacking: association with obesity, binge eating and psychological distress. *Int J Obes (Lond).* 2007;31(11):1722–1730
84. Decaluwé V, Braet C. Prevalence of binge-eating disorder in obese children and adolescents seeking weight-loss treatment. *Int J Obes Relat Metab Disord.* 2003;27(3):404–409
85. Decaluwé V, Braet C, Fairburn CG. Binge eating in obese children and adolescents. *Int J Eat Disord.* 2003;33(1):78–84
86. Van Vlierberghe L, Braet C, Goossens L, Rosseel Y, Mels S. Psychological disorder, symptom severity and weight loss in inpatient adolescent obesity treatment. *Int J Pediatr Obes.* 2008;1–9
87. Mellin AM, Neumark-Sztainer D, Story M, Ireland M, Resnick MD. Unhealthy behaviors and psychosocial difficulties among overweight adolescents: the potential impact of familial factors. *J Adolesc Health.* 2002;31(2):145–153
88. Erickson SJ, Robinson TN, Haydel KF, Killen JD. Are overweight children unhappy? Body mass index, depressive symptoms, and overweight concerns in elementary school children. *Arch Pediatr Adolesc Med.* 2000;154(9):931–935
89. Janssen I, Craig WM, Boyce WF, Pickett W. Associations between overweight and obesity with bullying behaviors in school-aged children. *Pediatrics.* 2004;113(5):1187–1194
90. Ackard DM, Neumark-Sztainer D, Story M, Perry C. Overeating among adolescents: prevalence and associations with weight-related characteristics and psychological health. *Pediatrics.* 2003;111(1):67–74
91. Barlow SE, Dietz WH. Obesity evaluation and treatment: expert committee recommendations. The Maternal and Child Health Bureau, Health Resources and Services Administration and the Department of Health and Human Services. *Pediatrics.* 1998;102(3). Available at: www.pediatrics.org/cgi/content/full/102/3/e29

92. Copperman N, Jacobson M. Medical nutrition therapy of overweight adolescents. *Adolesc Med.* 2003;14(1):11–20
93. Matheson DM, Hanson KA, McDonald TE, Robinson TN. Validity of children's food portion estimates: a comparison of 2 measurement aids. *Arch Pediatr Adolesc Med.* 2002;156(9):867–871
94. Schebendach J. The use of indirect calorimetry in the clinical management of adolescents with nutritional disorders. *Adolesc Med.* 2003;14(1):77–85
95. Celio AA, Bryson S, Killen JD, Barr Taylor C. Are adolescents harmed when asked risky weight control behavior and attitude questions? Implications for consent procedures. *Int J Eat Disord.* 2003;34(2):251–254
96. Epstein LH, Valoski A, Wing RR, McCurley J. Ten-year outcomes of behavioral family based treatment for childhood obesity. *Health Psychol.* 1994;13(5):373–383
97. Tsiros MD, Sinn N, Coates AM, Howe PR, Buckley JD. Treatment of adolescent overweight and obesity. *Eur J Pediatr.* 2008;167(1):9–16
98. Robinson TN. Behavioural treatment of childhood and adolescent obesity. *Int J Obes Relat Metab Disord.* 1999;23(suppl 2):S52–S57
99. Blair SN, Church TS. The fitness, obesity, and health equation: is physical activity the common denominator? *JAMA.* 2004;292(10):1232–1234
100. Wessel TR, Arant CB, Olson MB, et al. Relationship of physical fitness vs body mass index with coronary artery disease and cardiovascular events in women. *JAMA.* 2004;292(10):1179–1187
101. Becque MD, Katch VL, Rocchini AP, Marks CR, Moorehead C. Coronary risk incidence of obese adolescents: reduction by exercise plus diet intervention. *Pediatrics.* 1988;81(5):605–612
102. Epstein LH, Paluch RA, Gordy CC, Dorn J. Decreasing sedentary behaviors in treating pediatric obesity. *Arch Pediatr Adolesc Med.* 2000;154(3):220–226
103. Yanovski SZ, Yanovski JA. Drug therapy: obesity. *N Engl J Med.* 2002;346(8):591–602
104. Yanovski JA. Intensive therapies for pediatric obesity. *Pediatr Clin North Am.* 2001;48(4): 1041–1053
105. Inge TH, Krebs NF, Garcia VF, et al. Bariatric surgery for severely overweight adolescents: concerns and recommendations. *Pediatrics.* 2004;114(1):217–223
106. Garcia VF, Langford L, Inge TH. Application of laparoscopy for bariatric surgery in adolescents. *Curr Opin Pediatr.* 2003;15(3):248–255
107. Byrne TK. Complications of surgery for obesity. *Surg Clin North Am.* 2001;81(5):1181–1193, vii–viii
108. Schauer PR, Burguera B, Ikramuddin S, et al. Effect of laparoscopic Roux-en-Y gastric bypass on type 2 diabetes mellitus. *Ann Surg.* 2003;238(4):467–484
109. Lawson ML, Kirk S, Mitchell T, et al. One-year outcomes of Roux-en-Y gastric bypass for morbidly obese adolescents: a multicenter study from the Pediatric Bariatric Study Group. *J Pediatr Surg.* 2006;41(1):137–143; discussion 137–143
110. Nadler EP, Youn HA, Ren CJ, Fielding GA. An update on 73 US obese pediatric patients treated with laparoscopic adjustable gastric banding: comorbidity resolution and compliance data. *J Pediatr Surg.* 2008;43(1):141–146
111. Inge TH, Garcia V, Daniels S, et al. A multidisciplinary approach to the adolescent bariatric surgical patient. *J Pediatr Surg.* 2004;39(3):442–447; discussion 446–447
112. Strauss RS, Bradley LJ, Brolin RE. Gastric bypass surgery in adolescents with morbid obesity. *J Pediatr.* 2001;138(4):499–504
113. Siegel RJ, Cabeen WR Jr, Roberts WC. Prolonged QT interval: ventricular tachycardia syndrome from massive rapid weight loss utilizing the liquid-protein-modified-fast diet: sudden death with sinus node ganglionitis and neuritis. *Am Heart J.* 1981;102(1):121–122
114. Drott C, Lundholm K. Cardiac effects of caloric restriction-mechanisms and potential hazards. *Int J Obes Relat Metab Disord.* 1992;16(7):481–486
115. Sours HE, Frattali VP, Brand CD, et al. Sudden death associated with very low calorie weight reduction regimens. *Am J Clin Nutr.* 1981;34(4):453–461

116. Killen JD, Taylor CB, Hayward C, et al. Pursuit of thinness and onset of eating disorder symptoms in a community sample of adolescent girls: a three-year prospective analysis. *Int J Eat Disord.* 1994;16(3):227–238
117. Killen JD, Taylor CB, Hayward C, et al. Weight concerns influence the development of eating disorders: a 4-year prospective study. *J Consult Clin Psychol.* 1996;64(5):936–940
118. Neumark-Sztainer D, Wall M, Guo J, Story M, Haines J, Eisenberg M. Obesity, disordered eating, and eating disorders in a longitudinal study of adolescents: how do dieters fare 5 years later? *J Am Diet Assoc.* 2006;106(4):559–568
119. Austin SB, Kim J, Wiecha J, Troped PJ, Feldman HA, Peterson KE. School-based overweight preventive intervention lowers incidence of disordered weight-control behaviors in early adolescent girls. *Arch Pediatr Adolesc Med.* 2007;161(9):865–869
120. Anderson JW. Diet first, then medication for hypercholesterolemia. *JAMA.* 2003;290(4):531–533
121. US Department of Agriculture, US Department of Health and Human Services. *Nutrition and Your Health: Dietary Guidelines for Americans.* 4th ed. Washington, DC: US Department of Agriculture; 2000
122. Kimm SY. The role of dietary fiber in the development and treatment of childhood obesity. *Pediatrics.* 1995;96(5 pt 2):1010–1014
123. Belury MA, Mahon A, Banni S. The conjugated linoleic acid (CLA) isomer, t10c12-CLA, is inversely associated with changes in body weight and serum leptin in subjects with type 2 diabetes mellitus. *J Nutr.* 2003;133(1):257S–260S
124. Brown JM, McIntosh MK. Conjugated linoleic acid in humans: regulation of adiposity and insulin sensitivity. *J Nutr.* 2003;133(10):3041–3046
125. Simopoulos AP. Omega-3 fatty acids in inflammation and autoimmune diseases. *J Am Coll Nutr.* 2002;21(6):495–505
126. Pelkman CL, Fishell VK, Maddox DH, Pearson TA, Mauger DT, Kris-Etherton PM. Effects of moderate fat (from monounsaturated fat) and low-fat weight-loss diets on the serum lipid profile in overweight and obese men and women. *Am J Clin Nutr.* 2004;79(2):204–212
127. Epstein LH, Valoski A, Koeske R, Wing RR. Family-based behavioral weight control in obese young children. *J Am Diet Assoc.* 1986;86(4):481–484
128. Samaha FF, Iqbal N, Seshadri P, et al. A low-carbohydrate as compared with a low-fat diet in severe obesity. *N Engl J Med.* 2003;348(21):2074–2081
129. Sondike SB, Copperman N, Jacobson MS. Effects of a low-carbohydrate diet on weight loss and cardiovascular risk factors in overweight adolescents. *J Pediatr.* 2003;142(3):253–258
130. Gardner CD, Kiazand A, Alhassan S, et al. Comparison of the Atkins, zone, Ornish, and LEARN diets for change in weight and related risk factors among overweight premenopausal women: the A TO Z Weight Loss Study—a randomized trial [published correction appears in *JAMA.* 2007;298(2):178]. *JAMA.* 2007;297(9):969–977
131. Figueroa-Colon R, von Almen TK, Franklin FA, Schuftan C, Suskind RM. Comparison of two hypocaloric diets in obese children. *Am J Dis Child.* 1993;147(2):160–166
132. Bacon L, Keim NL, Van Loan MD, et al. Evaluating a "non-diet" wellness intervention for improvement of metabolic fitness, psychological well-being and eating and activity behaviors. *Int J Obes Relat Metab Disord.* 2002;26(6):854–865
133. Bacon L, Stern JS, Van Loan MD, Keim NL. Size acceptance and intuitive eating improve health for obese, female chronic dieters. *J Am Diet Assoc.* 2005;105(6):929–936
134. Bray GA, Blackburn GL, Ferguson JM, et al. Sibutramine produces dose-related weight loss. *Obes Res.* 1999;7(2):189–198
135. Berkowitz RI, Wadden TA, Tershakovec AM, Cronquist JL. Behavior therapy and sibutramine for the treatment of adolescent obesity: a randomized controlled trial. *JAMA.* 2003;289(14):1805–1812
136. Berkowitz RI, Fujioka K, Daniels SR, et al. Effects of sibutramine treatment in obese adolescents: a randomized trial. *Ann Intern Med.* 2006;145(2):81–90

137. García-Morales LM, Berber A, Macias-Lara CC, Lucio-Ortiz C, Del-Rio-Navarro BE, Dorantes-Alvárez LM. Use of sibutramine in obese Mexican adolescents: a 6-month, randomized, double-blind, placebo-controlled, parallel-group trial. *Clin Ther.* 2006;28(5):770–782

138. Chanoine JP, Hampl S, Jensen C, Boldrin M, Hauptman J. Effect of orlistat on weight and body composition in obese adolescents: a randomized controlled trial. *JAMA.* 2005;293(23):2873–2883

139. Freemark M, Bursey D. The effects of metformin on body mass index and glucose tolerance in obese adolescents with fasting hyperinsulinemia and a family history of type 2 diabetes. *Pediatrics.* 2001;107(4). Available at: www.pediatrics.org/cgi/content/full/107/4/e55

140. Kay JP, Alemzadeh R, Langley G, D'Angelo L, Smith P, Holshouser S. Beneficial effects of metformin in normoglycemic morbidly obese adolescents. *Metabolism.* 2001;50(12):1457–1461

141. Pratt JS, Lenders CM, Dionne EA, et al. Best practice updates for pediatric/adolescent WLS. *Obesity.* 2009; In press

HELPFUL WEB RESOURCES

Centers for Disease Control and Prevention: www.cdc.gov

Office of the Surgeon General: www.surgeongeneral.gov

President's Council on Physical Fitness and Sports: www.fitness.gov

American Academy of Pediatrics: www.aap.org

American Heart Association: www.americanheart.org

HealthierUS: www.healthierus.gov/steps

The Obesity Society: www.naaso.org

Adolesc Med 19 (2008) 406–420

Medical Interventions in Adolescent Obesity

Unab I. Khan, MD*[a,b], Monique Collier, MD[a]

Division of Adolescent Medicine, Departments of [a]Pediatrics and [b]Family and Social Medicine, Children's Hospital at Montefiore, Albert Einstein College of Medicine, 111 East 210th Street, Bronx, NY 10467, USA

Obesity results from an imbalance between energy intake and expenditure. Per recommendations made by the Expert Committee on the Assessment, Prevention, and Treatment of Child and Adolescent Overweight and Obesity,[1] obesity is defined as a BMI of ≥95th percentile for age and gender. The prevalence of obesity in the adolescent population has tripled over the past few decades, increasing from 5% in 1963–1970 to 17% in 2003–2004.[1,2] Adolescent obesity is a strong predictor of adult obesity, as well as its related comorbidities.[3] The likelihood of the persistence of obesity from childhood and adolescence to adulthood is related both to the severity of the obesity and to the age during childhood at which it presents. Obese adolescents have a 70% chance of remaining obese as adults.[4] Given the complexity of the disease, determination and use of appropriate and effective interventions to manage obesity can be challenging. This article will serve as an overview of the literature, evidence, and current recommendations pertaining to medical interventions for obese adolescents.

Several national surveys assess adolescent health behaviors and anthropometric measures, providing a cross-sectional overview of adolescent health status. Some surveys that assess dietary and physical activity behaviors include the National Health and Nutrition Examination Survey (NHANES), Growing Up Today Study (GUTS), and the Continuing Survey of Food Intake by Individuals (CSFII). Data from these surveys have been used to direct further studies evaluating the efficacy of interventions for weight loss.

DIET

To decrease the influence of increased energy intake in the imbalanced obesity equation, management has been directed toward dietary interventions. Interventions that focus on minimizing consumption of sugar-sweetened beverages (SSBs), appropriate daily fruit and vegetable consumption, balanced macronu-

*Corresponding author.
E-mail address: ukhan@montefiore.org (U. I. Khan).

 ISSN 1934-4287

trient intake, and consumption of a healthy breakfast are all part of the first and second stages of therapeutic dietary interventions recommended by the Expert Committee on the Assessment, Prevention, and Treatment of Child and Adolescent Overweight and Obesity.[1] The third and fourth stages of the expert committee's recommendations involve more comprehensive and multidisciplinary interventions for weight loss.[1] We will review the literature and evidence pertaining to many of these recommendations.

Soft drinks are the leading source of added sugars in the diets of adolescents.[5] The Growing Up Today Study showed that punch and soda were the top 2 contributors to total energy consumed by 9- to 14-year-olds.[6] By analyzing data from multiple surveys, investigators have shown that 73% of adolescent boys and 62% of adolescent girls consume carbonated soft drinks on any given day.[7] In addition, overweight and obese adolescents consume a greater proportion of their energy from SSBs than their nonoverweight peers.[8]

Given the significant negative impact of SSBs on nutritional status, interventions to eliminate and/or reduce adolescent consumption of SSBs represent excellent tools for decreasing energy intake. In a randomized, controlled trial of 103 adolescents aged 13 to 18 years, providing noncaloric beverages to case subjects versus controls decreased the consumption of SSBs by 82% in the case subjects. Although there was no difference in the mean BMI between the 2 groups, those in the upper tertile of BMI who received noncaloric beverages showed a significant decrease in BMI compared with those who did not. BMI decreased by 0.25 kg/m^2 for every serving per day of SSBs that was displaced.[9]

A longitudinal study that examined the relationship between beverage intake, BMI, and nutrient intake followed 2379 adolescent girls over a period of 10 years and monitored the consumption of 6 different types of beverages including milk, soda, fruit juice, fruit-flavored drinks, and coffee/tea. It was found that as soda consumption increased over the years, the BMI increased by 0.01 kg/m^2 for every 100 g of regular soda consumed. In addition, milk consumption decreased by 25% during the course of the study.[10]

Heavy consumption of SSBs among adolescents, their association with obesity, and their lack of nutritional value make their removal or decrease in the diets of adolescents the subject of multiple proposed obesity interventions.

Along with SSBs, carbohydrate consumption has progressively increased in adolescents.[6,8] Snack foods, which represent an average of 18% of energy intake among adolescents, consist of ~57% carbohydrates, 39% fat (15% saturated fat), and 6% proteins.[6] Thus, modification of macronutrient intake has become the focus of many dietary interventions for obesity.

Multiple clinical trials have evaluated the effect of low-carbohydrate, high-protein, and high-fat diets versus high-carbohydrate, low-fat, low-calorie diets on weight loss and obesity-associated morbidities in adults. Studies have shown that short-term weight loss was higher for participants on low-carbohydrate, high-protein diets compared with those on the high-carbohydrate, low-calorie diets.[11] However, at the 1-year follow-up, the weight loss was not different between the 2 groups.[11,12]

Studies of adolescents have had similar findings. In a randomized, controlled trial in obese adolescents aged 12 to 18 years, a low-carbohydrate diet was compared with a low-fat diet at 12 weeks.[13] Juices and sweetened beverages were omitted from the meal plan. There was a significantly greater decrease in weight in the low-carbohydrate group compared with those in the low-fat group despite the consumption of significantly more calories. This study shows that weight loss is not only associated with lower calorie consumption but also with the macronutrient composition of the diet. However, the role of low-carbohydrate diets in weight-loss programs for adolescents remains controversial.

High-protein diets have also become popular because of their ability to induce quick weight loss.[14] In addition, daily caloric intake with a high-protein, carbohydrate-restricted diet is generally self-limiting and rarely exceeds 6300 kJ/day (1500 kcal/day).[15] Therefore, diets with varying percentages of protein have been attractive options to explore as therapeutic obesity interventions.

A randomized, controlled trial in adults showed that at 6 months, participants on a high-protein diet lost significantly more weight compared with those in the group that received an average-protein diet.[16] After 12 months, the mean weight loss in the 2 groups was not significantly different. However, at 6 and 12 months, those in the high-protein-diet group showed lower intraabdominal fat as measured by waste circumference. This study shows that a high-protein diet not only enhances short-term weight loss but also provides better long-term maintenance of reduced intraabdominal fat stores and may help to prevent many of the morbidities associated with obesity.[16–19]

Specific commercial diets such as Atkins (carbohydrate restriction), zone (balanced macronutrients), Weight Watchers (caloric restriction), and Ornish (fat restriction) are becoming very popular among the general public. These diets provide specific guidelines, which makes them easier to understand and follow.[20–23] To date, there have been no randomized, controlled trials comparing the efficacy of the various commercial diets on weight loss in adolescents. A major concern has been the severe specific macronutrient restriction in adolescents who have not yet completed pubertal development and growth.

Studies have shown that these commercial diets reduce weight. However, the adherence rates have been consistently low.[24] Thus, to effectively manage obesity and achieve weight loss through dietary modifications, practical techniques to increase dietary adherence are necessary and are more important than the specific macronutrient composition of the diet.

In summary, modification of specific macronutrients may be effective in achieving short-term weight loss. However, the effectiveness of this approach for long-term weight loss has not been proven. In addition, the potential long-term risks of manipulation of macronutrients have not been studied. It is safe to say that manipulation of the macronutrient composition of the diet contributes to weight loss only if it influences caloric intake and can achieve total energy deficits. Hence, decreasing caloric intake seems to be a better predictor of sustained, long-term weight loss.

On the basis of review of the available literature, the easiest, safest, quickest, and most consistent intervention for producing weight loss in adolescents may be the elimination of SSBs from their diets. Although elimination of SSBs alone may not result in normalization of BMI in severely obese adolescents, it may serve as an effective initial dietary intervention.

PHYSICAL ACTIVITY

Another approach to resolving the imbalanced obesity equation is to influence the energy expenditure portion by increasing physical activity. The US Department of Agriculture and the Expert Committee on the Assessment, Prevention, and Treatment of Child and Adolescent Overweight and Obesity[1] have recommended that adolescents should participate in ≥60 minutes of moderate-intensity physical activity most days of the week.[1,25] Studies have shown that participation in school-based and extracurricular physical activities during adolescence significantly decreases the likelihood of obesity in young adulthood overweight.[26] However, recent Youth Risk Behavior Surveillance data indicate that only 72% of adolescent boys and 57% of adolescent girls meet these recommendations.[27] Also, data suggest that as few as 30% of teenagers are meeting the 60-minute guideline.[28,29] Hence there is an opportunity to use modification of adolescent physical activity as an intervention to manage obesity.

Increasing physical activity has important positive effects on health and body composition. However, studies evaluating the effect of physical activity on weight loss have not shown promising results in adults.[30,31] Results from randomized trials in children show positive effects of physical activity on decreasing fat mass and improving body composition by decreasing total body fat, but the effects are diminished after discontinuation of physical activity.[32,33]

The role of increased physical activity in weight maintenance has been studied in adults. With a survey of 5000 adults who maintained a 13.6-kg (30-lb) weight loss for at least 1 year, researchers found that although subjects had dissimilar diets, subjects expended ~11 760 kJ/week (2800 kcal/week).[30,34]

In summary, physical activity in isolation is not an effective intervention for weight loss. However, appropriate levels of physical activity can positively alter body composition by decreasing fat mass and also contribute to weight-loss maintenance. In addition, increased levels of physical activity during adolescence can help reduce persistence of adolescent obesity into adulthood, thereby reducing the adolescent's risk of developing obesity-related comorbidities. To sustain the desired positive health outcomes associated with physical activity, appropriate levels of physical activity must be consistent and persistent. However, discontinuation of physical activity will lead to weight regain and return of body composition to preintervention baseline.

BEHAVIORAL MODIFICATION

A persistent healthier lifestyle not only includes healthy eating and increasing physical activity but also healthier behaviors to achieve long-term weight loss and maintain a healthy weight.[35] Several strategies have been developed to achieve successful behavior change.[36] These strategies incorporate concepts from the transtheoretical model of change, social cognitive theory, and behavior-modification techniques. All these strategies help in identifying patients' readiness to make a behavioral change, goal setting, creating contracts, addressing barriers, and enlisting social support.[37]

Motivational interviewing is a well-known strategy for attaining lifestyle changes in weight-loss programs. Motivational interviewing identifies the patient's readiness for making a behavioral change and then uses the patient's own needs to promote a healthier change. To assess the effect of motivational interviewing on achievement of weight-loss goals, 55 obese, sedentary adults, enrolled in a weight-loss program, were randomly assigned to receive weekly motivational interviewing to decrease their ambivalence toward behavior change. Participants in the weight-loss program who received motivational interviewing lost significantly more weight and engaged in significantly greater physical activity than the participants who were not receiving motivational interviewing.[38]

A study that assessed the role of a motivational behavior coach on successful weight management in obese inner-city adolescents in a weight-loss program[39] revealed that a higher proportion of participants with a coach reported success in changing weight-related behaviors (50%) than those without a coach (37.5%). In addition, participants expressed that they could be more successful after a regimented weight-management program when receiving coaching on a consistent and regular basis and support from family members and friends.[39]

Cognitive behavioral therapy (CBT) is another strategy that helps in making healthy lifestyle changes. It is based on the premise that a problem persists because of certain dysfunctional cognitions and beliefs.[36,40] CBT uses techniques to modify behaviors by changing antecedents and consequences and combines them with cognitive techniques that help to identify, evaluate, and then restructure dysfunctional beliefs.[41] CBT also promotes the transfer of new skills and behaviors learned in therapy into everyday life and the maintenance of these changes across time.[36,42,43]

Tsiros et al[41] evaluated the effectiveness of a CBT program on improving body composition, diet, and physical activity in overweight and obese adolescents. In a 20-week randomized, controlled trial, the authors found that participants who were receiving CBT achieved significant improvements in weight, BMI, fat mass, abdominal fat, and hip circumference compared with those in the control group. In addition, there was reduction is total energy intake, specifically soft-drink consumption. It is interesting to note that CBT did not help to increase levels of physical activity.

These studies suggest the role of behavior-modification techniques in effectively modifying behavior and achieving weight-loss goals and can serve as useful adjuncts to the nutritional and physical activity interventions by facilitating patient adherence.

MULTIDISCIPLINARY WEIGHT-LOSS PROGRAMS

Simple education about health risks of obesity and routine counseling regarding diet and exercise are insufficient for preventing the seemingly inexorable increases in BMI observed in traditionally treated obese children.[44] In adults, obesity is now considered a chronic illness, with a steady weight loss of 5% to 10% being maintained over 2 years as an indicator for personal and programmatic success.[45,46] However, the long-term effects of weight-reduction programs in adults have been very disappointing.[47] It is encouraging that programs involving obese children and adolescents that use a multidisciplinary team approach[48–51] seem to be more successful than adult programs in maintenance of weight loss for 5 to 10 years.[52,53]

Using a multidisciplinary approach, individualizing nutritional counseling, and involving families in making lifestyle changes has been successful in pediatric obesity programs. Savoye et al[44] recruited interested 8- to 16-year-old English-speaking participants along with their caregivers to a multidisciplinary weight-loss program and compared them with participants who received traditional clinical weight-management counseling. There was a significant decrease in BMI, body fat, and insulin resistance in participants who attended the multidisciplinary program. In a randomized, controlled trial of 10- to 14-year-old obese Mexican American adolescents, those in the intensive intervention arm lost significantly more weight compared with those in the self-help group.[54] The 12-week intensive intervention consisted of individualized nutrition sessions, physical activity sessions 4 times per week, and motivational interviewing and positive role modeling. Hence, addressing the specific needs of the population being served increases the likelihood of program success.

Some researchers view obesity as a food addiction,[55] and treatment follows the same premise as other addiction specialties (ie, improvement of self-esteem).[56] In 46 inner-city girls, a celebrity lifestyle and fitness expert coached participants to attain improvement in self-esteem to help prevent consumption of trigger foods. Over the year, obese girls lost an average of 12.9 lb, and mean BMI decreased by 2.32 versus normal-weight girls. The authors found a positive correlation between weight loss and program participation.[57]

A recent meta-analysis reviewed the efficacy of randomized, controlled trials that compared pediatric lifestyle interventions to no treatment or information/education-only controls. Lifestyle interventions for pediatric obesity were found to be efficacious in the short-term with some evidence for extended persistence. The authors recommended further research to determine the optimal length and intensity of treatment required to produce enduring changes in weight status.[58]

Although successful results after family-based, multiprofessional behavioral treatment programs have been reported,[59–61] limited resources preclude such programs' availability in public health facilities.[62] There have been few reports of therapeutic programs for pediatric obesity in the primary care setting. A 3-year, nonrandomized clinical study that involved 3- to 18-year-olds showed that discussing obesity in individual and group meetings with participants and their families in an office setting could result in modest decreases in BMI.[63]

In pediatric obesity interventions, the reported attrition rate is high, ranging from 20% to 24%.[59,64] Parental involvement can play a critical role in the achievement of weight-loss goals. Studies have shown that for younger children, targeting and reinforcing behavioral changes in the parents and participants lead to more effective outcomes.[65,66] Similar results have been reported for younger and middle adolescents.[67] However, it has also been noted that parents represent the largest barrier to participation in youth weight-management programs.[68] Parental attitudinal issues include denial of their child's need for weight loss, unwillingness to talk with their child about weight, unwillingness to change the home environment to support their child's need for improved nutrition and exercise, inflexibility in making room in the family's schedule for the program, and inability to consider that they had some responsibility for their child's overweight status. Hence, parental engagement and involvement is key for attainment and maintenance of weight-loss goals.

Concern has been expressed regarding the impact of pediatric obesity interventions on self-esteem.[69] The results of studies observing the effects of obesity on self-esteem have been conflicting. Some have shown an inverse relationship between self-esteem and obesity,[70] whereas others have shown no significant association.[71] A study that followed obese adolescent girls over a period of 5 years showed that those with higher body satisfaction at baseline had smaller increases in their BMI 5 years later.[72] In a literature review of 21 studies that examined the relationship of self-esteem to weight loss, the authors found that 18 studies reported evidence of increases in self-esteem or components of self-esteem from before to after treatment. Of the studies that demonstrated positive improvements, 10 included control groups that did not experience equivalent improvements. Studies in younger children (7–11 years old) have shown uniformly positive changes in self-esteem, whereas those conducted in older children (12–18 years old) and mixed samples had more variable results.[73]

In summary, multidisciplinary weight-loss programs that provide individualized nutritional counseling and a physical activity component and use behavioral techniques to help adolescents achieve and maintain their weight-loss goals may be the best approach for dealing with the mounting epidemic of obesity. Although parental involvement should be a vital component of the approach to weight loss, especially for children and younger adolescents, the amount of parental involvement for middle and older adolescents' weight-control programs has still not been determined.

PHARMACOLOGIC THERAPY FOR OBESE ADOLESCENTS

Evidence from treating obese adults shows that moderate weight loss of 5% to 10% improves metabolic and cardiovascular risk factors and prevents progression to type 2 diabetes mellitus.[74–76] However, long-term data show that most patients who lose weight regain their lost weight within 5 years and that these disease-associated risk factors are reestablished.[77] As noncompliance with diet and exercise programs in the pediatric age group have been observed,[35] pharmacologic agents have been considered as adjuncts to improve compliance with lifestyle-modification recommendations.

Pharmacologic management is considered as the fourth stage of therapeutic interventions recommended by the Expert Committee on the Assessment, Prevention, and Treatment of Child and Adolescent Overweight and Obesity panel.[1] For initiation of pharmacologic management, patients should demonstrate failure to achieve weight-loss goals despite active involvement, have the maturity to understand the risks and benefits of the interventions, and should be willing to maintain the therapeutic lifestyle changes recommended by the weight-loss team. We agree with Dietz[78] that weight-loss medications should be given solely as an adjunct to behavior modification, family therapy, and increased activity.

At present, the US Food and Drug Administration (FDA) has approved 2 weight-loss drugs for use in adolescents. Orlistat can be prescribed to adolescents 12 years and older. The over-the-counter formulation is approved for patients aged 18 years and older.[79] Sibutramine is approved as a prescription medication for adolescents older than 16 years for up to 2 years. Table 1 provides a brief overview of each pharmacologic intervention.

Table 1.
Pharmacologic interventions for obesity in adolescents

Drug Name	Dosage	Common Adverse Effects	Notes
Orlistat	120 mg 3 times per d with meals	Gastrointestinal disturbance; steatorrhea; cholelithiasis; iron deficiency anemia; vitamin deficiencies	Decreases fat absorption; FDA-approved for 12- to 16-y-olds; over-the-counter formulation approved for 18 y and older; long-term efficacy not proven in adolescents
Sibutramine	5–10 mg daily; may titrate up to 15 mg/d	Hypertension; tachyarrhythmias; xerostomia; headaches	Appetite suppressant; long-term efficacy not proven in adolescents
Metformin	500 mg twice daily; may titrate up to 2000 mg/d	Gastrointestinal disturbance; can initiate ovulation; lactic acidosis in patients with renal insufficiency	Antihyperglycemic agent; improves insulin sensitivity; not FDA-approved for weight loss

Orlistat

Orlistat is a triacylglycerol lipase inhibitor that works in the intestinal lumen to reduce dietary fat absorption by up to 30%.[79] Because of this decrease in fat absorption, a daily vitamin to supplement the fat-soluble vitamins is recommended at least 2 hours after the use of orlistat.

Clinical trials in adults have shown effectiveness of orlistat in weight loss ranging from 1.3 to 3.3 kg for up to 4 years.[80–82] Because of its nonsystemic mechanism of action, orlistat seems to be an ideal pharmacologic option for adolescents, and multiple trials have been conducted to assess its safety and efficacy in obese adolescents.

In a randomized, placebo-controlled, multicenter trial, orlistat in addition to a hypocaloric diet, exercise, and behavior therapy in obese adolescents led to weight loss in the initial 12 weeks and then weight stabilization over a period of 1 year.[83] In another open-labeled, randomized, controlled trial, 12- to 16-year-old obese adolescents were put on orlistat in addition to nutritional and lifestyle-modification counseling. Again, those in the orlistat group had a significant decrease in BMI and weight than controls, but by 15 months, there was no significant difference in BMI between the 2 groups.[84]

Thus, orlistat in conjunction with diet, exercise, and behavior modification may help with weight loss in the initial phase. However, studies in adolescents have not shown its efficacy in the long-term.

Sibutramine

Sibutramine is a serotonin- and norepinephrine-reuptake inhibitor that increases satiety. Sibutramine has been found to be effective in the long-term management of obesity in adults.[85–87]

The safety and efficacy of sibutramine has been studied in adolescents. In a randomized, double-blind, placebo-controlled trial, 13- to 17-year-old obese adolescents were given sibutramine for 6 months followed by an open-label use for 7 to 12 months.[88] Adolescents in the sibutramine group lost significantly more weight, with greater reductions in hunger, than those in the placebo group. The mean weight loss in the sibutramine group at 1 year was 7.0 kg (10% BMI reduction), whereas those who switched from placebo to sibutramine at 7 months had a mean weight loss of 4.5 kg (6.4% BMI reduction). The difference in BMI between the 2 groups at 12 months was not significant, showing that weight loss plateaued at 6 months. Twenty-three subjects required dose reduction and 10 discontinued the medication because of elevated blood pressure. Subjects who showed compliance with the behavioral program as measured by keeping a food record and were treated with the drug achieved the greatest decrease in BMI.

In another randomized, controlled trial, the investigators observed the effects of sibutramine on weight and metabolic parameters.[89] Sixty-eight obese adolescents with a mean BMI of 37.5 kg/m^2 with no other medical complications were recruited and followed for 24 weeks. Adolescents in the sibutramine group had significantly more weight and BMI loss compared with those in the placebo group (3.6 vs 0.9 BMI loss). The adolescents in the sibutramine group also showed a significantly greater decrease in triglyceride and very low-density lipoprotein cholesterol levels compared with those in the placebo group. None of the subjects developed elevated blood pressure.

In a large multicenter, randomized, controlled trial, behavior therapy with sibutramine was studied against behavior therapy with placebo in 498 adolescents.[90] Participants (12–16 years of age) were recruited from 33 US centers and followed for 1 year. The attrition rate was high (24% in the treatment group and 38% in the placebo group). An intention-to-treat analysis showed that adolescents in the sibutramine-plus-behavior-therapy arm had a significantly greater decrease in weight (−6.35 kg) than those in the placebo-plus-behavior-therapy arm (+1.8 kg) and had a significant improvement in their metabolic profiles, with decreases in triglyceride levels and increases in high-density lipoprotein cholesterol levels.

Thus, sibutramine is effective in achieving weight loss in the short-term in adolescents. However, as with orlistat, its effect on maintenance of long-term weight-loss goals is still undetermined.

Metformin

Metformin is a biguanide oral hypoglycemic agent that has been approved by the FDA for the treatment of type 2 diabetes mellitus since 1995. Metformin improves insulin sensitivity in the peripheral organs, thereby decreasing plasma glucose in diabetic patients. Metformin is the drug of choice for overweight patients with type 2 diabetes mellitus and a first-line pharmacologic antidiabetic option for nonoverweight pediatric[91] and adult patients.

The effect of metformin on body weight in nondiabetic obese adults has been variable. A systematic review of randomized, controlled trials (duration: 15 days to 1 year) in populations without diabetes or polycystic ovary syndrome found insufficient evidence to consider metformin as a potential therapy for weight loss in overweight or obese adult subjects.[92] Also, meta-analyses have not supported consistent weight-reducing effects of metformin relative to placebo in diabetic or nondiabetic adult patients.[93]

Several well-designed studies have evaluated the effects of metformin on body weight and other metabolic parameters in the pediatric population. In a randomized, double-blind trial that evaluated metformin versus glimepiride in 285 subjects (aged 8–17 years) with uncontrolled type 2 diabetes mellitus, a significant difference was noted in the effects of metformin and glimepiride on mean BMI (-0.33 vs 0.26 kg/m^2) despite there being no differences between treatments with respect to glycemic parameters.[94] In other placebo-controlled trials in nondiabetic obese adolescents, a small but significant decrease in BMI was noted in the metformin group.[95–97] Despite promising results, metformin has not been approved by the FDA for weight loss in either the pediatric or adult population.

In summary, pharmacologic agents can be used carefully as adjuncts to proven interventions of obesity, including dietary and physical activity modification with behavioral support. Although initial data have seemed promising, most drugs have not shown beneficial effects on weight loss beyond 6 months in the adolescent literature. Also, patients taken off the medications regain most of the weight; therefore, these agents should not be considered to be the first line of therapy in the pediatric and adolescent populations.

REFERENCES

1. Barlow SE; Expert Committee. Expert committee recommendations regarding the prevention, assessment, and treatment of child and adolescent overweight and obesity: summary report. *Pediatrics*. 2007;120(suppl 4):S164–S192
2. Ogden CL, Carroll MD, Curtin LR, McDowell MA, Tabak CJ, Flegal KM. Prevalence of overweight and obesity in the United States, 1999–2004. *JAMA*. 2006;295(13):1549–1555
3. Freedman DS, Khan LK, Serdula MK, Dietz WH, Srinivisan SR, Berenson GS. The relation of childhood BMI to adult adiposity: the Bogalusa Heart Study. *Pediatrics*. 2005;115(1):22–27
4. Guo SS, Roche AF, Chumlea WC, Gardner JD, Siervogel RM. The predictive value of childhood body mass index values for overweight at age 35 y. *Am J Clin Nutr*. 1994;59(4):810–819

5. Guthrie JF, Morton JF. Food sources of added sweeteners in the diets of Americans. *J Am Diet Assoc.* 2000;100(1):43–51, quiz 49–50
6. Rockett HRH, Berkey CS, Field AE, Colditz GA. Cross-sectional measurement of nutrient intake among adolescents in 1996. *Prev Med.* 2001;33(1):27–37
7. French SA, Lin BH, Guthrie JF. National trends in soft drink consumption among children and adolescents age 6 to 17 years: prevalence, amounts, and sources. 1977/1978 to 1994/1998. *J Am Diet Assoc.* 2003;103(10):1326–1331
8. Troiano RP, Briefel RR, Carroll MD, Bialostosky K. Energy and fat intakes of children and adolescents in the United States: data from the National Health and Nutrition Examination Surveys. *Am J Clin Nutr.* 2000;72(5 suppl):1343S–1353S
9. Ebbeling CB, Feldman HA, Osganian SK, Chomitz VR, Ellenbogen SJ, Ludwig DS. Effects of decreasing sugar-sweetened beverage consumption on body weight in adolescents: a randomized, controlled pilot study. *Pediatrics.* 2006;117(3):673–680
10. Striegel-Moore RH, Thompson D, Affenito SG, et al. Correlates of beverage intake in adolescent girls: the national heart, lung, and blood institute growth and health study. *J Pediatr.* 2006; 148(2):183–187
11. Foster GD, Wyatt HR, Hill JO, et al. A randomized trial of a low-carbohydrate diet for obesity. *N Engl J Med.* 2003;348(21):2082–2090
12. Stern L, Iqbal N, Seshadri P, et al. The effects of low-carbohydrate versus conventional weight loss diets in severely obese adults: one year follow-up of a randomized trial. *Ann Intern Med.* 2004;140(10):778–785
13. Sondike SB, Copperman N, Jacobson MS. Effects of a low-carbohydrate diet on weight loss and cardiovascular risk factors in overweight adolescents. *J Pediatr.* 2003;142(3):253–258
14. St Jeor ST, Howard BV, Prewitt TE, Bovee V, Bazzarre T, Eckel RH. Dietary protein and weight reduction: a statement for healthcare professionals from the Nutrition Committee of the Council on Nutrition, Physical Activity, and Metabolism of the American Heart Association. *Circulation.* 2001;104(15):1869–1874
15. Freedman MR. *Popular Diets: A Scientific Review.* Washington, DC: US Department of Agriculture, Office of Research, Education, and Economics; 2000
16. Due A, Toubro S, Skov AR, Astrup A. Effect of normal-fat diets, either medium or high in protein, on body weight in overweight subjects: a randomized 1 year trial. *Int J Obes Relat Metab Disord.* 2004;28(10):1283–1290
17. Després JP, Moorjani S, Lupien PJ, Tremblay A, Nadeau A, Bouchard C. Regional distribution of body fat, plasma lipoproteins, and cardiovascular disease. *Arteriosclerosis.* 1990;10(4):497–511
18. Després JP. Dyslipidaemia and obesity. *Baillieres Clin Endocrinol Metab.* 1994;8(3):629–660
19. Kissebah AH, Krakower GR. Regional adiposity and morbidity. *Physiol Rev.* 1994;74(4):761–811
20. Atkins RC. *Dr. Atkins' New Diet Revolution.* New York, NY: Avon Books; 1998
21. Sears B. *The Zone: A Dietary Road Map.* New York, NY: HarperCollins; 1995
22. Ornish D. *EveryDay Cooking With Dean Ornish.* New York, NY: HarperCollins; 1997
23. Weight Watchers Publishing Group. *Weight Watchers New Complete Cookbook.* New York, NY: Macmillan Press; 1998
24. Dansinger ML, Gleason JA, Griffith JL, Selker HP, Schaefer EJ. Comparison of the Atkins, Ornish, Weight Watchers, and zone diets for weight loss and heart disease risk reduction: a randomized trial. *JAMA.* 2005;293(1):43–53
25. US Department of Health and Human Services, US Department of Agriculture. Dietary guidelines for Americans, 2005. Available at: www.health.gov/DietaryGuidelines/dga2005/document/default.htm. Accessed July 24, 2008
26. Menschik D, Ahmed S, Alexander MH, Blum RW. Adolescent physical activities as predictors of young adult weight. *Arch Pediatr Adolesc Med.* 2008;162(1):29–33
27. Kann L, Kinchen SA, Williams BI, et al. Youth risk behavior surveillance: United States, 1999. *MMWR CDC Surveill Summ.* 2000;49(5):1–32
28. Patrick K, Norman GJ, Calfas KJ, et al. Diet, physical activity, and sedentary behaviors as risk factors for overweight in adolescence. *Arch Pediatr Adolesc Med.* 2004;158(4):385–390

29. Pate RR, Freedson PS, Sallis JF, et al. Compliance with physical activity guidelines: prevalence in a population of children and youth. *Ann Epidemiol*. 2002;12(5):303–308
30. Hill JO, Wyatt HR. Role of physical activity in preventing and treating obesity. *J Appl Physiol*. 2005;99(2):765–770
31. Wing RR. Physical activity in the treatment of the adulthood overweight and obesity: current evidence and research issues. *Med Sci Sports Exerc*. 1999;31(11 suppl):s547–s552
32. Gutin B, Owens S, Okuyama T, Riggs S, Ferguson M, Litaker M. Effect of physical training and its cessation on percent fat and bone density of children with obesity. *Obes Res*. 1999;7(2):208–214
33. Owens S, Gutin B, Allison J, et al. Effect of physical training on total and visceral fat in obese children. *Med Sci Sports Exerc*. 1999;31(1):143–148
34. Klem ML, Wing RR, McGuire MT, Seagle HM, Hill JO. A descriptive study of individuals successful at long term maintenance of substantial weight loss. *Am J Clin Nutr*. 1997;66(2):239–246
35. Epstein LH, Myers MD, Raynor HA, Saelens BE. Treatment of pediatric obesity. *Pediatrics*. 1998;101(3 pt 2):554–570
36. Cooper Z, Fairburn CG, Hawker DM. *Cognitive-Behavioral Treatment of Obesity: A Clinician's Guide*. New York, NY: Guildford Press; 2004
37. American Academy of Pediatrics. Promoting physical activity. Available at: www.aap.org/family/physicalactivity/physicalactivity.htm. Accessed July 24, 2008
38. Carels RA, Darby L, Cacciapaglia HM, et al. Using motivational interviewing as a supplement to obesity treatment: a stepped-care approach. *Health Psychol*. 2007;26(3):369–374
39. Alm M, Soroudi N, Wylie-Rosett J, et al. A qualitative assessment of barriers and facilitators to achieving behavior goals among obese inner-city adolescents in a weight management program. *Diabetes Educ*. 2008;34(2):277–284
40. Duffy G, Spence SH. The effectiveness of cognitive self-management as an adjunct to a behavioural intervention for childhood obesity: a research note. *J Child Psychol Psychiatry*. 1993;34(6):1043–1050
41. Tsiros MD, Sinn N, Brennan L, et al. Cognitive behavioral therapy improves diet and body composition in overweight and obese adolescents. *Am J Clin Nutr*. 2008;87(5):1134–1140
42. Butler AC, Chapman JE, Forman EM, Beck AT. The empirical status of cognitive behavioral therapy: a review of meta-analyses. *Clin Psychol Rev*. 2006;26(1):17–31
43. Cooper Z, Fairburn CG. A new cognitive behavioural approach to the treatment of obesity. *Behav Res Ther*. 2001;39(5):499–511
44. Savoye M, Shaw M, Dziura J, et al. Effects of a weight management program on body composition and metabolic parameters in overweight children: a randomized controlled trial. *JAMA*. 2007;297(24):2697–2704
45. Goldstein DJ. Beneficial health effects of modest weight loss. *Int J Obes Relat Metab Disord*. 1992;16(6):397–415
46. Vidal J. Updated review on the benefits of weight loss. *Int J Obes Relat Metab Disord*. 2002;26(suppl 4):S25–S28
47. Crawford D, Jeffery RW, French SA. Can anyone successfully control their weight? Findings of a three year community-based study of men and women. *Int J Obes (Lond)*. 2000;24(9):1107–1110
48. Eliakim A, Kaven G, Berger I, Friedland O, Wolach B, Nemet D. The effect of a combined intervention on body mass index and fitness in obese children and adolescents: a clinical experience. *Eur J Pediatr*. 2002;161(8):449–454
49. Dao HH, Frelaut ML, Oberlin F, Peres G, Bourgeois P, Navarro J. Effects of a multidisciplinary weight loss intervention on body composition in obese adolescents. *Int J Obes Relat Metab Disord*. 2004;28(2):290–299
50. Braet C, Tanghe A, Bode PD, Franckx H, Winckel MV. Inpatient treatment of obese children: a multicomponent programme without stringent calorie restriction. *Eur J Pediatr*. 2003;162(6):391–396
51. Deforche B, de Bourdeaudhuij I, Debode P, et al. Changes in fat mass, fat-free-mass and aerobic fitness in severely obese children and adolescents following a residential treatment programme. *Eur J Pediatr*. 2003;162(9):616–622

52. Epstein LH, Valsoki AM, Kalarchian MA, Mc Curley J. Do children lose and maintain weight easier than adults: a comparison of child and parent weight changes from six months to ten years. *Obes Res.* 1995;3(5):411–417
53. Epstein LH. Methodological issues and ten-year outcomes for obese children. *Ann N Y Acad Sci.* 1993;699:237–249
54. Johnston CA, Tyler C, McFarlin BK, et al. Weight loss in overweight Mexican American children: a randomized, controlled trial. *Pediatrics.* 2007;120(6). Available at: www.pediatrics.org/cgi/content/full/120/6/e1450
55. Trotzky AS. The treatment of eating disorders as addiction among adolescent females. *Int J Adolesc Med Health.* 2002;14(4):269–274
56. High Voltage. *Energy Up! Shed Pounds, Get Fit, Gain Stamina, and Turn on Your Power With This Unique Program.* New York, NY: G.P. Putnam's Sons; 1997
57. Chehab LG, Pfeffer B, Vargas I, Chen S, Irigoyen M. "Energy Up": a novel approach to the weight management of inner-city teens. *J Adolesc Health.* 2007;40(5):474–476
58. Wilfley DE, Tibbs TL, Van Buren DJ, Reach KP, Walker MS, Epstein LH. Lifestyle interventions in the treatment of childhood overweight: a meta-analytic review of randomized controlled trials. *Health Psychol.* 2007;26(5):521–532
59. Epstein LH, Valsoki A, Wing RR, McCurley J. Ten-year follow-up of behavioral, family-based treatment for obese children. *JAMA.* 1990;264(19):2519–2523
60. Golan M, Crow S. Targeting parents exclusively in the treatment of childhood obesity: long-term results. *Obes Res.* 2004;12(2):357–361
61. Braet C, van Winckel M. Long-term follow-up of a cognitive behavioral treatment program for obese children. *Behav Ther.* 2000;31(1):55–74
62. Caprio S. Treating child obesity and associated medical conditions. *Future Child.* 2006;16(1): 209–224
63. Tanas R, Marcolongo R, Pedretti S, Gilli G. A family-based education program for obesity: a three-year study. *BMC Pediatr.* 2007;7:33
64. Savoye M, Berry D, Dzioura J, et al. Anthropometric and psychosocial changes in obese adolescents enrolled in a weight management program. *J Am Diet Assoc.* 2005;105(3):364–370
65. Wrotniak BH, Epstein LH, Paluch RA, Roemmich JN. Parent weight change as a predictor of child weight change in family-based behavioral obesity treatment. *Arch Pediatr Adolesc Med.* 2004;158(4):342–347
66. Epstein LH, Valoski A, Wing RR, McCurley J. Ten-year outcomes of behavioral family-based treatment for childhood obesity. *Health Psychol.* 1994;13(5):373–383
67. Brownell KD, Kelman JH, Stunkard AJ. Treatment of obese children with and without their mothers: changes in weight and blood pressure. *Pediatrics.* 1983;71(4):515–523
68. Eckstein KC, Mikhail LM, Ariza AJ, et al. Parents' perception of their child's weight and health. *Pediatrics.* 2006;117(3):681–690
69. O'Dea JA. Evidence for a self-esteem approach in the prevention of body image and eating problems among children and adolescents. *Eat Disord.* 2004;12(3):225–239
70. French SA, Story M, Perry CL. Self-esteem and obesity in children and adolescents: a literature review. *Obes Res.* 1995;3(5):479–490
71. Pesa JA, Syre TR, Jones E. Psychosocial differences associated with body weight among female adolescents: the importance of body image. *J Adolesc Health.* 2000;(26):330–337
72. van den Berg P, Neumark-Sztainer D. Fat 'n happy 5 years later: is it bad for overweight girls to like their bodies? *J Adolesc Health.* 2007;41(4):415–417
73. Lowry KW, Sallinen BJ, Janicke DM. the effects of weight management programs on self-esteem in pediatric overweight populations. *J Pediatr Psychol.* 2007;32(10):1179–1195
74. Dattilo AM, Kris-Etherton PM. Effects of weight reduction on blood lipids and lipoproteins: a meta-analysis. *Am J Clin Nutr.* 1992;56(2):320–328
75. Tuomilehto J, Lindstrom J, Eriksson JG, et al. Prevention of type 2 diabetes mellitus by changes in lifestyle among subjects with impaired glucose tolerance. *N Engl J Med.* 2001;344(18):1343–1350
76. Knowler WC, Barrett-Connor E, Fowler SE, et al. Reduction in the incidence of type 2 diabetes with lifestyle intervention or metformin. *N Engl J Med.* 2002;346(6):393–403

77. Wadden TA, Sternberg JA, Letizia KA, Stunkard AJ, Foster GD. Treatment of obesity by very low calorie diet, behavior therapy, and their combination: a five-year perspective. *Int J Obes (Lond).* 1989;13(suppl):239–246
78. Dietz WH. Pharmacotherapy for childhood obesity? Maybe for some. *Obes Res.* 1994;2(1): 54–55
79. Hvizdos KM, Markham A. Orlistat: a review of its use in the management of obesity. *Drugs.* 1999;58(4):743–760
80. Rössner S, Sjönström L, Noack R, Meinders AE, Noseda G. Weight loss, weight maintenance and improved cardiovascular risk factors after 2 years of treatment with orlistat for obesity. European Orlistat Obesity Study Group. *Obes Res.* 2000;8(1):49–61
81. Finer N, James WP, Kopelman PG, Lean ME, Williams G. One-year treatment of obesity: a randomized, double-blind, placebo-controlled, multicentre study of orlistat, a gastrointestinal lipase inhibitor. *Int J Obes Relat Metab Disord.* 2000;24(3):306–313
82. Torgerson JS, Hauptman J, Boldrin MN, Sjöström L. XENical in the prevention of diabetes in obese subjects (XENDOS Study): a randomized study of orlistat as an adjunct to lifestyle changes for the prevention of type 2 diabetes in obese patients [published correction appears in *Diabetes Care.* 2004;27(3):856]. *Diabetes Care.* 2004;27(1):155–161
83. Chanoine JP, Hampl S, Jensen C, Boldrin M, Hauptman J. Effect of orlistat on weight and body composition in obese adolescents: a randomized controlled trial. *JAMA.* 2005;293(23):2873–2883
84. Ozkan B, Bereket A, Turan S, Keskin S. Addition of orlistat to conventional treatment in adolescents with severe obesity. *Eur J Pediatr.* 2004;163(12):738–741
85. Walsh KM, Leen E, Lean ME. The effect of sibutramine on resting energy expenditure and adrenaline-induced thermogenesis in obese females. *Int J Obes Relat Metab Disord.* 1999; 23(10):1009–1015
86. James WPT, Astrup A, Finer N, et al. Effect of sibutramine on weight maintenance after weight loss: a randomized trial (STORM). *Lancet.* 2000;356(9248):2119–2125
87. Early JL, Apovian CM, Aronne LJ, et al. Sibutramine plus meal replacement therapy for body weight loss and maintenance in obese patients. *Obesity (Silver Spring).* 2007;15(6):1464–1472
88. Berkowitz RI, Wadden TA, Tershakovec AM, Cronquist JL. Behavior therapy and sibutramine for the treatment of adolescent obesity: a randomized controlled trial. *JAMA.* 2003;289(14): 1805–1812
89. Godoy-Matos A, Carraro L, Vieira A, et al. Treatment of obese adolescents with sibutramine: a randomized, double-blind, controlled study. *J Clin Endocrinol Metab.* 2005;90(3):1460–1465
90. Berkowitz RI, Fujioka K, Daniels SR, et al. Effects of sibutramine treatment in obese adolescents: a randomized trial. *Ann Intern Med.* 2006;145(2):81–90
91. Jones KL, Arslanian S, Peterokova VA, Park JS, Tomlinson MJ. Effect of metformin in pediatric patients with type 2 diabetes: a randomized controlled trial. *Diabetes Care.* 2002;25(1):89–94
92. Levri KM, Slaymaker E, Last A, et al. Metformin as treatment for overweight and obese adults: a systematic review. *Ann Fam Med.* 2005;3(5):457–461
93. Golay A. Metformin and body weight. *Int J Obes (Lond).* 2008;32(1):61–72
94. Gottschalk M, Danne T, Vlajnic A, Cara JF. Glimepiride versus metformin as monotherapy in pediatric patients with type 2 diabetes: a randomized, single-blind comparative study. *Diabetes Care.* 2007;30(4):790–794
95. Freemark M, Bursey D. The effects of metformin on body mass index and glucose tolerance in obese adolescents with fasting hyperinsulinemia and a family history of type 2 diabetes. *Pediatrics.* 2001;107(4). Available at: www.pediatrics.org/cgi/content/full/107/4/e55
96. Srinivasan S, Ambler GR, Baur LA, et al. Randomized, controlled trial of metformin for obesity and insulin resistance in children and adolescents: improvement in body composition and fasting insulin. *J Clin Endocrinol Metab.* 2006;91(6):2074–2080
97. Kay JP, Alemzadeh R, Langley G, D'Angelo I, Smith P, Holshouser S. Beneficial effects of metformin in normoglycemic morbidly obese adolescents. *Metabolism.* 2001;50(12):1457–1461

Adolesc Med 19 (2008) 421–430

Dietary Approaches to Healthy Weight Management for Adolescents: The New Moves Model

Dianne Neumark-Sztainer, PhD, MPH, RD*, Colleen Freeh Flattum, MS, RD, Mary Story, PhD, RD, Shira Feldman, MPH, RD, Christine A. Petrich, MEd

Division of Epidemiology and Community Health, School of Public Health, University of Minnesota, 1300 South Second Street, Suite 300, Minneapolis, MN 55454, USA

The high prevalence of obesity among adolescents is of public health concern given its physical and psychosocial consequences.[1] Although many factors contribute to the onset and maintenance of obesity, dietary behaviors play a major role. Dietary patterns that may increase risk for excessive weight gain in youth include large portion sizes,[2] low fruit and vegetable intake,[3] high consumption of sweetened beverages,[4,5] frequent consumption of fast foods,[6] and skipping breakfast.[7] Furthermore, dieting behaviors commonly used by adolescents may actually be contributing to excess weight gain. Frequent dieting and the use of unhealthy weight-control behaviors such as diet-pill use, self-induced vomiting, use of food substitutes, skipping meals for the purpose of weight loss, and fasting have been shown to predict weight gain and overweight status over time.[8] Dietary interventions aimed at obesity prevention in adolescents need to address these behaviors while taking into account both lifestyle and developmental issues of adolescents. Schools provide an excellent venue for reaching adolescents from diverse ethnic and low socioeconomic backgrounds who may not have easy access to interventions conducted within clinical or community settings. This article describes the dietary component of New Moves, a high school-based obesity-prevention program for adolescent girls to improve eating behaviors, as well as physical activity behaviors, body image, and overall self-esteem.

---

*Corresponding author.

E-mail address: neumark@epi.umn.edu (D. Neumark-Sztainer).

This study was supported by grant R01 DK063107 (Dr Neumark-Sztainer, principal investigator) from the National Institute of Diabetes and Digestive and Kidney Diseases, National Institutes of Health. The content is solely the responsibility of the authors and does not necessarily represent the official views of the National Institute of Diabetes and Kidney Diseases or the National Institutes of Health.

 ISSN 1934-4287

BACKGROUND

Studies have documented that dietary intakes of adolescents are far from ideal and are likely contributing to the tripling in the prevalence of obesity among adolescents over the past few decades.[9,10] In Project EAT (Eating Among Teens), a large population-based study of eating and weight among adolescents in the metropolitan area of the Twin Cities in Minnesota, we found that less than one third of adolescents ate ≥5 servings of fruits and vegetables on a daily basis.[10] Furthermore, fruit and vegetable intake tended to decline as adolescents got older.[11] Binge eating was reported by 17% of the adolescent girls and 8% of the adolescent boys, with higher percentages among overweight adolescents (21% and 12% among the overweight girls and boys, respectively).[12] Only 27% of the girls and 38% of the boys in middle school and high school ate breakfast every day.[7] Furthermore, we found that eating patterns such as breakfast skipping and binge eating longitudinally predicted overweight status in adolescents over a 5-year period.[13]

Adolescents concerned about their weight, particularly adolescent girls, often adopt unhealthy dieting and weight-control behaviors instead of making healthy dietary lifestyle changes. For example, in Project EAT, 57% of all adolescent girls, and 76% of those who were overweight, reported using unhealthy weight-control behaviors.[12] Several studies have shown that dieting and unhealthy weight-control behaviors are ineffective for long-term weight management in adolescents.[14–17] In Project EAT, we found that adolescent girls who dieted were at nearly twice the odds for being overweight 5 years later compared with nondieters, and those using unhealthy weight-control behaviors were at even greater risk, after adjusting for baseline weight status.[17] In examining why dieting leads to weight gain over time, we found that dieting was associated with increased binge eating among adolescent girls and boys, which, in turn, was associated with weight gain.[18] We also found that dieters were less likely to engage in behaviors found to help with long-term weight management, such as eating breakfast on a regular basis, compared with nondieters. In addition to being counterproductive to weight management, dieting behaviors have also been found to increase risk for disordered eating behaviors[16,17] and eating disorders[19] in adolescents.

Multiple factors influence dietary intake and eating patterns among adolescents, including socioenvironmental factors (eg, availability of healthy foods), personal factors (eg, perceived benefits of healthy eating), and behavioral factors (eg, goal setting). In an examination of factors associated with fruit and vegetable intake among adolescents participating in Project EAT, home availability of fruits and vegetables and taste preferences emerged as the most predictive of intake.[20] These findings emphasize the importance of addressing both socioenvironmental and individual-level factors within interventions aimed at improving dietary intake. Factors that influence unhealthy weight-control practices include weight pressures to be thin from family and friends and personal body dissatisfaction.[21,22] Body dissatisfaction is probably the strongest predictor of unhealthy weight-control practices and other disordered eating behaviors.[23,24] Interestingly, and of relevance to obesity-prevention intervention, more recent study findings suggest that body dissatisfaction predicts increased weight gain over time among overweight adolescent girls.[25] Our research from Project EAT suggests that body dissatisfaction does not motivate adolescents to engage in healthier behaviors, such as eating more fruits and vegetables or being more physically active, but, rather, to use unhealthy weight-control behaviors that are counterproductive to long-term weight management.[26]

On the basis of current knowledge, dietary interventions aimed at preventing and reducing adolescent obesity need to address dietary intake behaviors, such as increasing fruit and vegetable intake and decreasing sweetened-beverage intake. It is also essential to address eating patterns such as starting the day with breakfast, eating reasonable portion sizes, and paying attention to one's body's signs of hunger and satiety. Dietary interventions should also address weight-control practices, with an emphasis on avoiding short-term dieting and instead engaging in healthy eating behaviors that can be integrated into one's lifestyle. To enhance program effectiveness, dietary interventions should focus on socio-environmental, personal, and behavioral factors that influence dietary intake, eating patterns, and weight-control behaviors. Furthermore, given the multifactorial etiology of obesity, dietary interventions should be embedded within a more comprehensive approach that focuses on promoting physical activity, a balanced approach to eating (eg, meal regularity and moderation), psychological well-being, and a supportive physical and social environment.

In designing dietary interventions for obesity prevention in adolescents, it is also important to take lifestyle and developmental factors into account. Those who create programs need to consider adolescents' time schedules and competing activities such as school, work, extracurricular activities, and family responsibilities, because they have relevance for program attendance and participation. Interventions need to be implemented within an accessible facility and at convenient times for adolescents. The developmental stage of adolescents also needs to be considered in the design of interventions. Adolescents have increased autonomy in decision-making over their food choices but are often still reliant on their families. For example, given adolescents' increased purchasing power and independence in getting around, adolescents are often targeted with advertisements for fast-food restaurants. However, family meals are still important for the dietary intake of adolescents.[27–29] Thus, intervention designers must take into account adolescents' increased autonomy and developmental need for independence while encouraging parental support for healthy eating patterns. In working with adolescents from diverse ethnic and racial backgrounds, dietary-intervention designers also need to address cultural differences in food and eating behaviors and familial factors that influence these behaviors. Adolescent development, with its drastic physical, psychological, and social changes, also has implications for body-image concerns. Media messages regarding an "ideal appearance" can have a harmful impact on adolescents' body image at a period of life in which they are most vulnerable and when body image is an important part of their identity and self-esteem. Thus, dietary interventions for obesity prevention need to account for the sensitivity of body-image concerns and their centrality to adolescents' identity. Intervention designers need to ensure that messages do not inadvertently lead to increased body-image concerns that will place adolescents at risk for unhealthy weight-control and other disordered eating behaviors.

NEW MOVES: AN OVERVIEW

New Moves is a school-based obesity-prevention program for adolescent girls. The program's development was guided by findings from Project EAT and other studies, as discussed above, and by extensive formative assessments and pilot work.[30–34] We chose to focus on girls, given troubling research findings that have shown high levels of body-image concerns and disordered eating behaviors and low levels of physical activity among adolescent girls. Findings from our needs assessments and pilot work suggested that girls would feel more comfortable being physically active and discussing weight-related health issues in an all-girls environment. The underlying philosophy guiding the New Moves intervention is that if girls feel good about themselves and their bodies, then they will want to take care of their bodies through healthy eating, physical activity, and self-acceptance. Concepts and teaching strategies from both the obesity and eating-disorder fields were incorporated into the intervention because adolescent girls are at risk for a range of weight-related problems.

The New Moves study, a randomized, controlled, school-based trial funded by the National Institutes of Health, is currently testing whether high school girls participating in the New Moves intervention will significantly decrease their percentage of body fat compared with girls in a control group. The study is being conducted in 6 intervention and 6 control high schools in the metropolitan area of the Twin Cities in Minnesota. A total of 190 adolescent girls from 6 high schools (3 intervention and 3 control schools) participated in the study during the 2007–2008 school year. An additional 6 schools will participate in the program during the 2008–2009 school year. Inactive high schools girls who are overweight or at risk for becoming overweight as a result of sedentary lifestyles were targeted for inclusion in this study.

The New Moves intervention targets socioenvironmental (eg, peer support), personal (eg, body image), and behavioral (eg, goal setting) factors to bring about changes in eating and physical activity behaviors (see Fig 1). Specific behavioral objectives addressed in the program are listed in Table 1. New Moves includes an intensive intervention phase in which girls participate in daily activities as part of an all-girls physical education class. The class includes physical education ("Be Fit"), nutrition ("Be Fueled"), and social support/self-empowerment ("Be Fabulous") components. Four classes per week are devoted to physical activity

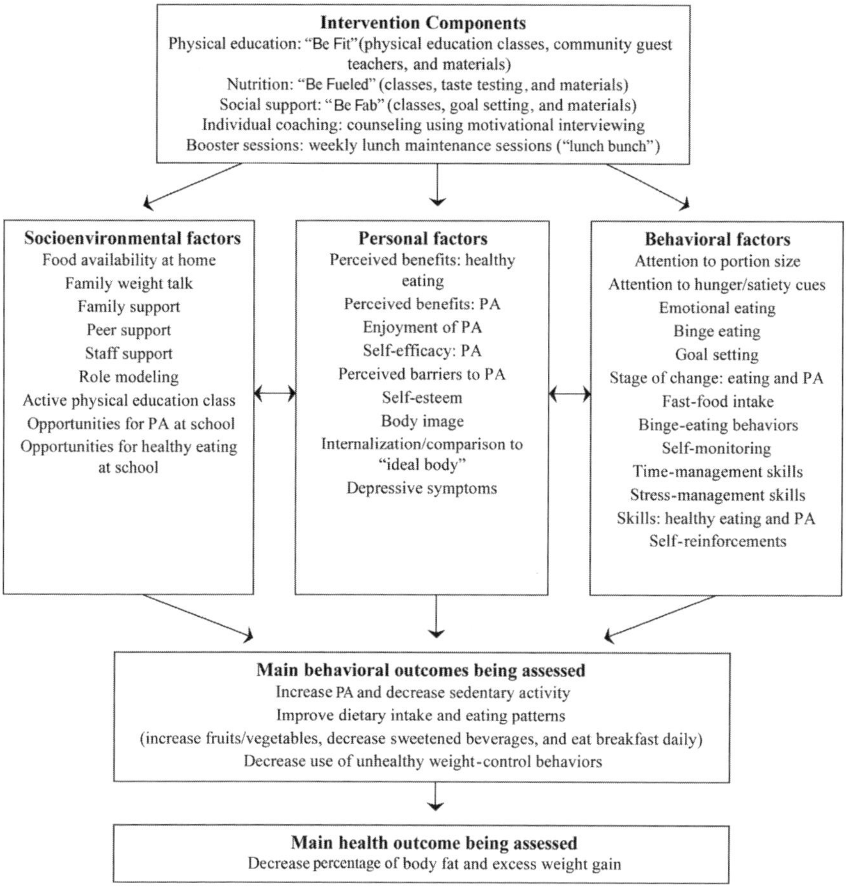

Fig 1. New Moves theoretical model of change based on Social Cognitive Theory. PA indicates physical activity.

and 1 class per week to either nutrition or social support. After the physical education class ends, the intervention includes a maintenance phase, with weekly meetings occurring over lunch at school. Individual counseling sessions are offered throughout both phases. A minimal parent-outreach component, which spans across both the physical education class and the maintenance phase, is also included. The intervention components are shown in Fig 2. Given that the focus of this article is on the New Moves dietary intervention, each of the intervention components that focus primarily on dietary behaviors are discussed in more detail below.

"Be Fueled" Nutrition Sessions

"Be fueled" classes take a nondieting approach toward healthy eating and weight management. The focus is on making sustainable behavior changes such as

Table 1
New Moves behavioral objectives

Aim to be physically active at least 1 h/d
Limit television/video watching to no more than 1 h/d
Eat at least 5 servings of fruits and vegetables each day; choose fruits and vegetables for snacks[a]
Limit pop/soda and other sweetened beverages; instead, drink noncaloric beverages[a]
Eat breakfast every day[a]
Pay attention to portion size and to your body's signs of hunger and fullness[a]
Avoid unhealthy weight-control practices[a]
Focus on your positive traits

[a] Dietary objectives.

paying attention to energy balance and portion size, drinking water instead of sweetened beverages, starting each day with a healthy breakfast, eating more fruits and vegetables, making healthy snack choices, having a well-balanced lunch, and making healthier choices at fast-food restaurants. Girls receive a teen magazine–styled workbook (GirlPages) with information and activities related to these behaviors. Interactive lessons focus on challenges that teenagers face in adopting healthy behaviors and specific ideas for implementing behavior change. Taste-testing a varicty of healthy foods is incorporated into the sessions.

Individual Sessions With a New Moves Coach

On the basis of our pilot work,[31] we determined that a group-class setting to deliver the New Moves intervention and behavior goals was not adequate for addressing the individual needs of the girls. Therefore, opportunities are provided for each participant to meet with a New Moves personal coach (ie, dietitian or health educator) for up to 7 individual sessions. Meetings last for ~20 minutes and are conducted at school, typically during a free period or before/after school. During these sessions, motivational interviewing techniques are used extensively. Motivational interviewing is a client-centered, collaborative, and directive approach to assist individuals in working through their ambivalence about behavior change and enhance intrinsic motivation.[35] Personal coaches establish a nonconfrontational and supportive climate in which the girls feel comfortable expressing their thoughts and feelings around behavior change. The coach is present primarily to identify barriers and boost motivation, thereby supporting each girl's autonomy and ability to make healthy lifestyle decisions. Each individual session follows a general interview format that includes open-ended questions designed to explore various issues related to the girls' individual dietary behaviors and goals. The individualized motivational interviewing format provides girls an opportunity to discuss dietary habits and goals with a counselor and complements the other New Moves group activities.

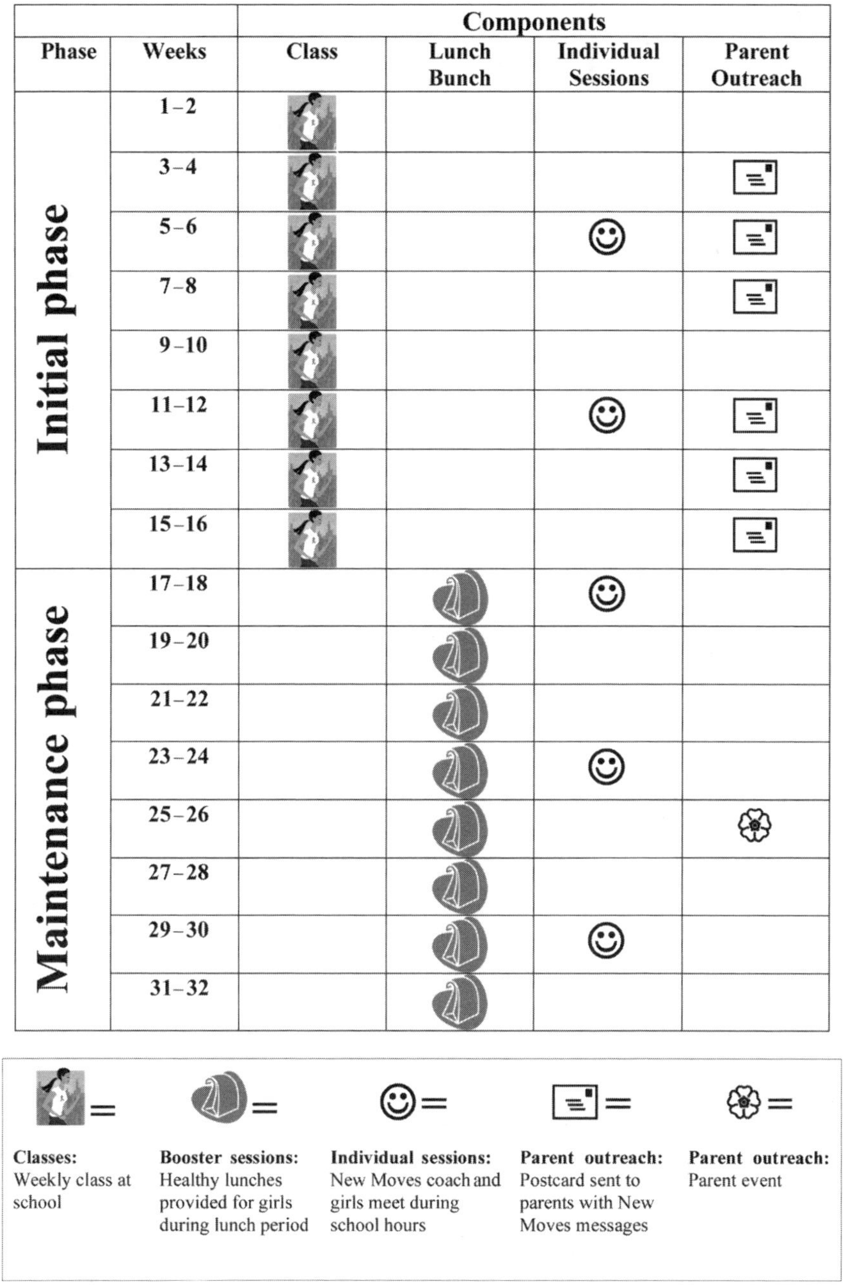

Fig 2. Intervention schedule during the initial and maintenance phases of the study.

Lunch Bunches

New Moves participants are invited to a weekly lunch get-together ("lunch bunch") once the physical education class ends, during the maintenance phase of New Moves. These booster sessions are held during the lunch period at school. A healthy lunch is provided with sandwiches, salads, or culturally diverse foods (eg, Ethiopian, Asian, or Mexican selections). Water or low-calorie beverages are served, as are side dishes such as fruit, vegetables, and low-fat snacks. Thus, the lunchtime sessions provide participants an environment in which girls can practice New Moves dietary goals of eating more fruits and vegetables, drinking water, and eating reasonable portion sizes. Each lunchtime session includes discussion of a topic relevant to the New Moves behavioral objectives, such as eating healthy over the holidays, making healthy choices at school, emotional eating, positive body image, stress management, staying fit with a busy schedule, and ways to be active while watching television. The sessions were designed to generate discussion on ways to identify and overcome common barriers for teenagers in making healthy choices. Although most of the sessions focus on activities specific to the New Moves objectives, some sessions address more general social and community-building activities in a less formal manner. The lunchtime meetings provide an opportunity for girls to eat a healthy lunch, receive social support, and connect with their New Moves classmates after the class is over.

Parent Outreach

Given the importance of parental support for healthy eating, physical activity, and a positive body image in adolescents, a parent-outreach component is also included in the New Moves intervention. However, budgetary constraints, potential sustainability within school systems, school cultures, and issues related to adolescent autonomy were also taken into account when developing the parental component. The result was a minimal parent intervention primarily aimed at fostering parental knowledge about New Moves and support for the program's philosophy. Throughout the intervention, parents of participating girls are sent 6 postcards with information about topics discussed in class. In addition, New Moves staff members are available to meet with parents at parent-teacher conferences in the fall. A Saturday "spa retreat" was held this past spring at a community center for New Moves participants and their parent, older sister, or other guardian. Girls and parents participate in activities such as making bath salts, receiving chair massages, and yoga. They were served a healthy lunch during which they heard a presentation about New Moves. They received a spa bag and a book about parenting teenagers to have a healthy weight and a positive body image.[36] This type of event provides an informal atmosphere for us to receive feedback about the class from both parents and teenagers.

CONCLUSIONS

Before completing the evaluation of the New Moves intervention, conclusions cannot be drawn as to whether the dietary approach being used will be effective in helping the girls make behavioral changes. Our early impressions are that the girls, teachers, and parents are very satisfied with the New Moves approach. However, we are also well aware of the difficulties inherent to behavioral change and weight management. If proven successful, it is our hope that the New Moves model will be incorporated within high schools. It seems that group education (eg, "Be fueled"), personal attention (eg, individual sessions with a New Moves coach), availability of healthy food options (eg, "lunch bunches"), and family involvement are important components of a dietary intervention for healthy weight management among adolescents.

REFERENCES

1. Daniels SR. The consequences of childhood overweight and obesity. *Future Child.* 2006;16(1): 47–67
2. Rolls BJ, Roe LS, Meengs JS, Wall DE. Increasing the portion size of a sandwich increases energy intake. *J Am Diet Assoc.* 2004;104(3):367–372
3. Striegel-Moore RH, Thompson DR, Affenito SG, et al. Fruit and vegetable intake: few adolescent girls meet national guidelines. *Prev Med.* 2006;42(3):223–228
4. French SA, Lin BH, Guthrie JF. National trends in soft drink consumption among children and adolescents age 6 to 17 years: prevalence, amounts, and sources, 1977/1978 to 1994/1998. *J Am Diet Assoc.* 2003;103(10):1326–1331
5. Ludwig DS, Peterson KE, Gortmaker SL. Relation between consumption of sugar-sweetened drinks and childhood obesity: a prospective, observational analysis. *Lancet.* 2001;357(9255):505–508
6. Bowman SA, Gortmaker SL, Ebbeling CB, Pereira MA, Ludwig DS. Effects of fast-food consumption on energy intake and diet quality among children in a national household survey. *Pediatrics.* 2004;113(1 pt 1):112–118
7. Timlin M, Pereira MA, Story M, Neumark-Sztainer D. Breakfast eating and weight change in a 5-year prospective analysis of adolescents: Project EAT (Eating Among Teens). *Pediatrics.* 2008;121(3). Available at: www.pediatrics.org/cgi/content/full/121/3/e638
8. Neumark-Sztainer D, Wall M, Haines J, Story M, Sherwood NE, van den Berg P. Shared risk and protective factors for overweight and disordered eating in adolescents. *Am J Prev Med.* 2007; 33(5):359–369
9. Ogden CL, Carroll MD, Curtin LR, McDowell MA, Tabak CJ, Flegal KM. Prevalence of overweight and obesity in the United States, 1999–2004. *JAMA.* 2006;295(13):1549–1555
10. Neumark-Sztainer D, Story M, Hannan PJ, Croll J. Overweight status and eating patterns among adolescents: where do youth stand in comparison to the *Healthy People 2010* objectives? *Am J Public Health.* 2002;92(5):844–851
11. Larson NI, Neumark-Sztainer D, Hannan PJ, Story M. Trends in adolescent fruit and vegetable consumption, 1999–2004: Project EAT. *Am J Prev Med.* 2007;32(2):147–150
12. Neumark-Sztainer D, Story M, Hannan PJ, Perry CL, Irving LM. Weight-related concerns and behaviors among overweight and non-overweight adolescents: implications for preventing weight-related disorders. *Arch Pediatr Adolesc Med.* 2002;156(2):171–178
13. Haines J, Neumark-Sztainer D, Wall M, Story M. Personal, behavioral, and environmental risk and protective factors for adolescent overweight. *Obesity (Silver Spring).* 2007;15(11):2748–2760
14. Stice E, Cameron RP, Killen JD, Hayward C, Taylor CB. Naturalistic weight-reduction efforts prospectively predict growth in relative weight and onset of obesity among female adolescents. *J Consult Clin Psychol.* 1999;67(6):967–974

15. Stice E, Presnell K, Shaw H, Rohde P. Psychological and behavioral risk factors for obesity onset in adolescent girls: a prospective study. *J Consult Clin Psychol.* 2005;73(2):195–202
16. Field AE, Austin SB, Taylor CB, et al. Relation between dieting and weight change among preadolescents and adolescents. *Pediatrics.* 2003;112(4):900–906
17. Neumark-Sztainer D, Wall M, Guo J, Story M, Haines J, Eisenberg M. Obesity, disordered eating, and eating disorders in a longitudinal study of adolescents: how do dieters fare five years later? *J Am Diet Assoc.* 2006;106(4):559–568
18. Neumark-Sztainer D, Wall M, Haines J, Story M, Eisenberg M. Why does dieting predict weight gain in adolescents? Findings from Project EAT-II: a five-year longitudinal study. *J Am Diet Assoc.* 2007;107(3):448–455
19. Patton GC, Selzer R, Coffey C, Carlin JB, Wolfe R. Onset of adolescent eating disorders: population based cohort study over 3 years. *BMJ.* 1999;318(7186):765–768
20. Neumark-Sztainer D, Wall MM, Hannan PJ, Story M, Croll J, Perry C. Correlates of fruit and vegetable intake among adolescents: findings from Project EAT. *Prev Med.* 2003;37(3):198–208
21. Paxton SJ, Schutz HK, Wertheim EH, Muir SL. Friendship clique and peer influences on body image concerns, dietary restraint, extreme weight-loss behaviors, and binge eating in adolescent girls. *J Abnorm Psychol.* 1999;108(2):255–266
22. Levine MP, Smolak L, Hayden H. The relation of sociocultural factors to eating attitudes and behaviors among middle-school girls. *J Early Adolesc.* 1994;14(4):471–490
23. Stice E, Shaw H. Eating disorder prevention programs: a meta-analytic review. *Psychol Bull.* 2004;130(2):206–227
24. Jacobi C, Hayward C, de Zwaan M, Kraemer HC, Agras WS. Coming to terms with risk factors for eating disorders: application of risk terminology and suggestions for a general taxonomy. *Psychol Bull.* 2004;130(1):19–65
25. van den Berg P, Neumark-Sztainer D. Fat 'n happy 5 years later: Is it bad for overweight girls to like their bodies? *J Adolesc Health.* 2007;41(4):415–417
26. Neumark-Sztainer D, Paxton SJ, Hannan PJ, Haines J, Story M. Does body satisfaction matter? Five-year longitudinal associations between body satisfaction and health behaviors in adolescent females and males. *J Adolesc Health.* 2006;39(2):244–251
27. Nicklas TA, Myers L, Reger C, Beech B, Berenson GS. Impact of breakfast consumption on nutritional adequacy of the diets of young adults in Bogalusa, Louisiana: ethnic and gender contrasts. *J Am Diet Assoc.* 1998;98(12):1432–1438
28. Larson NI, Neumark-Sztainer D, Hannan PJ, Story M. Family meals during adolescence are associated with higher diet quality and healthful meal patterns during young adulthood. *J Am Diet Assoc.* 2007;107(9):1502–1510
29. Neumark-Sztainer D, Hannan PJ, Story M, Croll J, Perry C. Family meal patterns: associations with sociodemographic characteristics and improved dietary intake among adolescents. *J Am Diet Assoc.* 2003;103(3):317–322
30. Neumark-Sztainer D, Story M. Recommendations from overweight youth regarding school-based weight control programs. *J Sch Health.* 1997;67(10):428–433
31. Neumark-Sztainer D, Story M, Hannan PJ, Rex J. New Moves: a school-based obesity prevention program for adolescent girls. *Prev Med.* 2003;37(1):41–51
32. Neumark-Sztainer D, Harris T, Story M. Beliefs and attitudes about obesity among teachers and school health care providers working with adolescents. *J Nutr Educ.* 1999;31(1):3–9
33. Neumark-Sztainer D, Story M, Coller T. Perceptions of secondary school staff toward the implementation of school-based activities to prevent weight-related disorders: a needs assessment. *Am J Health Promot.* 1999;13(3):153–156
34. Neumark-Sztainer D, Martin SL, Story M, iii. School-based programs for obesity prevention: what do adolescents recommend? *Am J Health Promot.* 2000;14(4):232–235
35. Rollnick SR, Miller WR. What is motivational interviewing? *Behav Cogn Psychother.* 1995;23: 325–334
36. Neumark-Sztainer D. *"I'm, Like, SO Fat!": Helping Your Teen Make Healthy Choices About Eating and Exercise in a Weight-Obsessed World.* New York, NY: Guilford Press; 2005

Adolesc Med 19 (2008) 431–449

Does Adolescent Media Use Cause Obesity and Eating Disorders?

Amy B. Jordan, PhD*[a], Emily K. Kramer-Golinkoff, BA[b], Victor C. Strasburger, MD, FAAP[c]

[a]*Annenberg Public Policy Center, University of Pennsylvania, 3620 Walnut Street, Philadelphia, PA 19104-6220, USA*

[b]*Marketing Communications, University of Pennsylvania Health System, 3600 Market Street, Suite 240, Philadelphia, PA 19104, USA*

[c]*Department of Pediatrics, University of New Mexico School of Medicine, Albuquerque, NM 87131, USA*

Concern over media use and the healthy development of adolescents has typically focused on issues such as the media's role in encouraging sexual behavior[1,2] and promoting aggressive solutions to conflicts.[3,4] More recently, attention has turned to the ways in which media may promote disordered eating in adolescents by encouraging children to be more sedentary and to consume more unhealthy foods while simultaneously conveying unrealistic thinness as the ideal for beauty. In this article, we examine the potential mechanisms underlying the relationship between adolescent media use and obesity and eating disorders. In doing so, we identify potential strategies that health care providers might use to promote healthier media diets.

OVERWEIGHT AND OBESITY IN ADOLESCENCE

Childhood obesity has been described as a "pandemic," perhaps justly given its wide geographic distribution and its impact on a high proportion of the population.[5] In the United States, >9 million children are at or above the 85th percentile for BMI,[6] a condition that puts them at risk for a host of medical problems including diabetes and joint abnormalities,[7] impaired physical functioning,[8] and social and psychological issues such as stigmatization and low self-esteem.[9]

After a sharp increase in prevalence of overweight through the 1980s and 1990s, the most recent National Health and Nutrition Examination Survey (NHANES) data suggest that rates of overweight among youth have leveled off. However, the

*Corresponding author.
E-mail address: ajordan@asc.upenn.edu (A. Jordan).

 ISSN 1934-4287

problem remains serious: more than one third (34.1%) of 12- to 19-year-olds are at or above the 85th percentile of the Centers for Disease Control and Prevention growth chart, according to data from the 2003–2006 survey.[10] The number climbs even higher for ethnic minority groups. Among adolescent girls in this sample, 44.5% of black and 37.1% of Mexican American girls are overweight or obese (compared with 31.7% of non-Hispanic white girls). Among boys, 40.5% of Mexican American boys are overweight (compared with 34.5% and 32.1% of non-Hispanic white and black boys, respectively).

Although public discourse about the problem of childhood obesity has increased, a recent study revealed low levels of parental recognition of or concern about children's overweight.[11] Unfortunately, weight problems are not typically something that youth "grow out of," as some parents might think. Overweight adolescents have a 70% chance of becoming overweight or obese adults.[12] The medical risks associated with carrying excess weight in adulthood are widely known and include not only heart disease, type 2 diabetes, and high blood pressure but also some forms of cancer.[13–15]

MEDIA USE AND OVERWEIGHT

Overweight in adolescence is thought to be the result of a confluence of genetic forces, parenting practices, lifestyle patterns, food choices, and environmental factors that result in a lack of physical activity, unhealthy eating patterns, or a combination of the two.[16] In the past 2 decades, researchers looking for modifiable contributors to overweight status have consistently found that youth who spend a great deal of time in front of a screen are significantly more likely to be overweight.

- A longitudinal study of 2223 adolescents found that those who watched >2 hours of television (TV) per day were twice as likely to be overweight at follow-up than adolescents who watched ≤2 hours.[17]
- In a national sample of 746 10- to 15-year-olds, watching TV for ≥5 hours/day increased the risk of being overweight nearly 5 times compared with those who viewed 0 to 2 hours/day.[18]
- In a cohort study of 2343 children aged 9 to 12 years, having a TV set in the bedroom was a significant risk factor for obesity, independent of physical activity or even total media time.[19]
- In addition, researchers have found that excessive TV viewing during childhood is associated with overweight in adulthood. Often, such research has involved large samples of children followed for up to 30 years. In the United Kingdom, a large-scale study of >10 000 5- to 10-year olds found that mean daily hours of TV viewed on weekends predicted a higher BMI at 30 years of age.[20] In New Zealand, a group of researchers followed 1000 unselected subjects from birth until 26 years of age and found that weeknight TV viewing between the ages of 5 and 15 years was strongly correlated with having higher BMIs as adults.[21] Similar studies have been conducted in Scotland,[22] Japan,[23] and the United States.[24,25]

Although we know more about the role of TV in childhood overweight,[18,26] it seems that all screen-based media deserve attention. Vandewater et al,[27] for example, found no relationship between weight status and TV viewing among adolescents and a significant but curvilinear relationship between weight status and electronic game play. Similarly, McMurray et al[28] found that although there was no significant effect of TV viewing on BMI in their sample of 10- to 16-year-olds, increased hours of video-game play enhanced the risk of overweight for both boys and girls. Several studies have also linked heavy computer use (>2 hours/day) to increased overweight in adolescents, particularly among girls.[29] TV is clearly not the only "sedentary" medium with which children spend time. A 2005 study by the Kaiser Family Foundation indicated that although TV viewing has remained stable among 8- to 18-year-olds, the use of video games and computers has increased significantly over time[30] (see Fig 1).

Widespread use of media and its potential contribution to overweight in adolescents have led researchers to attempt to understand mechanisms through which media use may affect adolescent BMI. These mechanisms include (1) the displacement of physical activity with sedentary leisure-time use, (2) the influence of media on dietary habits (ie, food choice and snacking while viewing), and (3) the erosion of children's sleep through nighttime use of media in the bedroom. We examine the evidence to support each proposed mechanism.

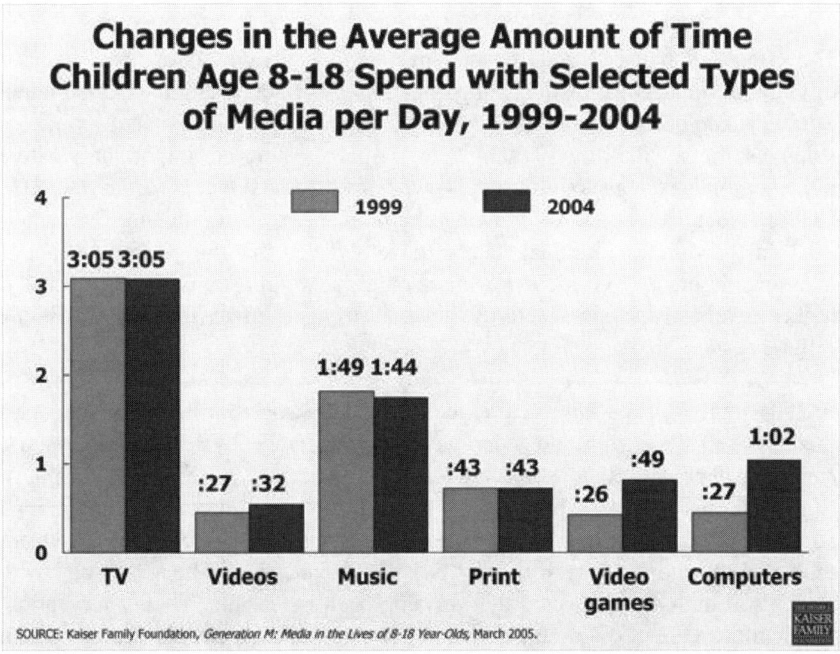

Fig 1. Reproduced with permission from Kaiser Family Foundation. Available at: facts.kff.org/chart.aspx?ch=443.

The Impact of Heavy Media Use on Physical and Sedentary Activity

Conventional wisdom suggests that watching TV, playing video games, and surfing the Web displace time that youth might spend running around, playing an organized sport, or otherwise "exercising" (and burning calories). However, the relationship is not always clear. Several studies of adolescents have found that physical activity is inversely associated with overweight status,[31] whereas other studies have found an inconsistent relationship[32] or no relationship.[33] Some have argued that the failure to find an association is an artifact of poor measures of physical activity.[34] A systematic review of research by Marshall et al[35] on the relationship between media use and physical activity showed little support for the displacement hypothesis. The current thinking is that sedentary children and adolescents will remain sedentary even if media are limited or removed.[36,37]

An alternative explanation is that that there are distinct behavioral pathways to obesity for physical activity and inactivity.[38] Clinical studies by Epstein et al[39] provided evidence that obese children targeted for reduction of sedentary behaviors (such as TV viewing and playing computer games) have similar or better long-term weight loss than children targeted for being more physically active. A review of interventions with adolescents revealed that such efforts typically combine sedentary behavior messages with other health information (eg, healthy eating and exercise), making it impossible to estimate the magnitude of the influences of sedentary behavior–reduction messages alone.[40]

The effects of physical activity and inactivity on weight status seem to have differential impacts for distinct subpopulations. The 2000 National Longitudinal Study of Adolescent Health (ADD Health) found that environmental influences (such as the availability of safe "play" space) exert an important positive influence on physical activity levels, whereas socioeconomic factors (such as lack of resources for safe TV-viewing alternatives) exert an influence on inactivity.[41] In addition, longitudinal surveys have revealed that the greatest impact of additional hours of TV/video viewing is on girls' weight status.[41,42] Conversely, higher levels of physical activity have a stronger effect for boys.[28] Ethnic differences are also apparent.[32,41]

A 2004 review of the empirical evidence of the association between sedentary media use (TV viewing and video-game playing) and physical fitness found a small but negative relationship between the 2 behaviors.[35] Several studies have suggested that the best possible scenario for preventing overweight among adolescents may be a combination of watching less TV per week and frequent moderate-to-vigorous physical activity.[32,38] Research by Robinson et al[43] with students at high risk indicated that this approach is feasible. Their intervention, the Stanford GEMS pilot, consisted of after-school dance classes and a 5-lesson program delivered to homes designed to reduce TV and video-game use. Compared with a control group (which received newsletters and health information lectures), 8- to 10-year-old black girls were more physically active and spent less time with media, including less time eating with the TV on.

Media's Influence on Dietary Habits

Adolescent use of media can affect food-intake habits via 2 distinct pathways. First, adolescents who are exposed to the steady stream of junk-food advertisements may be more likely to eat foods that are high in calories and low in nutrition. Second, children who eat with the TV on may be cued to eat (through habit or commercial suggestion) and may eat more mindlessly than children who do not combine eating with viewing.

Research by the Kaiser Family Foundation has shown that adolescents watch far more general audience and adult programs than children's programs and that this viewing exposes them to advertising that is neither federally regulated nor industry self-regulated.[44] According to their estimates, the average 13- to 17-year-old sees 17 food ads per day on TV and over the course of a year is exposed to 6000 food ads. Only 5% are for "healthy" foods such as dairy or fruit.

Several experimental studies have indicated that exposure to food ads makes young audiences more likely to prefer, request, and consume the advertised food. Although most of these studies have been conducted with younger children,[45,46] it seems likely that the advertisements are effective at producing behavior change in adolescents, too, particularly in light of the $11 billion spent per year on food marketing.[47] An experiment that assessed the impact of varying combinations of TV ads for unhealthy and healthy foods on children's dietary knowledge, attitudes, and intentions revealed that ads for nutritious foods (such as fruits and vegetables) do promote positive attitudes and beliefs concerning these foods, suggesting that food preferences do not always have to drift to the less nutritious variety.[48]

Some researchers argue that the content of media must be examined also. As pressure increases to reduce junk-food ad exposure on TV, more and more companies are paying for product placement in shows and movies. Coca Cola cups are ever-present in front of the *American Idol* judges (Fig 2). Burger King products are ubiquitous in the *Scooby Doo 2* movie, and McDonald's is featured in *Spy Kids*.[49] In addition, the portrayal of food consumption on programs popular with adolescents can be worrisome. One study of prime-time TV found that the prime-time diet, which consists mainly of fats, sweets, and alcohol, is not congruent with current dietary recommendations[50] (see Fig 3).

Several studies have suggested that teenagers who watch more TV tend to snack more frequently,[51,52] eat diets that are higher in fat,[53] drink more sodas,[54] eat more fast food,[52] and eat fewer fruits and vegetables.[55] In 1 study, TV viewing, in contrast to other media use such as music listening, significantly increased

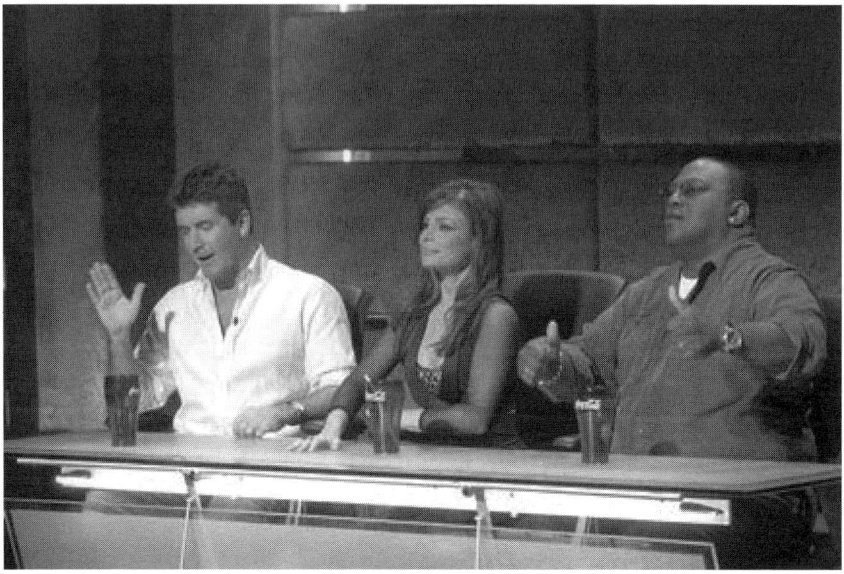

Fig 2. American Idol judges (from left to right): Simon Cowell, Paula Abdul, and Randy Jackson. (Photograph courtesy Ray Mickshaw/Fox.) Source: http://money.howstuffworks.com/product-placement6.htm.

food consumption among college-aged students.[56] In another study, children from families in which the TV was usually on during meals ate less healthy foods than those who did not, even when potential covariates such as socioeconomic factors were controlled.[57] Some explanations for the phenomena of excess caloric consumption during viewing have been offered. One argument is that advertisements for junk food cue children to want to eat while viewing or eat foods commonly advertised on TV. For instance, a recent study of 548 students in 5 public schools near Boston, Massachusetts, found that each hour increase in TV viewing resulted in an additional intake of 701.4 kJ/day (167 kcal/day), usually of foods advertised on TV.[53] Sugar-sweetened beverages, especially sodas and juices, seem to be the leading culprits in excess energy intake.[37] A second opinion is that TV viewing decreases internal signals of satiety or the feeling of fullness.[56] Finally, Coon et al set forth the intriguing notion that families who turn the television off during meals are "separating the act of eating from the world contained inside the television set, and to that extent there is a boundary between private family food culture and the food culture promoted on television."[57(p7)]

The Impact of Media on Sleep

A third potential mechanism underlying the media and overweight relationship may be that TV and other media use displaces or disturbs adolescents' sleep.

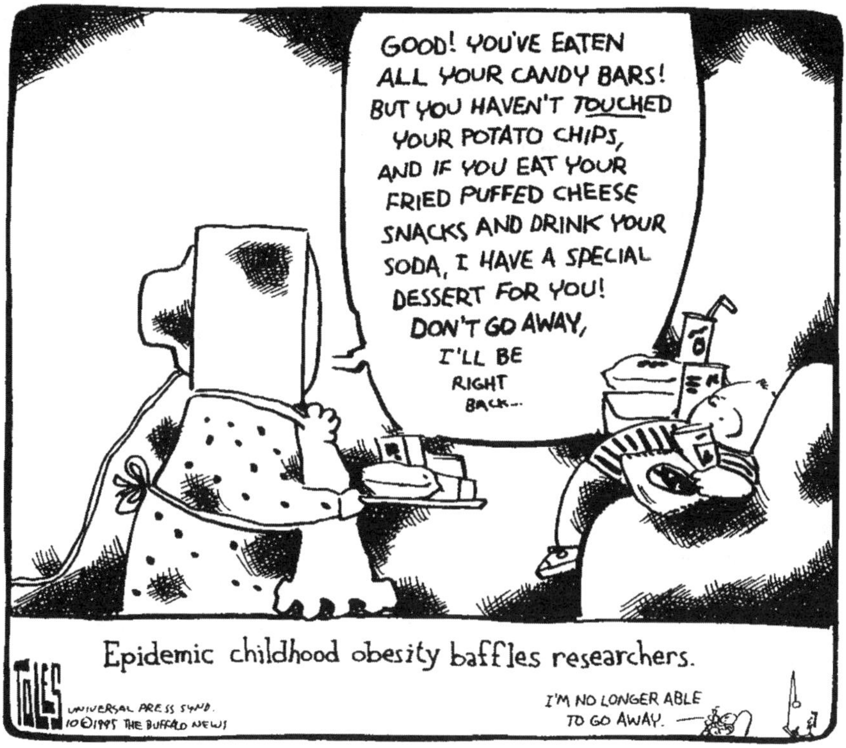
GOOD! YOU'VE EATEN ALL YOUR CANDY BARS! BUT YOU HAVEN'T TOUCHED YOUR POTATO CHIPS, AND IF YOU EAT YOUR FRIED PUFFED CHEESE SNACKS AND DRINK YOUR SODA, I HAVE A SPECIAL DESSERT FOR YOU! DON'T GO AWAY, I'LL BE RIGHT BACK...
Epidemic childhood obesity baffles researchers.
TOLES
UNIVERSAL PRESS SYND.
10©1995 THE BUFFALO NEWS
I'M NO LONGER ABLE TO GO AWAY.

Fig 3. TOLES (Reproduced with permission from Universal Press Syndicate).

Later bedtimes and less sleep are associated with greater risk for overweight among children.[58–60] One theory is that sleep deprivation alters food-consumption patterns. Short-sleeping college students, for example, were more likely to eat more small meals or snacks throughout the day than their long-sleeping peers, leading to the consumption of more calories.[61] Changes in food consumption that come from less sleep may be related to cortisol levels. One study found a negative association between amount of rapid-eye-movement sleep and cortisol levels and a positive association between cortisol levels and calories consumed.[62] In addition, sleep loss may produce stress for some individuals, which may lead to more snacking and a decrease in the consumption of typical meal-type foods.[63] In general, studies have indicated that sleep-deprived individuals are more likely to consume less healthy foods than those who get an adequate amount of sleep.[62] A second theory is that short sleep duration makes adolescents less able to be physically active or that tiredness leads to greater sedentary behavior, such as media use, perpetuating a cycle of inactivity.[64]

If short sleep cycles lead to greater unhealthy food consumption or less physical activity participation, is TV or other media use implicated in sleep disturbance? A cross-sectional study of adolescents in Belgium found that using media as a sleep aid is a common practice of adolescents. Those who reported using music, TV, and computer games more often as a sleeping aid slept fewer hours and were significantly more tired.[65] A longitudinal study of adolescents in New York found that extensive TV viewing during adolescence was significantly associated with the development of frequent sleep problems among youth who had not previously had frequent sleep problems. Most importantly, "adolescents with no history of frequent difficulty falling asleep who watch 3 hours or more of television per day may be twice as likely as those who watch less than 1 hour per day to experience frequent difficulty falling asleep by early adulthood."[66(p566)] Although more research is necessary to "connect the dots" between bedroom TVs, nighttime viewing, sleep disturbance, and adolescent overweight, this research path may offer an important clue into how excessive electronic media use affects weight status.

Recommendations

Concern over the relationship between excessive media use and childhood overweight has led many to call on health care providers to provide patients and their parents with strategies for developing healthier media-use patterns to prevent childhood obesity.[67,68] On the basis of this review, 2 strategies have the potential to be most effective at addressing the relationship between media and overweight status.

1. Nationally, two thirds of children over the age of 8 have TVs in their bedrooms.[30] Providers should recommend that TVs be eliminated completely from adolescents' bedrooms.[69] In addition, it must be recognized that the proliferation of new media, as well as the growing convergence of media platforms, means that parents must beware that children do not simply substitute one screen medium for another. Taking electronic media out of the bedroom may reduce the number of hours children spend in front of a screen; it may also improve sleep quality and increase sleep time, factors associated with weight status.

2. Four in 10 families have a TV set in the dining room or kitchen,[67] and the research reviewed above suggests that TV is often on while the family is eating meals together and when children are consuming snacks. This may increase the time children spend viewing, and it may undermine healthy eating habits. Disconnecting food intake from TV viewing may increase awareness of food consumption while also increasing family communication and decreasing total TV-watching time.

A systematic review by DeMattia et al[40] revealed a paucity of literature examining brief office interventions to address weight control. In a survey of 365 pediatricians, the most frequent barrier reported was a perceived lack of parental motivation or support for the recommendations to limit viewing.[70] One third of surveyed pediatricians said they lacked time to address media habits during well-child visits or felt that it was futile to try to affect patients' media habits. Perhaps asking parents 2 simple questions would allow health care providers to identify the youth who are most at risk for media use affecting weight status: (1) "Does your child have a TV set, video-game console, and/or computer in his or her bedroom?" and (2) "How much time per day does your child spend with screen media?"[69] An additional question could also be added about eating in front of the TV. When counseling patients, health care providers must keep in mind that TV and other media play a significant role in the day-to-day lives of families.[67] Altering access to media will surely meet resistance, and parents must be ready with alternative activities and willing to engage with children differently.

MEDIA USE AND EATING DISORDERS AMONG ADOLESCENTS

Despite increases in obesity rates among all age groups in the United States, the media's depiction of the "ideal" female body has steadily slimmed over the past 50 years.[71,72] In fact, Wiseman et al[73] found that more than half of American female beauty icons qualify as suffering from anorexia nervosa, according to their criteria. Along with the slimming down of media icons, there has been a concurrent increase in the prevalence of eating disorders, particularly among adolescent girls.[74] Research has shown that nearly 44% of teenaged girls believe themselves to be overweight, and 66% of teenaged girls purposefully attempt to lose weight, although most of them weigh in the normal range.[75–77] The desire to be thinner has been found among girls as young as 12 years of age, of which ~50% reported a desire to be thinner[78].

Female adolescents' heavy media consumption is associated with body dissatisfaction.[79,80] In 1 study, girls who wanted to look like media figures on TV, in the movies, or in popular magazines were twice as likely to be very concerned with their weight, become constant dieters, and engage in purging behavior.[81] In another study, 69% of girls admitted that their body ideal was affected by images in magazines, and 47% of girls claimed they wanted to lose weight as a result of these images.[82]

Adolescents who are dissatisfied with their bodies often go to unhealthy extremes in their efforts to become thinner. Experts estimate that ~0.5% of adolescent girls and young women in Western countries suffer from anorexia nervosa and ~2% suffer from bulimia nervosa.[83] They are among the ranks of the 8 million Americans with eating disorders, which includes 0.5% to 3% of the general population and 4% to 22% of college-aged women who engage in abnormal eating behaviors.[75]

Psychologically fragile adolescents, including those with low self-esteem, are particularly at risk for developing an eating disorder.[83] In addition, Martínez-González et al[83] found a correlation between girls' eating pathology and their parents' marital status. Girls whose parents separated or divorced suffered from an increased risk of developing an eating disorder. From this finding we infer that strong, stable family units have significant positive effects on children's and adolescents' psychological well-being.

In addition to psychological predictors of eating disorders, gender and ethnicity are associated with increased risk for eating disorders. The prevalence of eating disorders is consistently highest among white females from industrialized Western countries.[84] Studies repeatedly find that females experience more body dissatisfaction than do their male counterparts.[78] In fact, eating disorders occur >10 times as frequently among females than males.[84] The gender difference in the prevalence of body dissatisfaction and eating disorders is often attributed to our society's disproportionate emphasis on females' appearance and attractiveness.[85]

Despite the fact that eating disorders are reported less than half as frequently among blacks as whites, disordered eating patterns and body-image issues exist for blacks as well.[86] The disparity in prevalence of eating disorders between blacks and whites is often attributed to differences in body ideals. Black females tend to desire a more curvaceous, normal-weight figure than do white females. Botta[87] found that people of different ethnicities had varying levels of body dissatisfaction and dissimilar body ideals. However, despite frequent suggestions of immunity to media exposure, researchers have found that black females are indeed affected by media depictions of body ideals, albeit differently than their white counterparts.[86,87] Specifically, larger black females may be negatively affected by thin-promoting media and at risk for developing eating-disorder symptomatology.[86] However, thinner black females may also experience body dissatisfaction. The difference lies in the fact that efforts to gain weight to obtain one's ideal body size are not typically seen as disordered.[86]

Recent research has pointed to 3 dominant mechanisms through which the media transmit messages that construct and reinforce social norms for body ideals to females in particular. These mechanisms include the role of media in cultivating beliefs about beauty in early childhood; the resonance of thin-ideal messages in interpersonal interactions and cultural norms in adolescence; and the triggering of body dissatisfaction as adolescent girls pass through puberty and begin to diverge from media-inculcated norms of thinness.

Media Cultivate Beliefs About Beauty and Body Ideals in Early Childhood That May Be Asymptomatic Until Adolescence

Cultivation theory posits that through repeated exposure to unhealthily slim female bodies in the media, prepubescent children develop deeply entrenched beliefs and perceptions of societal body standards. In fact, Dohnt and Tiggemann[88] showed that children as young as 6 years of age absorb and espouse the belief that thinness is essential for beauty (the "thin ideal"). Thin-ideal internalization is the degree to which an individual adopts the thin body standard condoned by society and attempts to achieve this ideal herself.[89] The role of the media in the adoption and internalization of the thin ideal is suggested by the heavy media consumption reported by many girls. As they accumulate exposure to the thin ideal, children gradually learn and accept the notion that females must be ultra thin to be attractive and desired. In effect, repeated exposure to the thin ideal in the media gives children the building blocks to develop schema regarding body image. Ultimately, this may provide the foundation for later development of disordered eating, body dissatisfaction, or even eating disorders.

Children's acceptance of the thin ideal may not become overtly problematic until adolescence.[90] Researchers explain the delayed impact of children's beliefs about body ideals in 2 main ways. First, children tend to be naturally slim at young ages because of high levels of physical activity and a fast metabolism. Therefore, their bodies may actually mirror the ultra-trim, virtually fatless bodies of models and celebrities in the media. Second, the emphasis on extreme thinness in the media tends to focus on adult women. Thus, it is possible that children do not compare their own bodies to those of fully matured adults yet. According to Harrison and Hefne,[90] although children may not develop immediate body dissatisfaction from repeated exposure to thin-promoting media, research has suggested that heavy media consumption may have a more insidious, time-delayed effect. More specifically, accumulated exposure to the thin ideal likely informs children's development of schema surrounding body ideals, which can later serve as the groundwork for a lifelong unhealthy relationship with food and poor body image.

Media Messages Resonate With Interpersonal and Sociocultural Messages About Food, Exercise, and Beauty

Children do not grow up in an environment in which they subconsciously accept every mediated message they receive, of course. Rather, children's beliefs and perceptions of the world are informed by a multitude of factors, including interpersonal sources such as family members and peers. The sociocultural model, the second major mechanism of mediated message transmission to youth, suggests that young girls receive consistent messages about body ideals from many influential sources. These sources include the various forms of media and trusted people such as parents and friends. The ubiquity, pervasiveness, and varying channels of message transmission all serve to socialize children to unquestionably accept that thinness is essential to beauty.

Preadolescents who watched or read appearance-based media were more likely to engage in peer conversations about physical appearance, and conversations regarding appearance are associated with internalization of body ideals and body dissatisfaction.[82] Peers amplify the "appearance culture" wherein the media and peer influence function synergistically to socialize adolescent girls to adopt the thin ideal.

Children and adolescents receive messages from a wide variety of media forms, including magazines, music videos, video games, TV, and comic books, differently and for diverse reasons. In fact, Tiggemann examined both female undergraduates' TV and fashion-magazine consumption to evaluate if different forms of media had similar effects on audiences.[91] She found that fashion magazines and TV do not have similar effects on users. Although TV consumption was inversely associated with self-esteem and positively associated with BMI, fashion-magazine use was correlated with thin-ideal internalization. Thus, media have different effects on girls, in part because they use media in unique ways and for different purposes, such as entertainment, relaxation, or information.[92,93] In addition, various media portray women very differently, which likely affects the take-away message for adolescents about socially sanctioned female body ideals. For example, music videos often depict women merely as sexual figures whose entire worth is derived from their physical attractiveness and in relation to men.[94] Conversely, TV series and films more often provide a more realistic and complex image of women that are defined by more than their appearance.[93] Consequently, the messages children and adolescents receive from each medium as well as the correlation between "media use" and disordered eating, body dissatisfaction, or eating disorders vary tremendously on the basis of the nature of the content.

Physical Changes During Adolescence Make Media Messages More Powerful and Potentially Trigger Body Dissatisfaction

During childhood, heavy exposure to consistent messages socializes children to develop beliefs about body standards and lays the groundwork for future food and body-image issues. As children enter adolescence and undergo puberty, they experience bodily changes that make their schema surrounding body ideals more salient. Research has shown that adolescents often engage in social comparison with the idealized images of female bodies in the media, whereby they view themselves in contrast to others.[95] "Upward comparisons" may diminish an individual's sense of self-worth and are associated with depression.[96] As girls find their bodies increasingly diverging from the unhealthily slim bodies portrayed in the media as a result of new and redistributed fat from puberty, they may become dissatisfied with their own bodies and develop body-image distortion. Body-image distortion occurs when an individual has an inaccurate perception of his or her body size. It can be a predictor of severe body-image issues, including eating disorders.[78] "Teen girls are most at risk for developing eating disorders as they struggle with a body that is getting bigger in a culture that simultaneously sells them junk food and tells them they should be thin."[75(p159)] For example, a recent study found that girls who read fashion magazines in preadolescence were significantly more likely to report dieting 5 years later.[97]

Research has shown that body dissatisfaction and body-image disturbance often are precursors to the development of dangerous eating disorders such as bulimia and anorexia. The most powerful link between media and eating disorders appeared in a naturalistic study of teenaged girls in Fiji. Researchers studied >100 teenaged Fijian girls 3 years before and after the introduction of American TV shows. Only 3% reported vomiting to control their weight before American TV, but this figure rose to 15% afterward. In addition, three fourths of the girls reported feeling too fat, and those who watched TV at least 3 nights per week were 50% more likely to feel that way and 30% more likely to diet.[98] A study of 3000 Spanish 12-to 21-year-olds over a 19-month period found that those who read teen magazines had a doubled risk of developing an eating disorder.[83]

Recommendations

Health care providers can help mitigate the negative effects of media exposure on adolescents' body image and eating patterns by teaching parents and young children about the importance of a nutritional, balanced diet and physical activity for healthy psychological and physical development.[74] Pediatricians should also encourage youth to get involved in sports teams in their community or school. These opportunities allow young people to be physically active while having fun and socializing.[74] Beyond these general recommendations, health care providers can offer 3 suggestions for parents and adolescents concerned about disordered eating.

1. Encourage nightly family dinners, beginning while children are young and continuing through the teen years. Having a strong cultural identity may safeguard youth from the development of eating disorders.[74] The family dinner gives parents and young people the opportunity to connect, share their daily experiences with each other, and feel like they belong to a larger, supportive unit. Family meals also tend to be more nutritionally balanced than meals eaten in front of the TV.[57] At least 1 study has found that the practice of family dinners is a protective factor against eating problems, even after controlling for the effects of family support and communication.[99]

2. Emphasize the importance of an age-appropriate and time-restricted media diet. The American Academy of Pediatrics recommends a maximum of 1 to 2 hours of daily TV watching for children.[100] They also encourage parents to watch TV with their children to facilitate content-driven discussions. Furthermore, research has shown that when youth consume media targeted to older audiences, they are often exposed to appearance and dieting messages that can have harmful effects on their own body image and eating behaviors.[88,97] Age-appropriate media was not found to have an effect on children's body image or dieting awareness, which supports the idea that consuming appropriate media for limited amounts of time ideally in the company of a parent can significantly lessen the well-documented negative effects of media exposure on youths' relationship with food and body image.

3. Even with limitations for children regarding what types of media they can consume and for how long, neither parents nor health care providers can completely eradicate youths' exposure to thin-promoting media, which is pervasive and unavoidable. Pediatricians must encourage media education programs that can give parents and young people the tools to deconstruct the media images and messages about body image and eating. A recent evaluation of the Body Project, a National Institutes of Health–funded intervention based at the University of Texas, found that eating disorders were reduced by 61% for adolescent girls who were taught to understand the industry's efforts to manipulate their sense of beauty.[101] Girls Inc, the organization that created Girls Get the Message, creates educational programs to assist young females as they "confront subtle societal messages about their value and potential."[102] In particular, Girls Get the Message was designed to teach media literacy and "help girls recognize stereotypes in media and differentiate between those stereotypes and their own lives" (Girls Inc, 2007). Thus, it is critical that pediatricians address media literacy during their patients' young years and encourage schools to implement media education programs that teach them what constitutes a "healthy" body as opposed to the socially idealized body. Stinton and Birch[103] recommended that prevention efforts focus on deemphasizing appearance in an effort to ward off body dissatisfaction and disordered eating. In fact, a number of prevention messages have had documented positive effects on female adolescents' body image. These successful messages include: "Media images are not real"; "The ideal body changes through history and cultures"; and "Do not fall into the comparison trap."[76]

Pediatricians may be able to identify children and adolescents who are particularly vulnerable for development of disordered eating by asking meaningful questions about their media use. Reports of heavy consumption of appearance-oriented media in conjunction with concerning physical or psychological changes, such as weight gain, weight loss, or depressive symptomatology, among others, should alert pediatricians to the possibility of an abnormal body self-image or eating-disorder symptomatology.

CONCLUSIONS

Considerable data exist to justify the notion that the media make a significant impact on adolescents' eating habits and sedentary leisure-time use, leading to overweight and obesity. Media images also create ideals of beauty for adolescent girls, shaping the feelings they have about their own bodies and possibly contributing to the development of eating disorders among girls who feel they compare unfavorably with media role models. In this article we have suggested several ways in which health care providers can address adolescent media use and help parents cultivate healthier media habits in their children's lives. Research is needed to investigate the feasibility and efficacy of such brief interventions conveyed in clinical settings.

REFERENCES

1. Brown JD, L'Engle KL, Pardun CJ, Guo G, Kenneavy K, Jackson C. Sexy media matter: exposure to sexual content in music, movies, television, and magazines predicts black and white adolescents' sexual behavior. *Pediatrics*. 2006;117(4):1018–1027
2. Brown JD, Strasburger VC. From Calvin Klein to Paris Hilton and MySpace: adolescents, sex, and the media. *Adolesc Med State Art Rev*. 2007;18(3):484–507, vi–vii
3. Johnson JG, Cohen P, Smailes EM, Kasen S, Brook JS. Television viewing and aggressive behavior during adolescence and adulthood. *Science*. 2002;295(5564):2468–2471
4. Anderson CA, Dill KE. Video games and aggressive thoughts, feelings, and behavior in the laboratory and in life. *J Pers Soc Psychol*. 2000;78(4):772–790
5. Kimm S, Obarzanek E. Childhood obesity: a new pandemic of the new millennium. *Pediatrics*. 2002;110(5):1003–1007
6. Jordan AB. Preface. *Ann Am Acad Pol Soc Sci*. 2008;615:6–12
7. DeMattia L, Denney SL. Childhood obesity prevention: successful community-based efforts. *Ann Am Acad Pol Soc Sci*. 2008;615:83–99
8. Schwimmer JB, Burwinkle TM, Varni JW. Health-related quality of life of severely obese children and adolescents. *JAMA*. 2003;289(14):1813–1819
9. Williams J, Wake M, Hesketh K, Maher E, Waters E. Health-related quality of life of overweight and obese children. *JAMA*. 2005;293(1):70–76
10. Ogden CL, Carroll MD, Flegal KM. High body mass index for age among US children and adolescents, 2003–2006. *JAMA*. 2008;299(20):2401–2405
11. Eckstein KC, Mikhail LM, Ariza AJ, et al. Parents' perceptions of their child's weight and health. *Pediatrics*. 2006;117(3):681–690
12. Whitaker RC, Wright JA, Pepe MS, Seidel KD, Dietz WH. Predicting obesity in young adulthood from childhood and parental obesity. *N Engl J Med*. 1997;337(13):869–873
13. Saw SM, Rajan U. The epidemiology of obesity: a review. *Ann Acad Med Singapore*. 1997; 26(4):489–493
14. Must A, Jacques PF, Dallal GE, Bajema CJ, Dietz WH. Long-term morbidity and mortality of overweight adolescents: a follow-up of the Harvard Growth Study of 1922 to 1935. *N Engl J Med*. 1992;327(19):1350–1355
15. Freedman DS, Khan LK, Dietz WH, Srinivasan SR, Berenson GS. Relationship of childhood obesity to coronary heart disease risk factors in adulthood: the Bogalusa Heart Study. *Pediatrics*. 2001;108(3):712–718
16. Gable S, Lutz S. Household, parent, and child contributions to childhood obesity. *Fam Relat*. 2000;49(3):293–300
17. Kaur H, Choi WS, Mayo SM, Harris KJ. Duration of television watching is associated with increased body mass index. *J Pediatr*. 2003;143(4):506–511
18. Gortmaker SL, Must A, Sobol AM, Peterson K, Colditz GA, Dietz WH. Television viewing as a cause of increasing obesity among children in the United States, 1986–1990. *Arch Pediatr Adolesc Med*. 1996;150(4):356–362
19. Adachi-Mejia AM, Longacre MR, Gibson JJ, Beach ML, Titus-Ernstoff LT, Dalton MA. Children with a TV in their bedroom at risk for being overweight. *Int J Obes (Lond)*. 2007;31(4):644–651
20. Viner RM, Cole TJ. Television viewing in early childhood predicts adult body mass index. *J Pediatr*. 2005;147(4):429–435
21. Hancox RJ, Milne BJ, Poulton R. Association between child and adolescent television viewing and adult health: a longitudinal birth cohort study. *Lancet*. 2004;364(9430):257–262
22. Reilly JJ, Armstrong J, Dorosty AR, et al. Early life risk factors for obesity in childhood: cohort study. *BMJ*. 2005;330(7504):1357

23. Sugimori H, Yoshida K, Izuno T, et al. Analysis of factors that influence body mass index from ages 3 to 6 years: a study based on the Toyama cohort study. *Pediatr Int.* 2004;46(3):302–310
24. Davison KK, Marshall SJ, Birch LL. Cross-sectional and longitudinal associations between TV viewing and girls' body mass index, overweight status, and percentage of body fat. *J Pediatr.* 2006;149(1):32–37
25. O'Brien M, Nader PR, Houts RM, et al. The ecology of childhood overweight: a 12-year longitudinal analysis. *Int J Obes (Lond).* 2007;31(9):1469–1478
26. Andersen RE, Crespo CJ, Bartlett SJ, Cheskin LJ, Pratt M. Relationship of physical activity and television watching with body weight and level of fatness among children. *JAMA.* 1998; 279(12):938–942
27. Vandewater EA, Shim MS, Caplovitz AG. Linking obesity and activity level with children's television and video game use. *J Adolesc.* 2004;27(1):71–85
28. McMurray RG, Harrell JS, Deng S, Bradley CB, Cox LM, Bangdiwala SI. The influence of physical activity, socioeconomic status, and ethnicity on the weight status of adolescents. *Obes Res.* 2000;8(2):130–139
29. Schneider M, Dunton GF, Cooper DM. Media use and obesity in adolescent females. *Obesity.* 2007;15(9):2328–2335
30. Rideout V, Roberts DF, Foehr UG. *Generation M: Media in the Lives of 8–18 Year-Olds.* Menlo Park, CA: Kaiser Family Foundation; 2005. Available at: www.kff.org/entmedia/7251.cfm. Accessed September 26, 2008
31. Dowda M, Ainsworth BE, Addy CL, Saunders R, Riner W. Environmental influences, physical activity, and weight status in 8- to 16-year-olds. *Arch Pediatr Adolesc Med.* 2001;155(6):711–717
32. Stovitz SD, Steffen LM, Boostrom A. Participation in physical activity among normal- and overweight Hispanic and non-Hispanic white adolescents. *J Sch Health.* 2008;78(1):19–25
33. Lioret S, Maire B, Volatier JL, Charles MA. Child overweight in France and its relationship with physical activity, sedentary behavior and socioeconomic status. *Eur J Clin Nutr.* 2007; 61(4):509–516
34. Kohl HW 3rd, Hobbs KE. Development of physical activity behaviors among children and adolescents. *Pediatrics.* 1998;101(3 pt 2):549–554
35. Marshall SJ, Biddle SJ, Gorely T, Cameron N, Murdey I. Relationships between media use, body fatness and physical activity in children and youth: a meta-analysis. *Int J Obes Relat Metab Disord.* 2004;28(10):1238–1246
36. Jordan AB. Heavy television viewing and childhood obesity. *J Child Media.* 2007;1(1):45–54
37. Strasburger VC, Wilson BJ, Jordan AJ. *Children, Adolescents, and the Media.* 2nd ed. Thousand Oaks, CA: Sage; 2008
38. Gordon-Larsen P, Adair LS, Popkin BM. Ethnic differences in physical activity and inactivity patterns and overweight status. *Obes Res.* 2002;10(3):141–149
39. Epstein LH, Paluch RA, Gordy CC, Dorn J. Decreasing sedentary behaviors in treating pediatric obesity. *Arch Pediatr Adolesc Med.* 2000;154(3):220–226
40. DeMattia L, Lemont L, Meurer L. Do interventions to limit sedentary behaviours change behaviour and reduce childhood obesity? A critical review of the literature. *Obes Rev.* 2007; 8(1):69–81
41. Gordon-Larsen P, McMurray RG, Popkin BM. Determinants of adolescent physical activity and inactivity patterns. *Pediatrics.* 2000;105(6). Available at: www.pediatrics.org/cgi/content/full/105/6/e83
42. Crossman A, Sullivan DA, Benin M. The family environment and American adolescents' risk of obesity as young adults. *Soc Sci Med.* 2006;63(9):2255–2267
43. Robinson TN, Killen JD, Kraemer HC, et al. Dance and reducing television viewing to prevent weight gain in African-American girls: the Stanford GEMS pilot study. *Ethn Dis.* 2003;13(1 suppl 1):S65–S77
44. Gantz W, Schwartz N, Angelini JR, Rideout V. *Food for Thought: Television Food Advertising to Children in the United States.* Menlo Park, CA: Kaiser Family Foundation; 2007

45. Borzekowski DL, Robinson TR. The 30-second effect: an experiment revealing the impact of television commercials on food preferences of preschoolers. *J Am Diet Assoc.* 2001;101(1): 42–46
46. Chernin A. The effects of food marketing on children's preferences: testing the moderating roles of age and gender. *Ann Am Acad Pol Soc Sci.* 2008;615:102–118
47. Story M, Neumark-Sztainer D, French S. Individual and environmental influences on adolescent eating behaviors. *J Am Diet Assoc.* 2002;102(3 suppl):S40–S51
48. Dixon HG, Scully ML, Wakefield MA, White VM, Crawford DA. The effects of television advertisements for junk food versus nutritious food on children's food attitudes and preferences. *Soc Sci Med.* 2007;65(7):1311–1323
49. Linn S, Novosat CL. Calories for sale: food marketing to children in the 21st century. *Ann Am Acad Pol Soc Sci.* 2008;615:133–155
50. Byrd-Bredbenner C, Grasso D, Finckenor M. Nutrition messages on prime-time television programs. *Top Clin Nutr.* 2001;16(4):61–72
51. Snoek HM, van Strien T, Janssens JM, Engels RC. The effect of television viewing on adolescents' snacking: individual differences explained by external, restrained and emotional eating. *J Adolesc Health.* 2006;39(3):448–451
52. Utter J, Neumark-Sztainer D, Jeffery R, Story M. Couch potatoes or French fries: are sedentary behaviors associated with body mass index, physical activity, and dietary behaviors among adolescents? *J Am Diet Assoc.* 2003;103(10):1298–1305
53. Wiecha JL, Peterson KE, Ludwig DS, Kim J, Sobol A, Gortmaker SL. When children eat what they watch: impact of television viewing on dietary intake in youth. *Arch Pediatr Adolesc Med.* 2006;160(4):436–442
54. Giammattei J, Blix G, Marshak HH, Wollitzer AO, Pettitt DJ. Television watching and soft drink consumption: associations with obesity in 11- to 13-year-old schoolchildren. *Arch Pediatr Adolesc Med.* 2003;157(9):882–886
55. Krebs-Smith S, Cook A, Subar A, Cleveland L, Friday J, Kahle LL. Fruit and vegetable intakes of children and adolescents in the United States. *Arch Pediatr Adolesc Med.* 1996;150(1):81–86
56. Blass EM, Anderson DR, Kirkorian HL, Pempek TA, Price I, Koleini MF. On the road to obesity: television viewing increases intake of high-density foods. *Physiol Behav.* 2006; 88(4–5):597–604
57. Coon KA, Goldberg J, Rogers BL, Tucker KL. Relationships between use of television during meals and children's food consumption patterns. *Pediatrics.* 2001;107(1). Available at: www.pediatrics.org/cgi/content/full/107/1/e7
58. Sekine M, Yamagami T, Handa K, et al. A dose-response relationship between short sleeping hours and childhood obesity: results of the Toyama Birth Cohort Study. *Child Care Health Dev.* 2002;28(2):163–170
59. Chaput JP, Brunet M, Tremblay A. Relationship between short sleeping hours and childhood overweight/obesity: results from the "Quebec en Forme" Project. *Int J Obes (Lond).* 2006; 30(7):1080–1085
60. Agras WS, Hammer LD, McNicholas F, Kraemer HC. Risk factors for child overweight: a prospective study from birth to 9.5 years. *J Pediatr.* 2004;145(1):20–25
61. Hicks RA, McTighe S, Juarez M. Sleep duration and eating behaviors in college students. *Percept Mot Skills.* 1986;62(1):25–26
62. Wells TT, Cruess DG. Effects of partial sleep deprivation on food consumption and food choice. *Psychol Health.* 2006;21(1):79–86
63. Oliver G, Wardle J. Perceived effects of stress on food choice. *Physiol Behav.* 1999;66(3): 511–515
64. Nelson MC, Gordon-Larsen P. Physical activity and sedentary behavior patterns are associated with selected adolescent health risk behaviors. *Pediatrics.* 2006;117(4):1281–1290
65. Eggermont S, Van den Bulck J. Nodding off or switching off? The use of popular media as a sleep aid in secondary-school children. *J Paediatr Child Health.* 2006;42(7–8):428–433

66. Johnson JG, Cohen P, Kasen S, First MB, Brook JS. Association between television and sleep problems during adolescence and early adulthood. *Arch Pediatr Adolesc Med.* 2004;158(6): 562–568
67. Jordan AB, Hersey JC, McDivitt JA, Heitzler CD. Reducing children's television-viewing time: a qualitative study of parents and their children. *Pediatrics.* 2006;118(5). Available at: www.pediatrics.org/cgi/content/full/118/5/e1303
68. Jordan AB, Robinson TN. Children, television viewing, and weight status: summary and recommendations from an expert panel meeting. *Ann Am Acad Pol Soc Sci.* 2008;615:119–132
69. Strasburger VC. First do no harm: why have parents and pediatricians missed the boat on children and media? *J Pediatr.* 2007;151(4):334–336
70. Gentile DA, Oberg C, Sherwood NE, et al. Well-child visits in the video age: pediatricians and the American Academy of Pediatrics' guidelines for children's media use. *Pediatrics.* 2004; 114(5):1235–1241
71. Anderson PM, Butcher KE. Childhood obesity: trends and potential causes. *Future Child.* 2006;16(1):19–45
72. Harrison K. Does interpersonal attraction to thin media personalities promote eating disorders? *J Broadcast Electron Media.* 1997;41(4):478–500
73. Wiseman CV, Gray JJ, Mosimann JE, Ahrens AH. Cultural expectations of thinness in women: an update. *Int J Eat Disord.* 1992;11(1):85–89
74. Derenne JL, Beresin EV. Body image, media, and eating disorders. *Acad Psychiatry.* 2006; 30(3):257–261
75. Brown JD, Witherspoon EM. The mass media and American adolescents' health. *J Adolesc Health.* 2002;31(6 suppl):153–170
76. Durkin SJ, Paxton SJ, Wertheim EH. How do adolescent girls evaluate body dissatisfaction prevention messages? *J Adolesc Health.* 2005;37(5):381–390
77. Centers for Disease Control and Prevention. Youth Risk Behavior Surveillance: United States, 2007. *MMWR Morb Mortal Wkly Rep.* 2008;57(SS-4):1–36. Available at: www.cdc.gov/HealthyYouth/yrbs/pdf/yrbss07_mmwr.pdf. Accessed July 8, 2008
78. Jung J, Peterson M. Body dissatisfaction and patterns of media use among preadolescent children. *Fam Consum Sci Res J.* 2007;36(1):40–54
79. Cusumano DL, Thompson JK. Media influence and body image in 8–11-year-old boys and girls: a preliminary report on the multidimensional media influence scale. *Int J Eat Disord.* 2001;29(1):37–44
80. Harrison K, Cantor J. The relationship between media consumption and eating disorders. *J Commun.* 1997;47(1):40–67
81. Field AE, Camargo CA, Taylor CB, Berkey CS, Colditz GA. Relation of peer and media influences to the development of purging behaviors among preadolescent and adolescent girls. *Arch Pediatr Adolesc Med.* 1999;153(11):1184–1189
82. Clark L, Tiggemann M. Appearance culture in nine- to 12-year-old girls: media and peer influences on body dissatisfaction. *Soc Dev.* 2006;15(4):628–643
83. Martínez-González MA, Gual P, Lahortiga F, Alonso Y, de Irala-Estévez J, Cervera S. Parental factors, mass media influences, and the onset of eating disorders in a prospective population-based cohort. *Pediatrics.* 2003;111(2):315–320
84. Pritts SD, Susman J. Diagnosis of eating disorders in primary care. *Am Fam Physician.* 2003;67(2):297–304
85. Drogosz LM, Levy PE. Another look at the effects of appearance, gender, and job type on performance-based decisions. *Psychol Women Q.* 1996;20(3):103–116
86. Gentles KA, Harrison K. Television and perceived peer expectations of body size among African American adolescent girls. *Howard J Commun.* 2006;17(1):39–55
87. Botta RA. The mirror of television: a comparison of black and white adolescents' body image. *J Comm.* 2000;50(3):144–161
88. Dohnt HK, Tiggemann M. Body image concerns in young girls: the role of peers and media prior to adolescence. *J Youth Adolesc.* 2006;35(2):135–145

89. Thompson SH, Corwin SJ, Sargent RG. Ideal body size beliefs and weight concerns of fourth-grade children. *Int J Eat Disord.* 1997;21(3):279–284
90. Harrison K, Hefne V. Media exposure, current and future body ideals, and disordered eating among preadolescent girls: a longitudinal panel study. *J Youth Adolesc.* 2006;35(2):146–156
91. Tiggemann M. Media exposure, body dissatisfaction and disordered eating: television and magazines are not the same! *Eur Eat Disord Rev.* 2003;11(5):418–430
92. Rubin AM. Media uses and effects: a uses-and-gratifications perspective. In: Bryant J, Zillmann D, eds. *Media Effects: Advances in Theory and Research.* Hillsdale, NJ: Lawrence Erlbaum Associates; 1994:417–436
93. Arnett JJ. Adolescents' uses of media for self-socialization. *J Youth Adolesc.* 1995;24(5):519–533
94. Tiggemann M, Pickering AS. Role of television in adolescent women's body dissatisfaction and drive for thinness. *Int J Eat Disord.* 1996;20(2):199–203
95. Botta R. Television images and adolescent girls' body image disturbance. *J Commun.* 1999; 49(2):22–41
96. Heinberg LJ, Thompson JK. Body image and televised images of attractiveness: a controlled laboratory investigation. *J Soc Clin Psychol.* 1995;14:325–338
97. van den Berg P, Neumark-Sztainer D, Hannan PJ, Haines J. Is dieting advice from magazines helpful or harmful? Five-year associations with weight-control behaviors and psychological outcomes in adolescents. *Pediatrics.* 2007;119(1). Available at: www.pediatrics.org/cgi/content/full/119/1/e30
98. Becker AE, Borwell MP, Herzog DB, Hamburg P, Gilman SE. Eating behaviours and attitudes following prolonged exposure to television among ethnic Fijian adolescent girls. *Br J Psychol.* 2002;180:509–514
99. Fulkerson JA, Story M, Mellin A, Leffert N, Neumark-Sztainer D, French SA. Family dinner meal frequency and adolescent development: relationships with developmental assets and high-risk behaviors. *J Adolesc Health.* 2006;39(3):337–345
100. American Academy of Pediatrics, Committee on Public Education. Children, adolescents, and television. *Pediatrics.* 2001;107(2):423–426
101. Stice E, Marti CN, Spoor S, Presnell K, Shaw H. Dissonance and healthy weight eating disorder prevention programs: long-term effects from a randomized efficacy trial. *J Consult Clin Psychol.* 2008;76(2):329–340
102. Girls Inc. Girls Inc media literacy. Available at: www.girlsinc.org/about/programs/media-literacy.html. Accessed July 7, 2008
103. Stinton MM, Birch LL. Individual and sociocultural influences on pre-adolescent girls' appearance schemas and body dissatisfaction. *J Youth Adolesc.* 2006;35(2):157–167

Adolesc Med 19 (2008) 450–474

Bariatric Surgery in Adolescents: Mechanics, Metabolism, and Medical Care

Pamela J. Murray, MD, MHP*

Department of Pediatrics, Children's Hospital of Pittsburgh and University of Pittsburgh School of Medicine, 3705 Fifth Avenue, Pittsburgh, PA 15213-2583, USA

Obesity is a major medical problem and public health crisis. Extreme and super obesity (Table 1) are increasing at even greater rates than are overweight and obesity. Evidence-based interventions to decrease the weight of adolescents or adults have yielded only modest results. Sustained weight loss for >1 year, after combinations of behavioral, pharmacologic, and nutritional approaches, rarely exceeds 5 kg.[1–3]

Increasing numbers of adolescents and young adults have sought and will continue to seek and receive bariatric surgery. Clinicians who care for such youth will be asked to evaluate, consult, and guide them and their families about the potential risks and benefits of bariatric surgery. Practitioners will also see an increasing number of young adults who have undergone bariatric surgical procedures who will be requesting follow-up care or presenting with problems that may be related to the procedure. At this time, clinicians can prepare by becoming familiar with the current literature and common clinical practices.

The earliest recipients of bariatric surgery were individuals with extremely high BMI and multiple comorbidities who received open and drastic malabsorptive surgical procedures. Operative techniques and equipment have improved, and surgery no longer is considered a last resort. Younger individuals with lower BMIs who wish to prevent and reverse comorbidities, desire a higher quality of life, wish for normal longevity, and want to avoid the likely trajectory of escalating obesity and its complications now are candidates for bariatric surgery. Outcome data from these young adults will be a more applicable source of information for adolescents who are also making queries about bariatric surgery than earlier data from older adults.

The objectives of this review are to describe current procedures and outcomes in adults and, when available, adolescents. Metabolic effects of bariatric surgery

*Corresponding author.
E-mail address: murraypj@upmc.edu (P. J. Murray).

 ISSN 1934-4287

Table 1
Definitions of weight categories

Category	BMI, kg/m^2
Underweight	<19
Ideal	19–24.9
Overweight	≥25
Obese (class 1)	≥30
Severe (class 2) obesity	≥35
Extreme or morbid obesity (class 3)	≥40
Super obese	≥50

will be described and special considerations for adolescents will be discussed with reference to guidelines that may assist in the evaluation of this age group.

OBESITY

Sixteen percent of US children and adolescents are obese and have a BMI of >95th percentile for their age and gender; >11% are at >97th percentile.[4] One half to three quarters of obese adolescents will be obese adults.[5] Multidisciplinary weight-reduction programs for adolescents have modest success at best and a high rate of recidivism. Although a 5% to 10% weight reduction will often decrease some of the common comorbidities, most obese people do not achieve sustained modest weight loss. In studies of adults, and in smaller studies of adolescents, bariatric surgery has produced significant and durable weight loss of 50% to 80% of excess body weight (initial weight minus ideal body weight), with improvement and frequently resolution of medical comorbidities.[6–8] Bariatric surgery offers a single and permanent intervention that can address multiple chronic morbidities.

In a recent review,[1] a multidisciplinary group of experts made recommendations for the treatment of child and adolescent overweight and obesity. They proposed a comprehensive and staged approach to treatment beginning with prevention ("Prevention Plus"), advancing to "structured weight management," expanding to "comprehensive multidisciplinary intervention," and embracing "tertiary care intervention" when indicated. Although attempting to be "evidence based" in their recommendations, the lack of quality evidence left the conclusions of this expert group "evidence influenced." They adapted adolescent and adult data by guarded extrapolation and correlation, and although many recommendations are untested, they still were proposed as "best-practice" recommendations. The proposed tertiary care interventions endorsed medication-supplemented behavioral interventions and consideration of bariatric surgery for adolescents who comply with the 2004 consensus guidelines[9] listed in Table 2.

Table 2
Criteria for bariatric surgery for adolescents

- Structured behavioral weight-loss program for 6 mo
- Failed to reduce weight substantially
- Demonstrated ability to adhere to diet, exercise, medical, and supplementation routines
- Close to physiologic/structural maturity
- Bone age of 13 y in girls, 15 y in boys
- Severely obese (BMI ≥40) with serious comorbidities or BMI ≥50 with "less-severe" comorbidities
- Demonstrate commitment (cooperation) with comprehensive medical and psychological evaluations before and after surgery
- Avoid pregnancy for 1 y after surgery
- Be capable and willing to adhere to nutritional guidelines after surgery
- Provide informed assent to surgical treatment
- Demonstrate decisional capacity
- Have a supportive family environment

Source: Inge TH, Krebs NF, Garcia VF, et al. *Pediatrics*. 2004;114(1):217–223.

MECHANICS OF BARIATRIC SURGERY

The first jejunoileal bypass was performed in 1954 (Fig 1a). This procedure produced dramatic weight loss by malabsorption with consequent diarrhea, dumping, and nutritional deficiencies, and operative mortality rates were significant (Table 3). The surgical options widened with the introduction of a predecessor of the Roux-en-Y gastric bypass (RYGB), in which a 30-mL gastric pouch was attached downstream to the ileum. The currently popular RYGB procedure causes weight loss by a combination of both malabsorptive and restrictive mechanisms (Figs 1e and 2 upper).

In the 1980s, staplers were introduced for gastroplasty, producing weight loss by restricting gastric volume rather than rerouting the gastric contents. This concept has been modified with the currently popular and prevalent procedure of adjustable gastric band (AGB) placement (Figs 1f and 2 lower). Advances in laparoscopic instruments, visualization, and experience have enabled surgeons to perform the array of bariatric surgical procedures with fewer operative complications. Current operative techniques that are anatomically restrictive include the AGB, vertical banded gastroplasty, intragastric balloon, and laparoscopic sleeve gastroplasty (Fig 1b). A second group of operations combines elements of gastric restriction with rerouting and bypassing some part of the small intestine and producing selective malabsorption; commonly performed are the RYGB and biliopancreatic diversion (Fig 1c) with or without duodenal switch (Fig 1d). Gastric sleeve resection falls somewhere between the 2 categories; it is less commonly performed, but it produces RYGB levels of weight loss and is easier to convert to one of the other operations, if needed. AGB and RYGB[10] are the 2 procedures currently being evaluated in adolescents (http://clinicaltrials.gov/

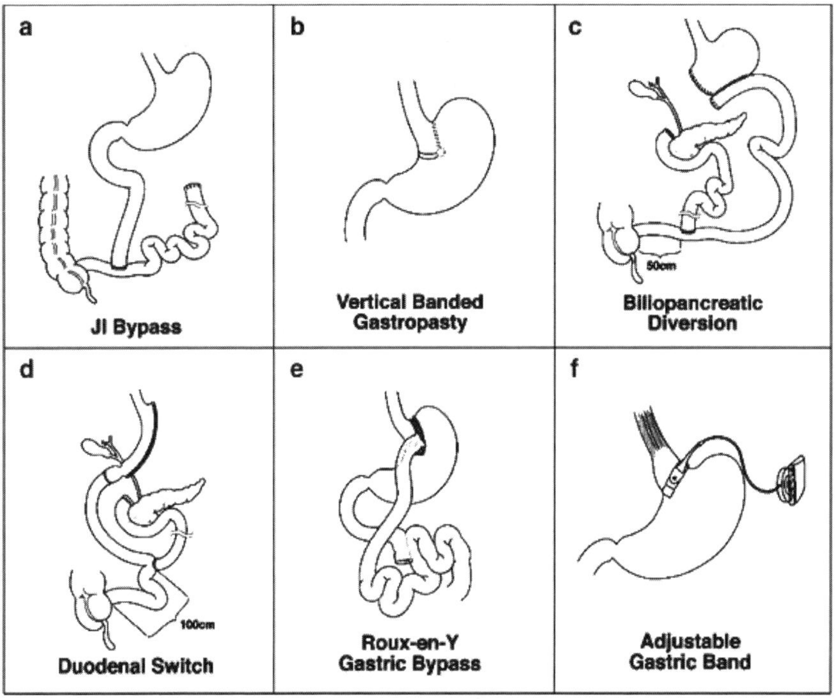

Fig 1. Surgical procedures used in bariatric surgery. (Reproduced with permission from Torpy JM, Burke A, Glass RM. *JAMA*. 2005;294[15]:1986.)

ct2/show/NCT00447590 and http://clinicaltrials.gov/ct2/show/NCT00474318). Because the AGB procedure involves a device, the Lap-Band, which is not yet approved by the US Food and Drug Administration for use in adolescents, is only available experimentally in the United States; it has had more widespread use in adults and adolescents in Europe and Australia. The pros and cons of these 2 surgical approaches are listed in Tables 4 and 5. It is believed that all procedures have metabolic as well as mechanical consequences and that gut hormones and neuroendocrine pathways are altered as a result of the operations.

OUTCOMES

Morbidity and Mortality in Adults

Concerns about bariatric surgery have been focused on surgical morbidity and mortality, weight-loss outcomes and sustainability, and other health consequences.[6–8] Randomized clinical trials comparing surgeries[11–14] or surgical to medical treatment[15] have been rare. Some of the best comparative data come from the prospective case-controlled Swedish Obesity Study[16] of >4000 adults with a median BMI of 41 kg/m^2 that compared morbidity and mortality in the 50% of subjects who received bariatric surgery with the matched controls who

Table 3
Complications known to occur after bariatric surgery

Immediate and Short-term (Surgical)	Medium-term	Long-term
• Bleeding • Bowel obstruction • Intestinal leakage at anastomosis sites • Wound infections • Thromboembolic events • Persistent nausea • Vomiting (anastomotic stenosis or stricture) • Plugging • Dehydration • Hypokalemia • Hypomagnesia • Thiamine deficiency • Vitamin D deficiency	• Heartburn/vomiting • Band problems: slippage, infection, port and tube problems • Dumping • B_{12} and iron deficiencies • Anastomotic ulceration • Hyperinsulinemic hypoglycemic nesidioblastosis	• More band problems • Pill esophagitis • Gallstones • Hernias • Vitamin and mineral deficiencies • Weight regain/loss failure

did not. Mean follow-up was almost 11 years, and only 3 patients were lost to follow-up (71% female; mean age at surgery: 47 years). There were fewer deaths in the surgery group than in the nonsurgical group, with myocardial infarctions and cancer accounting for most deaths. However, the surgery group had more deaths resulting from infection and "sudden" cardiac death. Ten-year weight loss averaged 25% of total weight in subjects who had gastric-bypass procedures, 16% with vertical banded gastroplasty, and 14% after gastric banding. Reoperations or conversion surgeries unrelated to postoperative complications occurred in 17%, 21%, and 31% of the patients in each group, respectively.

Improvements in morbidity[17] included a decrease in diabetes, cardiovascular risk factors and symptoms, sleep apnea, and joint pain and improved health-related quality of life. After a mean follow-up of 7 years, Adams et al[18] analyzed data from 8000 pairs of consecutive patients who had RYGB and matched severely obese controls (84% female; mean age at surgery: 39.5 years). They found a 40% reduction in the overall mortality rate in the bariatric-surgery group, especially of deaths resulting from coronary artery disease, diabetes, and cancer. However, death rates from accidents, poisonings, and suicide were 58% higher in the surgery group. Excess deaths resulting from "preventable" causes are of particular concern for young populations in which the rate of accidental death is high and the suicide rate is increasing.

Outcomes in Adolescents

Most studies of adolescents have been modest in size and reported short-term to medium-term (1- to 6-year) outcomes.[14,19–23] Studies reporting longer

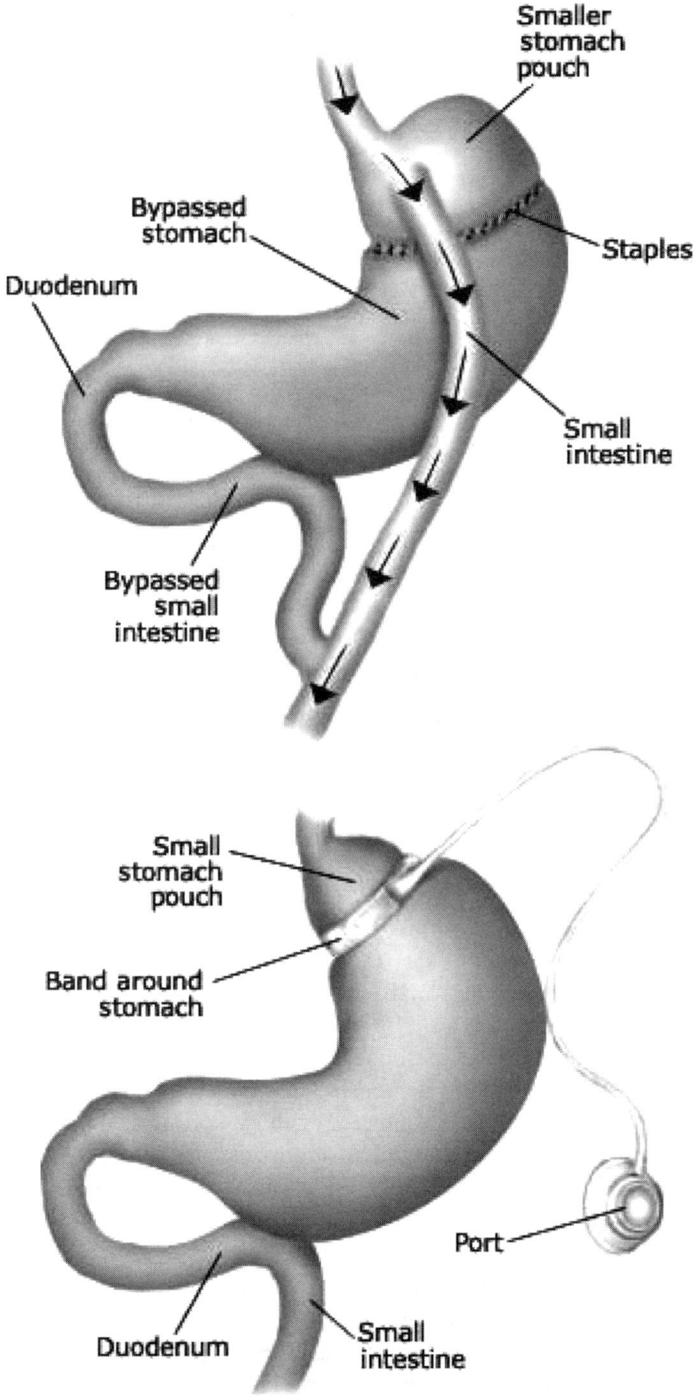

Fig 2. Surgical procedures used in bariatric surgery: gastric bypass (upper) and AGB placement (lower). Available at: http://jama.ama-assn.org/cgi/content/full/294/15/1986.

Table 4
AGB (Lap-Band) procedure: pros and cons

Pros	Cons
• Extensive and longer-term international experience • Simple and quick initial placement • Minimal hospital time • Low mortality rates • Minimal nutritional consequences resulting from malabsorption • Removable • Gradual but ongoing losses over ≥2–3 y • No disruption to gastrointestinal conduit (no cutting, stapling, or rerouting) • Adjustable • Rapid recovery: return to work in ~1 wk • Return to vigorous exercise in ~4–6 wk	• Apparatus needed for lifetime • Vomiting and undernutrition • Scarring and fibrosis from sutures and band • Revision or conversion can be complex and complicated • Complications that increase over time (~2%/y): slippage and erosion • Unknown effect of patient growth on fit and function of band • Require ongoing visits and adjustments • Access to a skilled provider • Body-image and privacy concerns raised by percutaneous access and needles • Effect of alcohol, pizza, soda pop, and irritants on esophagus • Esophageal dysfunction risks • Ability to increase caloric intake by ingestion of sweets that are not band-restricted • Limited experience in youth • Less total weight loss in the medium-term and long-term • Very long-term outcomes are not known • Revision, replacement, wreckage • Investigational device exemption to limited sites, for limited numbers • Long-term costs; insurance coverage for adjustment

follow-up have had sizeable "loss-to-follow-up" rates, and some used procedures that have gone out of favor. As with adults, weight loss with gastric banding is slower than with RYGB, but the percentage of excess weight lost (52%–70%) is closer to that usually achieved with RYGB.[19,23,24] The 1-year longitudinal follow-up of Lawson et al[25] from the multicenter Pediatric Bariatric Study Group (2006) demonstrated a 37% reduction in BMI 1 year after RYGB in 30 individuals compared with 12 nonsurgical controls whose BMIs decreased 3%. As with adults, insulin resistance, diabetes, triglyceride levels, obstructive sleep apnea, depression, and health-related quality of life all improved after surgery.

The Washington State Health Care Authority[26] (www.hta.hca.wa.gov) commissioned a report to evaluate bariatric surgery in pediatric patients that was updated most recently in 2007. Data from 17 studies with a total of 553 pediatric patients were included in their analysis. Strengths of the available (almost all retrospective) studies included data collection from consecutive (nonselected) patients and

Table 5
RYGB: pros and cons

Pros	Cons
• Most experience in adolescents • Relatively high volume and longer duration of adult experience • Weight loss is rapid • Adolescent outcome data are available • Weight loss sustained over 10 y • No adjustments needed • Impressive improvement and cure rates for diabetes mellitus, insulin resistance, PCOS, obstructive sleep apnea, and hypertension • Low mortality rates in experienced centers	• Difficult to reverse • Surgical learning curve (50–100 operations) to minimize complications • Surgical complications (at anastomoses) • Marginal ulcers (increase with nonsteroidal antiinflammatory drugs, smoking, alcohol) • Internal hernias are long-term risk • 10% revision rate • Deficiencies of B-complex vitamins • Risk of decreased fat-soluble vitamin absorption • Increased parathyroid hormone; poor calcium absorption • Need for careful and sufficient protein intake • Difficult for vegetarians because of fiber intolerance • Dumping and diarrhea • Malnutrition requiring revision • Pregnancy nutritional complications

the data and surgeries' origins in academic medical centers. Weaknesses included the lack of rigorous design or controls and limited long-term follow-up. Similarities to the adult literature include the heavier subject weights in RYGB series compared with the laparoscopic gastric-band reports. In almost all areas there was weak evidence based on long-term follow-up and moderate evidence based on short-term (1-year postsurgery) outcomes of weight loss and improvement of comorbidities to support bariatric surgery in adolescents. There was insufficient evidence to assess relative safety of interventions, cost comparisons, and evaluation for any of the above-mentioned according to patient subgroup classification. Given the limitations of the data, both operative approaches led to clinically significant weight loss and resolution of hypertension. The Washington State Health Care Authority proposed a national surgical registry to collect data to facilitate answering these critically important outcome questions. Because of the current data limitations and lack of long-term follow-up, the report concluded that it would not support, at the time of writing, payment for bariatric surgery for adolescents younger than 18 years.

Holterman et al[27] published 9-month outcomes for the first ten 14- to 17-year-old morbidly obese girls in the Food and Drug Administration–approved trial for laparoscopic AGB placement. Their mean BMI was 50 kg/m^2 and excess weight was 171 lb. Many comorbidities were previously undiagnosed, including depression (3), sleep apnea (3), hypertension (6), dyslipidemia (7), insulin resistance

(9), metabolic syndrome (9), ultrasound diagnosis of fatty liver (9), biopsy-proven steatohepatitis (4 of 5 biopsies), asthma (2), gastroesophageal reflux disease (GERD) (3), and impaired quality of life (8 by patient report and 10 by parent report). As anticipated, the operations and hospital stays were short (45 minutes and 23 hours, respectively).

Complications observed in the 10 subjects included dehydration in 2 and the need for 1 pouch dilatation and 1 port revision. At the 9-month follow-up, all had lost weight with a mean of 30% excess weight lost. Fifty percent had a BMI of <40 kg/m^2 at 9 months. Other measured outcomes demonstrated resolution of hypertension and metabolic syndrome and improved insulin resistance, depression, and quality of life scores.

Another outcome series of adolescent laparoscopic gastric-banding recipients was published by Nadler et al.[28] The mean preoperative weight (298 lb) and BMI (48 kg/m^2) were similar to those in other reports. Fifty-four of the 73 patients were female; mean age was 15.8 years. Mean operative time was 35 minutes. The reported percentage of excess weight lost was 35% at 6 months, 57% at 1 year, and 61% at 2 years (n = 16). Mechanical/surgical complications included band slippage, hiatal hernia, gastric perforation after band replacement, wound infection, and port leakage. Nutritional complications included mild hair loss (14), iron deficiency (13), and vitamin D deficiency (4). Medical complications included GERD (3), cholelithiasis (2), and nephrolithiasis (1).

CANDIDATE SELECTION AND GUIDELINES

The 2004 consensus guidelines[9] communicated the expert opinion of a multidisciplinary group that came together to influence the emerging field of adolescent bariatric surgery. At the time, ~3000 bariatric surgical procedures were thought to have been performed on adolescents since 1996, representing <1% of the total number of bariatric procedures. Indications for bariatric surgery in adults are a BMI of 35 kg/m^2 with major comorbidities or a BMI of 40 kg/m^2 without comorbidities. A more cautious and conservative cutoff was recommended for adolescents: a BMI of 40 kg/m^2 with comorbidities or 50 kg/m^2 without comorbidities. Adolescent-specific concerns that influenced the caution of the statement included recognition of the possibilities of coercion, the subtleties of consent and assent, a recognition that 20% to 30% of obese adolescents will not be obese adults, the lack of published peer-reviewed data to support mortality reduction, and the lack of longer-term outcome data including cumulative risks and the need for revision.

The document outlined a clear procedure for evaluating available candidates (Table 2). More recently, Xanthakos and Inge[29] reevaluated the BMI cutoffs for bariatric surgery in adolescents in response to an analysis of current pediatric data sets for the prevalence of extreme obesity and cardiovascular and metabolic risk factors by Freedman et al.[5] Cardiovascular risk factors are present in 59% of children and adolescents with a BMI at >99th percentile; all youth with a BMI of >99th percentile remain obese as adults, and obese adults have a fourfold relative risk of death at age 50. They built the evidence to make the bariatric-surgery cutoff at the 99th percentile, thus proposing to lower the adolescent weight cutoffs to the standard adult levels that fit that evidence and statistically based threshold.

A multidisciplinary team should evaluate adolescent candidates for bariatric surgery.[29,30] The team should include adolescent obesity evaluation and management experts, health professionals from psychology, nutrition, and physical activity instruction, and bariatric-surgery experts with specialized adolescent training and experiences. A consultative team including pediatric subspecialists in adolescent medicine, endocrinology, pulmonology, cardiology, orthopedics, gastroenterology, and ethics should be engaged. Comprehensive medical and psychological evaluations, including a diagnostic mental health evaluation, individual patient and parent interviews, an assessment of the coping skills of the adolescent and the severity of psychosocial comorbidities, and an assessment of the ability of the adolescent and his or her family unit to comply with the postoperative regimen, are expected. A patient review board should make specific recommendations for or against bariatric surgery considering health compromise, failure of other treatment options, and whether the patient has decisional capacity for understanding and assent. Contraindications or exclusions for surgery are listed in Table 6.

A recent study by Schilling et al[31] retrospectively examined national trends in adolescent bariatric surgery from 1997 to 2003 by using a national surgical database. There was a fivefold increase in surgeries between 1997 and 2003. Eighty-five percent of bariatric procedures on adolescents were performed in adult hospitals with high annual volumes of such procedures. Gastric bypass is increasingly the procedure of choice, and length of stay decreased from 4.5 to <2.8 days. Only 6 hospitals performed >6 operations annually on adolescents.

Table 6
Conditions that exclude a candidate from surgery

- Medically correctable cause of obesity
- Substance use problem in past year
- Medical, psychiatric, or cognitive condition that significantly impairs the patient's ability to adhere to postoperative dietary or medication regimens
- Current lactation
- Pregnancy
- Planned pregnancy in 2 y
- Inability or unwillingness to consider or comprehend the procedure, medical consequences, and need for lifelong medical surveillance

Although the consensus statement clearly set a higher standard for adolescent bariatric procedures, and the review by Spear also endorsed pediatric bariatric surgery specialty centers, few of these centers currently exist, and it seems that the specialized adult centers have branched into the adolescent bariatric surgical arena.[32]

Psychiatric problems are prevalent among bariatric surgical candidates.[33–36] Adult outcomes show that some psychiatric problems will improve after surgery, but for any individual this is a challenging part of the assessment for surgical suitability. Underlying psychiatric problems and the psychological comorbidities of severe obesity may confound the assessments of motivation and the ability to follow the changes in eating behavior that are necessary for long-term success.

Neuroendocrine, skeletal, and psychosocial maturation of the adolescent surgical candidate could each be affected by the existing overnutrition and the malnutrition and undernutrition consequent to successful bariatric surgery.[37] Severely overweight individuals may have undiagnosed micronutrient malnutrition. Anorexia and starvation have a negative effect on brain development that is active throughout early and midadolescence. Early puberty and large stature are common among obese early adolescents, but their physical maturity does not accelerate their developmental or cognitive maturity. A "mature" bone age usually ensures that 95% of adult stature is attained. A delayed bone age suggests the need for additional evaluation of endocrinologic and other causes of obesity. Pregnancy is contraindicated during the postsurgical period of rapid weight loss because of concerns for fetal development. However, pregnancies are common after bariatric surgery, because physiologic fertility improves and changes in social encounters and sexual behaviors occur.

METABOLIC AND PHYSIOLOGIC EFFECTS OF BARIATRIC SURGERY

Endocrine: Insulin and Glucose

Over the past 2 decades, numerous outcome studies and systematic reviews[7,38–41] have demonstrated and confirmed that glucose homeostasis improves after bariatric surgery. As with other bariatric-surgery weight-loss outcomes, surgeries with a malabsorptive component such as RYGB are more effective at "curing" type 2 diabetes mellitus than restrictive techniques. Schauer et al[42] and others[41] subsequently have reported that blood glucose levels normalize before there is much weight loss or fat reduction. Increased attention has focused on the endocrine aspects of the gut and its role in glucose homeostasis and how bariatric surgery might alter the hormonal milieu of severely obese patients.[43] Alterations in the gut anatomy that bypass the proximal small intestine and the fundus of the stomach may alter satiety, hunger, and insulin secretion. Other possible factors that contribute to the improvement of glucose control after bariatric surgery include the exclusion of the foregut or duodenum, which signals aspects of glucose-insulin interactions. Further down the gut, altered absorption of nutrients and changes in free fatty acids may have direct effects on insulin and glucose action, endothelial integrity, and blood pressure and influence other comorbidities. Fat-derived peptides including tumor necrosis factor α, leptin, resisten, adiponectin, and interleukin (IL) 1 and IL-6 have been observed in animal models to play a role in the changes in metabolism and physiology that may contribute to the resolution of diabetes in humans as well.

The Diabetes Prevention Program trial[44] demonstrated that in individuals with impaired glucose tolerance, moderate weight loss and increased physical activity reduces the progression to type 2 diabetes mellitus. The role of the weight loss alone or the effect on people with normal glucose metabolism is less clear. Short-term caloric restriction (or the establishment of negative energy balance) quickly improves abnormal glucose and insulin homeostasis. This is likely to be true for bariatric-surgery weight loss also, during which rapid metabolic improvements can be demonstrated, with some modulation once weight stabilizes. For example, blood pressure levels drop early after surgery and then increase when the weight stabilizes. In 1 study,[45] liposuction removed 9 to 10 kg of subcutaneous fat from 8 subjects with normal glucose metabolism and 7 with type 2 diabetes mellitus; neither glucose nor insulin parameters changed. Levels of gut hormones and inflammatory factors also were not altered. Negative energy balance and loss of body fat and mass work together to change these parameters in a desirable direction. These observations are compatible with the impressive metabolic changes after bariatric-surgery weight loss.

Sleep Architecture and Function

Sleep-architecture disturbances, including obstructive sleep apnea, have been a long-recognized serious comorbidity of severe obesity. The consequences are known to negatively influence cardiorespiratory physiology and daytime functioning and to interfere with the restorative aspects of sleep. Obstructive sleep apnea is an independent risk factor for cardiovascular and metabolic comorbidities, acting through the autonomic nervous system, increasing sympathetic activity, altering endothelial function, and increasing insulin resistance. Inflammatory cytokines tumor necrosis factor α, IL-1β, and IL-6 influence sleep regulation, and increased levels are thought to contribute to sleepiness and fatigue. Recently, additional associations between sleep disturbances and polycystic ovarian syndrome (PCOS) have been recognized beyond the role of weight alone.[46] PCOS is a common finding among women with severe obesity, further compounding the importance and influence of this problem.

Dixon et al[47] wrote a report of 313 consecutive patients with a mean BMI of 46 in Australia who eventually had an AGB placement. Sleep was evaluated by preoperative standardized questionnaires and clinical assessment repeated 12 months after bariatric surgery. Fifty-nine percent of the men and 45% of the women had sleep disturbance, >10 times the community rate. Mean weight loss was 48% of excess body weight, and mean BMI was 35 kg/m^2 at 12 months. Questionnaire responses indicated marked improvement after bariatric surgery in all areas, with only 14% reporting habitual snoring and 2% having observed sleep apnea versus 82% and 33%, respectively, before surgery.

Kalra et al[48] recently reported data from 19 adolescents (mean age: 16.5 years; mean BMI: 60 kg/m^2; 66% female) who had overnight polysomnogram sleep studies performed before and after (mean: 0.91 years; mean weight loss: 66.4 kg) gastric-bypass surgery (laparoscopic RYGB). Fourteen (74%) had obstructive sleep apnea before surgery, and 5 had a severe apnea-hypoxia index (>15 events per hour). Mean apnea-hypoxia index before surgery was 20.5 events per hour and decreased to 1.9 events per hour after bariatric-surgery weight loss; only 16% had normal sleep efficiency before surgery, whereas 83% had normal sleep efficiency after bariatric-surgery weight loss.

Gastrointestinal

When GERD has been evaluated before and after bariatric surgery, mixed outcomes have been reported, with the least favorable outcomes in banding procedures. Some of this is accounted for by stomach prolapse. Nonsteroidal antiinflammatory drug use and the presence of chronic and erosive gastroesophageal disease may also contribute to the lack of resolution of GERD. Vitamin preparations taken postoperatively may be another contributor to persistent symptoms. Specific recommendations to take chewable or crushable formulations may minimize post–bariatric-surgery “vitamin esophagitis.” An optimized angle of the gastroesophageal junction after surgery may structurally prevent reflux of stomach acids into the esophagus. Dixon and O’Brien[49] reported from their growing series of gastric-band recipients that 48 (16%) of 274 consecutive patients had a history of reflux esophagitis requiring regular therapy. Patients were mostly female with a median age of 39 years and a 1-year weight loss of 49% of excess body weight. Three quarters resolved all GERD symptoms after surgery, and an additional 14% reported improvement.

Pulmonary

From their series of laparoscopic AGB placements in 296 consecutive Australian patients, Dixon et al[50] reported that of 32 patients with asthma (preoperative mean BMI: 46 kg/m^2; mean age at surgery: 39 years; mean weight loss at 12 months: 49% of excess body weight), the mean asthma score was 44.5 (range: 0–100) before surgery and 14.3 1 year after the bariatric procedure. Asthma rate differentials may be even greater and more severe for the adolescent population. For those with the most severe disease and symptoms, steroid medications may exacerbate weight gain.

Cardiovascular

Reported outcomes suggest that some of the cardiovascular morbidity associated with extreme obesity may be reversible with bariatric-surgery weight loss. Multiple cardiovascular risks and morbidities have been described for severely obese adults, with variable reversibility after bariatric-surgery weight loss. Willens et al[51] evaluated cardiac function before and after bariatric surgery in adults and demonstrated decreases in left ventricular (LV) mass but no changes in posterior wall or septal thickness or in LV end-diastolic septal thickness. Recent studies of bariatric surgery in adults have demonstrated decreased mortality rates,[16,18] with one third to one half of the difference accounted for by cardiovascular deaths.

The adolescent heart and myocardium seem to have more plasticity in response to weight loss over a modest amount of time. A study by Ippisch et al[52] evaluated data from 38 adolescents (aged 13–19 years; 29 female; 85% white) who had testing of cardiac function before and after (mean follow-up: 10 months) bariatric surgery (laparoscopic RYGB). Mean preoperative BMI was 60 kg/m^2, and postoperative BMI was 40 kg/m^2. Before surgery, 25% of these adolescents had concentric LV hypertrophy, a high-risk cardiac finding, and only 36% had normal LV geometry. After bariatric-surgery weight loss, there was significant improvement in relative LV wall thickness, end-diastolic septal thickness, end-diastolic LV wall thickness, and a decrease in heart rate and systolic blood pressure, and 79% had normal LV geometry.

Ippisch et al[52]commented that the adolescents had an average indexed LV mass of 54 g/m. In hypertensive adults, an LV mass of >51 g/m is associated with a more than fourfold risk of future adverse cardiac events. Multiple parameters suggest a reduction on cardiac workload with bariatric-surgery weight loss, including the decrease in heart rate and systolic blood pressure. Possible confounders may be behavioral (increased exercise) or metabolic (decreased sleep apnea, decreased inflammatory markers, decreased androgen levels in PCOS, decreased lipids, decreased hypertension, and improved glucose/insulin metabolism and fat distribution).

Renal

Relatively little has been written about the effect of severe obesity on renal function, although some renal lesions are known to occur more often in the obese population. Renal disease is critically consequent to the common comorbidities of diabetes and hypertension. Navarro-Diaz et al[53] reported on renal function and parameters before and 24 months after bariatric surgery in 61 adults (37 female; mean age: 41 years; mean BMI: 54 kg/m^2) and 24 (15 women) normal-weight (mean BMI: 23.5 kg/m^2) controls. Obese subjects had significantly higher systolic and diastolic blood pressures, increased creatinine clearance, proteinuria, albuminuria, and microhematuria compared with normal-weight controls. In the first 12 months after bariatric surgery, systolic and diastolic blood pressures, creatinine clearance, proteinuria, albuminuria, and hematuria decreased. Renal hyperfiltration has been recognized in obese individuals and is thought to be a part of the complex processes that contribute to hypertension and a factor in the development of irreversible renal damage. Thus, bariatric-surgery weight loss is accompanied with a reversal of these parameters known to be associated with progressive comorbidities.

Polycystic Ovarian Syndrome

Despite its high and growing population prevalence and its potential response or resolution with bariatric surgery, there have been just a few reports that focused on PCOS and bariatric surgery.[54,55] Weight loss improves clinical, biochemical, and functional problems associated with PCOS. Recognition has been given recently to low quality of life ratings in adolescents[56] and a high prevalence of sleep disturbances in women with PCOS. Other medical and metabolic comorbidities are well established in the literature.

Escobar-Moreale et al[55] reported on the experience of 17 women who had PCOS among 36 consecutive premenopausal women undergoing bariatric surgery in Spain. Only 7 of the 17 had been previously diagnosed. Twelve were reevaluated 7 to 26 months (mean: 12 months) after surgery. Among other reasons, subjects' use of oral contraceptives after surgery made them ineligible for reevaluation. Clinical and biochemical parameters of hyperandrogenism and insulin sensitivity improved in 11 of 12 women. Regular menses returned for all 12, and 10 had luteal values of progesterone compatible with ovulation. Hirsutism, which is often a considerable concern of adolescents, also improved. Eid et al[54] reported that in a series of 24 women with PCOS, normal menses returned at a mean of 3.4 months after bariatric surgery. The impressive resolution of signs, symptoms, and ovulatory function are a reminder of the importance of continuously addressing preconceptional counseling and contraceptive care for this population (Table 7).

Gynecology

Miller et al[57] reviewed issues in bariatric surgery and adolescent gynecology and cited the experience of the Cincinnati, Ohio, team that is the academic leader of the multisite clinical trial currently (2007–2011) evaluating bariatric-surgery outcomes in adolescents compared with an older 25- to 35-year-old cohort. (http://clinicaltrials.gov/ct2/show/NCT00474318). Obesity is known to influence growth, puberty, menstrual function, and fertility. Anovulation associated with obesity is associated with oligomenorrhea, dysfunctional uterine bleeding, iron deficiency, anemia, and increased risk of endometrial cancer from unopposed estrogen exposure. Weight loss from bariatric surgery is associated with regular ovulatory menses, improved fertility, and an increased rate of pregnancy.[58]

Table 7
Gynecologic and contraceptive concerns for the bariatric-surgery patient

- High frequency of unplanned pregnancies after surgery
- Good perinatal outcomes compared with women at preoperative weight
- Importance of preconception care and correction of any deficiencies
- Decreased efficacy of some contraceptives at higher weights
- Weight gain on Depo-Provera
- Resolution of menstrual disorders
- Late identification of pregnancy
- Risk of gestational diabetes
- Post–bariatric-surgery patients are still usually obese
- Risk of thromboembolic events influenced by weight and mobility
- Bone development and density
- Consider intraoperative Mirena intrauterine system

Nutritional, contraceptive, and preconceptional counseling is important to address regularly and repeatedly before surgery and during the post–bariatric-surgery period of ongoing weight loss, particularly for adolescents, who have high rates of unintended pregnancy. Supplementation with folic acid, iron, and B-complex vitamins (Table 8) will decrease fetal risk. Other obstetric risks are decreased with weight loss, and improved obstetric outcomes are observed.[59] Pregnancies "against medical advice" have occurred while the patient is still

Table 8
Nutritional supplementation after bariatric surgery

Recommended supplements
- High-potency oral chewable multivitamins daily, including folic acid
- Calcium citrate oral (1000 mg/d in 2–3 divided doses)
  - or calcium lactate 1200–1500 mg/d in 2–3 divided doses
- Elemental iron (ferrous) 65 mg/d orally for menstruating females
  - Do not take with calcium
  - Addition of 500 mg of vitamin C may promote absorption
- Vitamin D 800–1200 IU/d
  - Especially in Northern and cloudy climates and for dark-skinned people

Supplements to consider
- Vitamin B_1, 10–50 mg/d orally for 6 mo
- Vitamin B_{12}, may have extra need if on metformin
  - 500 μ g/d orally
  - or 1000 μ g/mo intramuscularly
- Ferrous sulfate or gluconate (325–650 mg/d) after mixed procedures or if iron depleted

Medication regimen advice
- Avoid bedtime dosing
- Medication no more than 2 times per day if possible
- Consider some medications on a nondaily basis (eg, iron and calcium) if they help simplify the regimen
- Guidelines on caloric and fluid supplementation needed for those with high physical activity
- Crush or chew tablets to minimize esophagitis

losing weight rapidly, and a novel approach has been to insert a levonorgestrel intrauterine system (Mirena) at the time of the bariatric surgery. This system offers excellent contraception and decreased uterine bleeding for up to 5 years and avoids the excess medical risks of thromboembolic events, hypertension, and dyslipidemia that may occur with systemic estrogen and progestin use in the obese patient.

Musculoskeletal Health and Growth

Overweight children have a slightly earlier puberty and height growth spurt than do normal-weight adolescents. The proposed "minimum age" for bariatric-surgery consideration has been 13 years for girls and 15 years for boys on the basis of physiologic maturity, bone growth maturation, and height potential of 14 years (for both genders) on the basis of physical and developmental maturation concerns. Most bariatric surgery on adolescents to date has been performed at the older end of the spectrum (16- and 17-year-olds). The effect of surgery and weight loss compared with no surgery and severe obesity on bone and integumentary parameters is not known. This is an area in which it may be less valid to extrapolate the experience of the older young adults, because the balance of metabolic activity in bones differs; bone becomes more dense and grows as longitudinal growth is completed in the midteens, and bone metabolism is active but morphology is relatively stable by the mid-20s. Some of the poor diet choices and malnourishment of the severely obese teenager can result in alterations in calcium metabolism. Other factors that promote bone-density accumulation include weight-bearing exercise and adequate estrogen levels. Exercise is diminished and estrogen cycling and levels may be altered from chronic anovulation in the very obese teenager. Other physical activity factors may also negatively influence muscle, ligament, and joint maturation. Poor tone and strength accompany lack of exercise, but obese adolescents do not have the degree of degenerative joint problems commonly found in obese adults. Thus, prevention of joint damage and disability argue for relatively early intervention.

Nutrition

Macronutrient and micronutrient processing are altered with bariatric surgery. Malinowski[37] described the common and reported nutritional and metabolic perturbations. Before surgery, some individuals already have micronutrient deficits from nutrient-poor food choices, excess uterine bleeding, lack of dairy, and lack of sun exposure. Once engaged in care and anticipating bariatric surgery, nutritional consultation, and supplementation are recommended. The first 4 items in Table 8 are frequently recommended for female adolescents. The next group is recommended after surgery to avoid preventable micronutrient deficiencies. Because of the decreased overall caloric intake after surgery, attention to sufficient (60 g/day) protein consumption is warranted.

Immediately before surgery candidates will be on a liquid diet. A general scheme for advancing food postoperatively is listed in Table 9. Certain foods are known

Table 9
Eating guidelines after bariatric surgery

- Immediately after surgery: intravenous multivitamins daily
- Week 1: clear liquids
- Weeks 2–3: liquids and soft foods
- Weeks 3–4: soft and semisolid foods
- Weeks 4–5: regular foods in small quantities
- Weeks 4–16: gradually introduce more solids
- Identify connection between food intake (volume) and fullness
- Identify hunger, satiety, and "contentment"
- Develop ability to stop eating
- Calculate portion size and meal components
- Take small bites
- Chew long and a lot
- Plan for eating in different situations

to cause nausea and vomiting in restrictive-procedure recipients. Frequent culprits are high-protein foods, fiber, iron, red meat, bread, white chicken, and chocolate. Eating later in the day may cause additional reflux symptoms. Most nutritional deficits occur in the first year after bariatric surgery, but some can develop or continue as chronic problems. Adequate protein ingestion can be a challenge, and hypoalbuminemia can be found after malabsorptive procedures when accompanied by rapid weight loss and severe diarrhea. Hyperphagia, muscle wasting, and edema may develop and require rapid diagnosis and treatment. Fat malabsorption is a major contributor to desired weight loss after bypass procedures, with excess stool losses of calories and fat-soluble vitamins occurring when there is too little functioning small intestine. These complications should be rare in the more conservative surgical techniques used in adolescents. Micronutrient deficiencies occur because of disruptions in the sites or physiology of absorption or inadequate intake. Limited gastric tissue, acid secretion, and gastric, biliary, and pancreatic enzymes all play a role. For the clinician it is important to become familiar with the signs and symptoms of nutritional deficiencies not usually seen in countries with adequate food supplies.

Iron deficiency occurs in ~50% of menstruating bariatric-surgery patients. Multiple factors contribute to its high frequency: decreased stomach acid, decreased organic heme intake, and shorter absorptive stretches of duodenum and proximal jejunum.[60] Fatigue, pallor, pica, nail abnormalities, exercise intolerance, and excess menstrual losses may accompany iron deficiency. Long-term supplementation is advised, with some individuals requiring larger doses to replenish and sustain levels. Absorption of supplemental iron is improved with vitamin C ingestion for acidity, avoidance of simultaneous calcium and dairy, and use of short-acting ferrous preparations.

Folate is another critical nutrient and plays a unique preventive role in women; a deficiency of folate contributes to an increased risk of neural tube defects in their offspring. Folate intake may be compromised after surgery by undernutrition, and absorption and enteropathic reabsorption may be undermined by a shortened small intestine and decreased biliary enzymes. Supplementation is recommended before and after surgery for all women of reproductive age.

Mental Heath and Mood Disorders

The full spectrum of psychiatric disorders is encountered in bariatric-surgery patients, and in some individuals treatment for psychiatric problems with atypical antipsychotic medication has escalated the obesity problem. For some adolescents, the evaluation before bariatric surgery provides the patient with the first opportunity to get his or her psychiatric disorder diagnosed and treated.

Kalarchian et al[61] performed standardized independent psychiatric diagnostic assessments of 288 adults who were seeking bariatric surgery. Subjects were 83% female with a mean BMI of 52 kg/m^2 and mean age of 46 years. More than one third (38%) of them met criteria for a current Axis 1 diagnosis, and two thirds had an axis 1 diagnosis in their lifetime. Axis 1 diagnoses independently positively correlated with BMI. The most frequently diagnosed Axis 1 condition "ever experienced" was depression (45%) and "current" was anxiety (24%). Lifetime substance abuse was reported by 33% of individuals, and current use was reported by 2%. Lifetime eating disorder was reported by 30% and currently by 16%. Twenty-nine percent of the adults seeking bariatric surgery had a current Axis 2 diagnosis, with the following subtypes most frequent: avoidant (internalizing) (17%), obsessive-compulsive (fearful) (8%), paranoid (6%), borderline (5%), and antisocial (3%).

Kim et al[36] reported on the psychological status of a series of 14- to 21-year-olds who were undergoing evaluation for bariatric surgery. Diagnosis of a psychiatric disorder in their lifetime was made in 22 of the 25 patients. Depression (68%) was the most common; 59% were currently receiving treatment. A spectrum of abnormal eating behaviors had prevalence rates from 20% to 50%. Tobacco smoking was endorsed by 20%, but other drug use was rare, in contrast to some of the adult-derived data.

Most adult-oriented bariatric-surgery programs require a mental health assessment, and the guidelines for bariatric surgery in adolescents place this assessment at the beginning of their evaluation pathway. This is an opportunity to identify and treat mental illness and to review medication use that may be compounding obesity, such as atypical antipsychotic medications or valproic acid. For adolescents, we would anticipate a lower lifetime prevalence of mental health disorders, because of the limited time to accumulate the problems, and may see different proportions and prevalence in the array of disorders. The relatively high prevalence and underdiagnosis of anxiety disorders described by Kalarchian et al[61] in adults is supported by the author's clinical experience with adolescents and young adults. Ongoing clinical assessment and care of mental health problems during and after weight loss are recommended and may be a major contributing factor for those who fail to lose weight or regain weight after bariatric surgery. The interrelationships and causality of the experiences of trauma, stigma, abuse, mood disorders, substance use, and personality characteristics in the individual and family context of obesity are complex and may provide additional insights about the psychoneuroendocrine web that regulates mood, behavior, satisfaction, satiety, hunger, and happiness.

EATING DISORDERS AND BODY IMAGE

Binge eating is frequently extinguished after bariatric surgery, although the feeling of "loss of control" may persist in relationship to other eating behaviors including night eating, grazing, and "uncontrolled eating" that may still be prevalent.[62] Uncontrolled eating was found to be more common in those who were young, female, and had a high level of dissatisfaction with body appearance.[61] Grazing may be an eating pattern that is facilitated by the anatomy after bariatric surgery, which can accommodate continuous eating of small amounts of food. Greater risk may exist for those individuals with emotional and environmental facilitators: loneliness, isolation, and inactivity. At the other end of the eating-behavior spectrum, postsurgical refusal to eat or "postsurgical eating-avoidance disorder" and other variants have been described.[63] After bariatric surgery, refusal to eat becomes a greater nutritional and metabolic liability than in an anatomically intact individual, with potentially life-threatening nutritional and metabolic consequences.

Emotional-cognitive-behavioral integration differs among younger, middle, and older adolescents. Body-image value and vulnerability and peer relationships and responses are core concepts in adolescent development. The influences of early extreme obesity and earlier treatment are open for study, because earlier timing of bariatric surgery may prove to be a benefit or a barrier to better long-term outcomes. Given what we know about the trajectory of these developmental domains, attention to eating behaviors and body image in the young patient after bariatric surgery may be especially critical for longer-term success. Plastic surgeries including abdominoplasty, body contouring, arm and thigh lifts, and, most frequently, breast-reduction surgery have become common procedures after bariatric surgery in adults. Some plastic surgeons have developed expertise in these operations, and patients exploring these options are advised to find surgeons with extensive, specific experience. There is no current literature specifically addressing this in adolescents and young adults, although more descriptive series on outcomes are anticipated given the increased popularity of bariatric surgery in younger populations.

CONCLUSIONS

There has been hesitation among the nonsurgical community to endorse bariatric surgery as an option for severe and more extreme obesity.[64] However, given the ineffectiveness of all other interventions and the growing experience with bariatric surgery in adolescents and young adults, bariatric surgery is included in the endorsed staged-treatment model developed by obesity experts.[1,9,65] Pediatric obesity centers will need to collaborate with the most experienced bariatric surgeons to develop pediatric/adolescent bariatric surgeons with sufficient expertise and experience. Issues of disparities and equity do not escape this arena.[66] Ethnic and racial minorities and patients in lower socioeconomic groups face additional burdens in accessing individual and community prevention and intervention programs. Minority youth and those living in poverty in the United States have higher levels of severe obesity than more-advantaged peers. Cultural competency of programs and providers and attention to the economic and insurance challenges that disproportionately affect these populations are critical and long-term considerations.

Currently, adolescents seeking bariatric surgery will find opportunities to have skilled and experienced surgeons perform RYGB. Access to AGB placement for adolescents in the United States, however, is limited to a small number of centers approved for experimental use and committed to careful long-term follow-up. Successful outcomes, if we extrapolate from adult data, will lead to significant and largely sustained weight loss. Many of these youth will still meet criteria for obesity after substantial weight loss. Nonetheless, the morbidities and mortality associated with obesity increase at higher BMIs. Early intervention may provide more resolution of comorbidities because of the plasticity of the younger organism and its parts. There is a lack of randomized, controlled trials to support medical versus surgical treatment and limited studies to compare different surgical approaches; creative methodologies and coordinated efforts are necessary to answer the most pressing questions.

What we choose to do with adolescents in the upcoming decades will reflect what we learn from the current bariatric-surgery recipients in their young adult years.[67] The optimal age, weight, and procedure for each individual that will be most likely to produce better health, longer life, and a high quality of life should be informed by data, but individual preferences will be influenced by personal contacts, the media, esthetics, and insurance. The policies of some health centers and bariatric surgery "centers of excellence" encourage transparency about outcomes, and the Internet and inquisitive patient-consumers can promote better decision-making. The popularity, publicity, and pricing have made surgery an attractive option for earlier intervention. Careful, consistent, and collaborative collection of and access to data about presurgical assessment, surgical details, and long-term postsurgical experience are critical if we want to be able to inform and affect individuals' decisions about obesity treatment options and optimize the outcomes and safety of patients.[67]

Ultimately, we would like to not need bariatric surgery for adolescents or adults, but this is not realistic. We have several contemporary generations that are unlikely to lose their excess weight safely and sustainably to prevent serious morbidity, and they are at high risk for premature death. The impact of early and protracted obesity has metabolic, psychological, personal, and interpersonal impacts that may be only partially reversible. We have both a cultural and metabolic milieu that has overridden energy balance and the balance of hunger and satiety meant to regulate energy intake. One day we may better understand and control this interaction. Until then, bariatric surgery is a useful intervention.

ACKNOWLEDGMENTS

Special appreciation goes to Cassandra Ward for her typing and bibliographic assistance and Susan Coupey for her editing and assistance above and beyond the call of duty.

REFERENCES

1. Spear BA, Barlow SE, Ervin C, et al. Recommendations for treatment of child and adolescent overweight and obesity. *Pediatrics.* 2007;120(suppl 4):S254–S288
2. Berkowitz RI, Fujioka K, Daniels SR, et al. Effects of sibutramine treatment in obese adolescents: a randomized trial [summary for patients in *Ann Intern Med.* 2006;145(2):I16]. *Ann Intern Med.* 2006;145(2):81–90
3. Shai I, Schwarzfuchs D, Henkin Y, et al. Weight loss with a low-carbohydrate, Mediterranean, or low-fat diet. *N Engl J Med.* 2008;359(3):229–241
4. Ogden CL, Carroll MD, Flegal KM. High body mass index for age among US children and adolescents, 2003–2006. *JAMA.* 2008;299(20):2401–2405
5. Freedman DS, Mei Z, Srinivasan SR, Berenson GS, Dietz WH. Cardiovascular risk factors and excess adiposity among overweight children and adolescents: the Bogalusa Heart Study. *J Pediatr.* 2007;150(1):12–17, e2
6. Maggard MA, Shugarman LR, Suttorp M, et al. Meta-analysis: surgical treatment of obesity [summary for patients in *Ann Intern Med.* 2005;142(7):I55]. *Ann Intern Med.* 2005;142(7):547–559
7. Buchwald H, Avidor Y, Braunwald E, et al. Bariatric surgery: a systematic review and meta-analysis. *JAMA.* 2004;292(14):1724–1737
8. Buchwald H, Estok R, Fahrbach K, Banel D, Sledge I. Trends in mortality in bariatric surgery: a systematic review and meta-analysis. *Surgery.* 2007;142(4):621–632; discussion 632–635
9. Inge TH, Krebs NF, Garcia VF, et al. Bariatric surgery for severely overweight adolescents: concerns and recommendations. *Pediatrics.* 2004;114(1):217–223
10. Inge TH, Zeller M, Harmon C, et al. Teen-longitudinal assessment of bariatric surgery: methodological features of the first prospective multicenter study of adolescent bariatric surgery. *J Pediatr Surg.* 2007;42(11):1969–1971
11. Bessler M, Daud A, Kim T, DiGiorgi M. Prospective randomized trial of banded versus nonbanded gastric bypass for the super obese: early results. *Surg Obes Relat Dis.* 2007;3(4): 480–484
12. Himpens J, Dapri G, Cadière GB. A prospective randomized study between laparoscopic gastric banding and laparoscopic isolated sleeve gastrectomy: results after 1 and 3 years. *Obes Surg.* 2006;16(11):1450–1456
13. Olbers T, Björkman S, Lindroos A, et al. Body composition, dietary intake, and energy expenditure after laparoscopic Roux-en-Y gastric bypass and laparoscopic vertical banded gastroplasty: a randomized clinical trial. *Ann Surg.* 2006;244(5):715–722

14. Angrisani L, Lorenzo M, Borrelli V. Laparoscopic adjustable gastric banding versus Roux-en-Y gastric bypass: 5-year results of a prospective randomized trial. *Surg Obes Relat Dis*. 2007;3(2): 127–132; discussion 132–133
15. Dixon JB, Strauss BJ, Laurie C, O'Brien PE. Changes in body composition with weight loss: obese subjects randomized to surgical and medical programs. *Obesity*. 2007;15(5):1187–1198
16. Sjöström L, Narbro K, Sjöström CD, et al. Effects of bariatric surgery on mortality in Swedish obese subjects. *N Engl J Med*. 2007;357(8):741–752
17. Sjöström L. Surgical intervention as a strategy for treatment of obesity. *Endocrine*. 2000;13(2): 213–230
18. Adams TD, Gress RE, Smith SC, et al. Long-term mortality after gastric bypass surgery. *N Engl J Med*. 2007;357(8):753–761
19. Al-Qahtani AR. Laparoscopic adjustable gastric banding in adolescent: safety and efficacy. *J Pediatr Surg*. 2007;42(5):894–897
20. Nadler EP, Youn HA, Ginsburg HB, Ren CJ, Fielding GA. Short-term results in 53 US obese pediatric patients treated with laparoscopic adjustable gastric banding. *J Pediatr Surg*. 2007; 42(1):137–141
21. Silberhumer GR, Miller K, Kriwanek S, Widhalm K, Pump A, Prager G. Laparoscopic adjustable gastric banding in adolescents: the Austrian experience. *Obes Surg*. 2006;16(8):1062–1067
22. Yitzhak A, Mizrahi S, Avinoach E. Laparoscopic gastric banding in adolescents. *Obes Surg*. 2006;16(10):1318–1322
23. Fielding GA, Duncombe JA. Laparoscopic adjustable gastric banding in severely obese adolescents. *Surg Obes Relat Dis*. 2005;1(4):399–405; discussion 405–407
24. Dillard BE 3rd, Gorodner V, Galvani C, et al. Initial experience with the adjustable gastric band in morbidly obese US adolescents and recommendations for further investigation. *J Pediatr Gastroenterol Nutr*. 2007;45(2):240–246
25. Lawson ML, Kirk S, Mitchell T, et al. One-year outcomes of Roux-en-Y gastric bypass for morbidly obese adolescents: a multicenter study from the Pediatric Bariatric Study Group. *J Pediatr Surg*. 2006;41(1):137–143; discussion 137–143
26. Treadwell J, Sun F, Bruening W, et al. Bariatric surgery in pediatric patients. Available at: www.hta.hca.wa.gov/documents/pbs_executive_summary.pdf. Accessed September 19, 2008
27. Holterman AX, Browne A, Dillard BE 3rd, et al. Short-term outcome in the first 10 morbidly obese adolescent patients in the FDA-approved trial for laparoscopic adjustable gastric banding. *J Pediatr Gastroenterol Nutr*. 2007;45(4):465–473
28. Nadler EP, Youn HA, Ren CJ, Fielding GA. An update on 73 US obese pediatric patients treated with laparoscopic adjustable gastric banding: comorbidity resolution and compliance data. *J Pediatr Surg*. 2008;43(1):141–146
29. Xanthakos SA, Inge TH. Surgical management of severe obesity in adolescents. *UpToDate* [serial online]. 2008;16.2. Available at: www.uptodate.com/home/content/topic.do?topicKey=pedigast/17895. Accessed September 22, 2008
30. Xanthakos SA, Daniels SR, Inge TH. Bariatric surgery in adolescents: an update. *Adolesc Med Clin*. 2006;17(3):589–612
31. Schilling PL, Davis MM, Albanese CT, Dutta S, Morton J. National trends in adolescent bariatric surgical procedures and implications for surgical centers of excellence. *J Am Coll Surg*. 2008; 206(1):1–12
32. Tsai WS, Inge TH, Burd RS. Bariatric surgery in adolescents: recent national trends in use and in-hospital outcome. *Arch Pediatr Adolesc Med*. 2007;161(3):217–221
33. Wadden TA, Sarwer DB, Fabricatore AN, Jones L, Stack R, Williams NS. Psychosocial and behavioral status of patients undergoing bariatric surgery: what to expect before and after surgery. *Med Clin North Am*. 2007;91(3):451–469, xi–xii
34. Norris L. Psychiatric issues in bariatric surgery. *Psychiatr Clin North Am*. 2007;30(4):717–738
35. Zeller MH, Roehrig HR, Modi AC, Daniels SR, Inge TH. Health-related quality of life and depressive symptoms in adolescents with extreme obesity presenting for bariatric surgery. *Pediatrics*. 2006;117(4):1155–1161

36. Kim RJ, Langer JM, Baker AW, Filter DE, Williams NN, Sarwer DB. Psychosocial status in adolescents undergoing bariatric surgery. *Obes Surg*. 2008;18(1):27–33
37. Malinowski SS. Nutritional and metabolic complications of bariatric surgery. *Am J Med Sci*. 2006;331(4):219–225
38. Sjöström L, Lindroos AK, Peltonen M, et al. Lifestyle, diabetes, and cardiovascular risk factors 10 years after bariatric surgery. *N Engl J Med*. 2004;351(26):2683–2693
39. Ferchak CV, Meneghini LF. Obesity, bariatric surgery and type 2 diabetes: a systematic review. *Diabetes Metab Res Rev*. 2004;20(6):438–445
40. Cunneen SA. Review of meta-analytic comparisons of bariatric surgery with a focus on laparoscopic adjustable gastric banding. *Surg Obes Relat Dis*. 2008;4(3 suppl):S47–S55
41. Meneghini LF. Impact of bariatric surgery on type 2 diabetes. *Cell Biochem Biophys*. 2007; 48(2–3):97–102
42. Schauer PR, Burguera B, Ikramuddin S, et al. Effect of laparoscopic Roux-en Y gastric bypass on type 2 diabetes mellitus. *Ann Surg*. 2003;238(4):467–484
43. Neary NM, Small CJ, Bloom SR. Gut and mind. *Gut*. 2003;52(7):918–921
44. Knowler WC, Barrett-Connor E, Fowler SE, et al. Reduction in the incidence of type 2 diabetes with lifestyle intervention or metformin. *N Engl J Med*. 2002;346(6):393–403
45. Klein S, Fontana L, Young VL. Absence of an effect of liposuction on insulin action and risk factors for coronary heart disease. *N Eng J Med*. 2004;350(25):2549–2557
46. Tasali E, Van Cauter E, Ehrmann DA. Relationships between sleep disordered breathing and glucose metabolism in polycystic ovary syndrome. *J Clin Endocrinol Metab*. 2006;91(1):36–42
47. Dixon JB, Schachter LM, O'Brien PE. Sleep disturbance and obesity: changes following surgically induced weight loss. *Arch Intern Med*. 2001;161(1):102–106
48. Kalra M, Mannaa M, Fitz K, et al. Effect of surgical weight loss on sleep architecture in adolescents with severe obesity. *Obes Surg*. 2008;18(6):675–679
49. Dixon JB, O'Brien PE. Gastroesophageal reflux in obesity: the effect of lap-band placement. *Obes Surg*. 1999;9(6):527–531
50. Dixon JB, Chapman L, O'Brien P. Marked improvement in asthma after Lap-Band surgery for morbid obesity. *Obes Surg*. 1999;9(4):385–389
51. Willens HJ, Chakko SC, Byers P, et al. Effects of weight loss after gastric bypass on right and left ventricular function assessed by tissue Doppler imaging. *Am J Cardiol*. 2005;95(12):1521–1524
52. Ippisch HM, Inge TH, Daniels SR, et al. Reversibility of cardiac abnormalities in morbidly obese adolescents. *J Am Coll Cardiol*. 2008;51(14):1342–1348
53. Navarro-Díaz M, Serra A, Romero R, et al. Effect of drastic weight loss after bariatric surgery on renal parameters in extremely obese patients: long-term follow-up. *J Am Soc Nephrol*. 2006;17(12 suppl 3):S213–S217
54. Eid GM, Cottam DR, Velcu LM, et al. Effective treatment of polycystic ovarian syndrome with Roux-en-Y gastric bypass. *Surg Obes Relat Dis*. 2005;1(2):77–80
55. Escobar-Morreale HF, Botella-Carretero JI, Alvarez-Blasco F, Sancho J, San Millán JL. The polycystic ovary syndrome associated with morbid obesity may resolve after weight loss induced by bariatric surgery. *J Clin Endocrinol Metab*. 2005;90(12):6364–6369
56. Trent ME, Rich M, Austin SB, Gordon CM. Quality of life in adolescent girls with polycystic ovary syndrome. *Arch Pediatr Adolesc Med*. 2002;156(6):556–560
57. Miller RJ, Xanthakos SA, Hillard PJ, Inge TH. Bariatric surgery and adolescent gynecology. *Curr Opin Obstet Gynecol*. 2007;19(5):427–433
58. Roehrig HR, Xanthakos SA, Sweeney J, Zeller MH, Inge TH. Pregnancy after gastric bypass surgery in adolescents. *Obes Surg*. 2007;17(7):873–877
59. Wax JR, Cartin A, Wolff R, Lepich S, Pinette MG, Blackstone J. Pregnancy following gastric bypass surgery for morbid obesity: maternal and neonatal outcomes. *Obes Surg*. 2008;18(5): 540–544
60. Love AL, Billett HH. Obesity, bariatric surgery, and iron deficiency: true, true, true and related. *Am J Hematol*. 2008;83(5):403–409

61. Kalarchian MA, Marcus MD, Levine MD, et al. Psychiatric disorders among bariatric surgery candidates: relationship to obesity and functional health status. *Am J Psychiatry*. 2007;164(2): 328–334; quiz 374
62. Colles SL, Dixon JB, O'Brien PE. Grazing and loss of control related to eating: two high-risk factors following bariatric surgery. *Obesity*. 2008;16(3):615–622
63. Segal A, Kinoshita Kussunoki D, Larino MA. Post-surgical refusal to eat: anorexia nervosa, bulimia nervosa or a new eating disorder? A case series. *Obes Surg*. 2004;14(3):353–360
64. Flum DR, Khan TV, Dellinger EP. Toward the rational and equitable use of bariatric surgery. *JAMA*. 2007;298(12):1442–1444
65. Lau DC, Douketis JD, Morrison KM, et al. 2006 Canadian clinical practice guidelines on the management and prevention of obesity in adults and children. *CMAJ*. 2007;176(8):S1–S13
66. Flum DR, Salem L, Elrod JAB, Dellinger PD, Cheadle A, Chan L. Early mortality among Medicare beneficiaries undergoing bariatric surgical procedures. *JAMA*. 2005;294(15):1903–1908
67. Courcoulas AP, Flum DR. Filling the gaps in bariatric surgical research. *JAMA*. 2005;294(15): 1957–1960

Adolesc Med 19 (2008) 475–497

The Metabolic Syndrome: A Gathering Challenge in a Time of Abundance

Lee A. Bricker, MD[a], Donald E. Greydanus, MD, FAAP*[b]

Departments of [a]Internal Medicine and [b]Pediatrics, Michigan State University/Kalamazoo Center for Medical Studies, 1000 Oakland Drive, Kalamazoo, MI 49008-1284, USA

The metabolic syndrome (also known as dysmetabolic syndrome, MetS, Reaven syndrome, syndrome X, and insulin-resistance syndrome) is a well-recognized and all-too-frequently encountered condition of modern life, with staggering economic consequences.[1–5] The terms "insulin-resistance syndrome," "dysmetabolic syndrome," "MetS," and "metabolic syndrome" are generally used interchangeably throughout this review. This syndrome is one of the most complex and heterogeneous of metabolic maladies. It has become an intrusive part of life in much of the modern world, and its consequences are so grave and widespread that it can truly be described as a plague, a multifaceted source of misery and debility, afflicting ever younger children and youth.[6]

The syndrome is, in many ways, a byproduct of modern civilization, resulting in particular from overfeeding, sedentary lifestyle, and inattention to relatively basic aspects of good health practices. In association with certain genetic and ethnic factors, it is increasingly associated with serious morbidity, particularly cardiovascular disease, polycystic ovarian syndrome (PCOS), and diabetes mellitus.[7] It is proving to be largely resistant to weight-management efforts and requires a complex constellation of variably effective pharmacologic and other interventions. However, these interventions, thus far, have done little to ease the high prevalence of this syndrome.

Severe insulin resistance, the early β-cell failure that accompanies it, and frank type 2 diabetes are developing earlier in life than previously appreciated, especially in sedentary youth and physically inactive schoolchildren, with cardiovascular disease following in parallel.[8,9] More than 2 decades ago, Reaven[10] recognized and described the importance of insulin resistance in human disease. Reaven clarified the concept that truncal obesity, with or without diabetes, is associated with defective insulin action that requires increasing production of

*Corresponding author.
E-mail address: greydanus@kcms.msu.edu (D. E. Greydanus).

 ISSN 1934-4287

insulin to overcome it.[10] The resulting hyperinsulinemia brings with it, directly or indirectly, cardiovascular and other complications.[11] Affected youth who ultimately fail to make sufficient endogenous insulin, even in much larger amounts than normal, develop type 2 diabetes mellitus.

Insulin resistance is manifested differently in liver, muscle, and fat; these tissues are involved together in a complex interlocking orchestration of events associated with glucose intolerance, hypertension, β-cell failure, hyperinsulinemia, frank diabetes mellitus,[12] dyslipidemia, and release of inflammatory and procoagulant factors into the circulation.

METABOLIC SYNDROME AND THE ADOLESCENT

It has been estimated that >1 million 12- to 19-year-old adolescents in the United States have the metabolic syndrome; this involves 4.2% overall and 6.1% of male adolescents and 2.1% of female adolescents.[13] Findings from the 1988–1994 Third National Health and Nutrition Examination Survey (NHANES) suggest that 4% of adolescents and nearly 30% of overweight adolescents in the United States have MetS.[13] The prevalence is higher in obese youth versus overweight youth and is lowest in normal-weight youth.[14] A review of the 1999–2000 NHANES suggests an overall MetS prevalence in American adolescents of 6.4% (9.1% in boys and 3.7% in girls).[15] The trend of recent research suggests that MetS has its origins in in utero life as well as childhood and adolescence.[16,17]

Table 1 identifies specific features for the metabolic syndrome and reflects World Health Organization (WHO) criteria, although various criteria for MetS definition have been used by different researchers including the National Cholesterol

Table 1
WHO criteria for metabolic syndrome

Central obesity
Waist/hip ratio
Men, >0.90
Women, >0.85
BMI >30 kg/m^2
Triglyceride level >150 mg/dL (1.69 mmol/L)
HDL cholesterol
Men, <35 mg/dL (0.9 mmol/L)
Women, <39 mg/dL (1.0 mmol/L)
Blood pressure
Systolic, ≥140 mm Hg
Diastolic, ≥90 mm Hg
Fasting glucose level ≥110 mg/dL (6.1 mmol/L)
Microalbuminuria
Urine albumin excretion rate ≥20 mg/min, or
Albumin/creatinine ratio ≥30 mg/g

Education Program Adult Treatment Panel III, American Association of Clinical Endocrinologists (AACE), European Group for the Study of Insulin Resistance (EGIR), and the Research Group on Diabetes and Chronic Illnesses (REGODCI).[18–22] MetS prevalence depends on the criteria used for its diagnosis. For example, a prevalence of 6.5% is noted with the Adult Panel III criteria, 7.7% with the AACE data, 4.5% with the WHO data, 3.8% with the EGIR data, and 7.8% with the REGODCI data.[21] A prevalence of 4.5% (1.1 million adolescents aged 12–17 years in 2006) is noted when using the pediatric International Diabetes Federation criteria; this involves 6.7% of male versus 2.1% of female adolescents and is highest among Mexican American adolescents at 7.1%.[23] Authors of a review of the world literature from 1950 to 2007 noted an increasing incidence of features of the metabolic syndrome related to obesity that have also been noted in children and adolescents in developing countries, where malnutrition is still a public health menace.[24]

Many different definitions for MetS have been used by researchers, and a standard definition for use in pediatrics and adolescent medicine that recognizes ethnic-specific variations would be beneficial for both researchers and clinicians.[25,26] For example, using different MetS definitions has resulted in prevalence rates for obese adolescents ranging from 12% to 44%.[27] Recent research on adolescents by Jolliffee and Janssen[28] was based on linking MetS classification to health-based Adult Treatment Panel III and International Diabetes Federation adult criteria. The authors noted that MetS has nearly doubled in prevalence over the past decade and suggested a prevalence of 7.6% (on the basis of the Adult Treatment Panel III data) and 9.6% (on the basis of new International Diabetes Federation adolescent data) in American adolescents 12 to 19 years of age.[28]

It should also be noted that the very existence of a specific syndrome termed the “metabolic syndrome” for children and adolescents remains controversial.[13,29–31] The debate centers on whether well-known clusters of risk factors for diabetes and cardiovascular diseases used in adults can be successfully applied to children and adolescents with inherent metabolic changes caused by puberty.[32] Do these risk factors of obesity, hyperlipidemia, hypertension, hyperglycemia, and others as noted in this review actually constitute a specific syndrome? Should screening start in children and adolescents for a specific syndrome called the “metabolic syndrome?” If parents and adolescents are told about this “syndrome,” will it result in improved lifestyle changes by parents for their children and by adolescents for themselves?[30] Is there a specific syndrome that is unique to adolescents and different from that seen in adults? Is seeking to define a metabolic syndrome useful or just a distraction from clinically helping these children and adolescents?[33] Research continues for a single underlying factor for MetS in adolescents that would also support a single definition.[25,26,34]

To provide a broad view of these features, research from the adult literature as well as that reflective of research on youth is provided in this discussion. It is important for clinicians to be aware of basic features of this syndrome that will develop in various combinations in childhood, adolescence, and adulthood. The existence of these various features is well known. The readers of this article can decide for themselves if lumping them into a specific term is helpful. Let the debate continue, and let clinicians continue to care for these at-risk youth. In this regard, understanding the underlying pathophysiology is important. We start with specific tissues and cells (ie, the liver, brain and central nervous system, adipose tissue, and the β cell) that are involved in these various features and provide a broad swath of supportive literature.

The Liver

When even greatly expanded rates of insulin production ultimately cannot keep pace with demand, the often prodigious insulin levels that result are nonetheless relatively insufficient and cannot keep the liver's output of glucose suppressed. This, in turn, results in impaired carbohydrate tolerance and a rising output of glucose from the liver. This occurs in association with rising glucagon levels that errantly stimulate hepatic glucose production,[35,36] further disrupting the body's glucose-disposal abilities.

Coupled with these events in the liver may be progressive pancreatic β-cell failure. Truncal obesity, associated with even minor impairment in fasting glucose tolerance (~110–125 mg/dL), reflects large reductions in β-cell mass and function[37,38] brought about by apoptosis and the chronic intoxicating effects of a sustained high-glucose environment on the β cell.[38] Added to this is the role played by impaired insulin sensitivity, with reduced glucose disposal and glycogen synthesis, in skeletal muscle that requires high concentrations of insulin to overcome it.[39]

Hepatosteatosis (ie, fatty liver, hepatic steatosis, nonalcoholic steatohepatosis, nonalcoholic fatty liver disease [NAFLD]) is a phenomenon in which the liver assumes the role of an auxiliary fat-storage site and is found often in patients with metabolic syndrome with or without diabetes; it can advance to frank cirrhosis.[40–42] NAFLD is a risk factor for large-vessel disease,[43] and subjects maintaining diets rich in carbohydrate seem to be at greater risk than those on other diets.[44,45] It is closely associated with failing β-cell function.[46]

Brain and Central Nervous System

In the fasting state, most tissue glucose disposal occurs independent of insulin in the brain and central nervous system. Non–insulin-mediated tissue glucose uptake is greater in patients with type 2 diabetes than in normal subjects. With basal hepatic glucose production increased in these patients, the parallel elevation of non–insulin-mediated glucose-disposal rates in the brain may be a compensatory effect moderating the impairment in insulin efficiency and protecting the brain against hypoglycemia. This protection, associated with conscious recognition of falling glucose, may fail in insulin-treated diabetic patients.[47] The ways in which the body protects against hypoglycemia are multiple and complex.[48,49] The brain's role in influencing factors such as appetite, satiety, and other aspects of glucose metabolism is under intense study, with different levels of insulin resistance and responses to hyperinsulinemia noted in lean and overweight individuals.[50]

Adipose Tissue

Detection of obesity (including abdominal obesity) is an important step in recognizing MetS in adolescents, and use of waist/height ratio is an important index for identifying children and adolescents with a high risk for metabolic and cardiovascular risks associated with MetS.[51–53] Maternal abdominal obesity increases risks for MetS in her offspring.[54] Patients with the insulin-resistance syndrome are often (but not always) obese, with the excess adiposity disproportionately distributed in the splanchnic (visceral) region, in contrast to areas such as buttocks and thighs. On physical examination, these youth have an increased BMI and a high ratio of circumferences of waist-to-hip. These simple anthropometric measures are, in fact, powerful indicators of the presence of the syndrome and, as such, carry prognostic implications.[55]

Moreover, in recent years it has been recognized that visceral fat is itself a true endocrine organ, secreting a class of agents known as adipokines. These several hormones, involved in many physiologic systems, may act to improve insulin sensitivity, to diminish it, or to enhance inflammation or hypercoagulability and operate in part by signaling mechanisms in the central nervous system.[56] They include adiponectin, leptin, resistin, tumor necrosis factor α (TNF-α), visfatin, and interleukin 6.[57]

Adiponectin is a family of several molecular species with similar activity. They are secreted by adipose tissue in amounts inversely related to adipose tissue mass and are diminished in type 2 diabetes.[58] Adiponectin deficiency may also vary among ethnic groups (eg, more problematic in Pima Indians). When present in high concentrations, adiponectin protects against vascular disease,[59] apparently independent of the degree of glycemic control; also, when deficiency exists, there is a high correlation with insulin resistance. As shown in Table 2, it is directly associated with various beneficial metabolic effects. It seems to act through stimulation of adenosine monophosphate kinase activity in liver and muscle, leading to enhanced glucose disposal and free fatty acid (FFA) uptake and oxidation[60] in insulin-sensitive tissues. It also exerts a suppressive effect on inflammation and atherogenesis in vascular endothelial cells. The means of making adiponectin available for therapy or of increasing its synthesis and/or action in obesity and type 2 diabetes are under current investigation.

Table 2
Consequences of insulin resistance in body tissues

I. Liver
- A. Reduced storage of glucose
- B. Increased hepatic glucose production, hyperglycemia[141,155,156]

II. Non–insulin-mediated tissue glucose uptake
- A. Elevated in type 2 diabetes
- B. Compensates for decreased peripheral insulin effect[39]

III. Muscle
- A. Insensitivity to insulin, reduced glucose-disposal rates
- B. Reduced glycogen synthesis

IV. Adipose tissue
- A. Hydrolysis of stored fat
- B. Increased FFAs
- C. Impaired islet-cell function[157]
- D. Adipokines
  - 1. Adiponectin
    - Improves insulin sensitivity in skeletal muscle and liver
    - Increased fatty acid oxidation in liver and muscle
    - Diminished circulating FFA and fat uptake by liver and muscle
    - Increased adenosine monophosphate kinase activity in liver and muscle
    - Decreased vascular inflammation
    - Antiatherogenic properties[158]
    - Future exogenous administration holds promise for management
  - 2. Leptin
    - Signaling mechanism to the brain regarding nutrient intake
    - Effect decreases as obesity increases
    - Future exogenous administration holds promise
  - 3. Resistin
    - Directly correlates with insulin resistance
    - Apparent association with cardiovascular inflammatory factors
  - 4. Tumor necrosis factor α, interleukin 6
    - Proinflammatory; correlates directly with insulin resistance
    - Predictive of diabetes type 2 and cardiovascular disease
  - 5. Angiotensin II
    - Hypertension; vascular and cardiovascular remodeling
  - 6. Inflammatory and procoagulant factors
    - Angiotensin II, transforming growth factor β, plasminogen activator inhibitor type 1 (PAI-1)[159]
    - Hypercoagulable disorders, large-vessel atherosclerosis
    - C-reactive protein

V. The β cell
- A. Apoptosis
- B. Amyloid infiltration
- C. Glucose intoxication

VI. Vascular endothelium and cardiovascular system
- A. Endothelial dysfunction
- B. Pathogenic effects of inflammatory and procoagulant factors
- C. Microalbuminuria

VII. The ovary
- A. PCOS
- B. Hyperandrogenism
- C. All other features of insulin-resistance syndrome

Leptin is a 167 amino acid peptide secreted by fat cells in proportion to their mass.[61] It is an important signaling mechanism to the brain regulating nutrient intake. Morbid obesity develops in the total absence of leptin in humans.[62] These uncommon aleptinemic patients frequently also have hypogonadotropic hypogonadism and severe insulin resistance but are without diabetes; exogenous leptin has been shown to benefit these patients.[61,63] Resistance to leptin at the hypothalamic level is evidently far more common than is true leptin deficiency, with increasing obesity associated with decreasing effectiveness, rather than insufficient levels of the hormone, in moderating food intake. This defect, however, has been shown to be remediable in some overweight individuals by administration of exogenous leptin.[64]

Leptin treatment has decreased triglyceride levels and improved glucose disposal in a subset of patients with lipodystrophy, a rare entity displaying selective loss of both subcutaneous and visceral fat, elevated triglyceride levels, diabetes, and hepatomegaly.[65] The possible future use of leptin as a management modality for other patients with insulin-resistance syndrome remains under investigation. In a mouse model, coadministration of recombinant adiponectin and leptin abolished insulin resistance,[66] which is an observation with potential therapeutic implications.

Resistin, a cysteine-rich adipokine, contrasts with adiponectin in that its levels correlate directly with elevated insulin resistance and specific vascular risk factors. Resistin levels parallel several markers of inflammation, BMI, and white blood cell count in patients without diabetes or cardiovascular disease.[67] Research is underway to correlate white blood cell counts with risks for development of MetS in adolescents.[68]

Tumor necrosis factor α, visfatin, and interleukin 6 are proinflammatory factors that correlate positively with increased visceral fat content and hyperinsulinemia.[69] Infiltrated with macrophages in obesity, affected adipose tissue produces these inflammatory cytokines that aggravate insulin resistance, the former by interfering with adiponectin synthesis and by stimulating fatty acid release from adipocytes[70,71]; the latter is by less-certain mechanisms but is well correlated with risk of type 2 diabetes and myocardial infarction.[72] Adipose tissue is also known to produce and release the procoagulant factor plasminogen activator inhibitor 1 (PAI-1) as well as other inflammatory factors including angiotensin II[73] and immunomodulating factors.

The β Cell

The consequences of progressive insulin resistance, as described above, create escalating demands on the β cell to keep up with the body's needs. Significant hyperinsulinemia, often at several-fold elevations of normal concentrations, nonetheless cannot stem the tide of vascular consequences that develop even in individuals without frank diabetes; this hyperinsulinemia has its own separate sequelae as well, as noted below. In the large subset of insulin-resistant patients at risk for development of type 2 diabetes, various factors seriously augment that risk; these factors include physical inactivity, high-calorie diet, increasing age, and genetic and ethnic factors. When the β-cell mass, stretched to its maximum, can no longer keep up with demand, carbohydrate intolerance develops, opening the possibility of all the added complications of diabetes mellitus.

Apoptosis is a principal mechanism responsible for the loss of β cells,[74] occurring together with amyloid infiltration into them. Glucose itself plays a role in intoxicating and damaging the β cell, setting up a vicious cycle in which hyperglycemia, resulting from progressive β-cell failure, progressively despoils β-cell function, aggravating that failure.[75] Fatty acids can also stimulate insulin resistance[76] and, with oxidative stress, are also involved in bringing about β-cell damage in those with diabetes.[77]

The Cardiovascular System

The insulin-resistance syndrome is a macrovascular disease equivalent. Abdominal (visceral) obesity, in conjunction with hypertension, dyslipidemia, hyperglycemia, oxidative stress, and wide-spread glycosylation, leads to lipid deposition, inflammation, endothelial dysfunction, and their composite end results of heart disease, cerebrovascular accident, and other large-vessel atherosclerosis.[78] Obesity itself is not a requirement in this chain of events but makes these end results more likely. In susceptible individuals these changes may begin early in life.[79] Despite genetic and ethnic factors, attempts at modifying lifestyle may be the best solution now available for management; however, shepherding the successful implementation of lifestyle changes remains a critical challenge for the clinician caring for these youth.

The consequences of insulin-resistance syndrome on the toll of coronary artery disease are grave, with the risk rising sharply in proportion to the number of risk factors (Table 3) that are present.[80] Not all are necessarily present together in a given individual, but all of those present tend to reinforce each other in a cascade of progressive morbidity and mortality. The presence of MetS in childhood and adolescence predicts cardiovascular disease as an adult.[81] Several of these factors are briefly considered below.

Dyslipidemia is a complex factor in the metabolic syndrome. Its components are elevated small, dense low-density lipoprotein (LDL) levels, elevated triglyceride levels, and depressed levels of high-density lipoprotein (HDL). These commonly occur together in the metabolic syndrome. An elevated small, dense LDL level is a serious risk factor that may occur independently, unrelated to insulin resistance, in primary hypercholesterolemia, primary hypothyroidism, and obstructive liver disease. Absent other factors, an elevated small, dense LDL level is a powerful predictor of early vascular disease. When presenting as a part of the

Table 3
Clinical features in metabolic syndrome associated with endothelial dysfunction and coronary artery disease[160]

Visceral obesity
Sedentary lifestyle
Hyperglycemia and type 2 diabetes
Hypertriglyceridemia and elevated FFA flux
Low HDL levels
Hypercoagulability and defective fibrinolysis
Endothelial dysfunction
Hypertension
Microalbuminuria
Elevated small, dense LDL levels
Elevated C-reactive protein levels
Hyperuricemia
Obstructive sleep apnea
PCOS

combined dyslipidemia in metabolic syndrome, elevated levels of small, dense LDL contribute heavily to the problematic convergence of unwanted results. These results include increased FFA release from adipose tissue into the liver with resulting increases in triglyceride and very low-density lipoprotein (VLDL) synthesis, some of which may be retained in liver (see above), producing fatty liver.

Triglyceride-rich LDL and HDL particles become a preferred substrate for hepatic lipoprotein lipase, and in large amounts these particles overwhelm the enzyme and so reduce its triglyceride-digesting activity. This, in turn, leads to reduced clearance of small, dense LDLs with its attendant enhanced atherogenicity and possible microvascular implications. Triglyceride-rich lipoproteins induce removal of cholesterol from HDL to VLDL via a cholesterol-ester transfer protein, augmenting the fraction of LDL that is classified as subclass B (ie, atherogenic small, dense LDL).[82]

The combined hyperlipidemia (VLDL plus small, dense LDL) in metabolic syndrome has similarities to those lipid patterns seen in familial combined dyslipidemia, a separate primary entity also associated with early coronary artery disease.[83] When circulating levels of VLDL triglyceride are elevated, they may saturate lipoprotein lipase. When, in addition, there is circulating postprandial hyperchylomicronemia from a high-fat meal, the inhibited lipoprotein lipase is unable to hydrolyze the high levels of accompanying triglycerides. Such postprandial hyperlipemia is a known associate of endothelial dysfunction[84,85] and is a likely separate high-risk dyslipidemic event in the metabolic syndrome.

Hypertension is defined as a blood pressure of ≥130/85 mm Hg, although more liberal criteria have been set forth by some experts (see Table 1). Blood pressure measurement in routine clinical practice is an important part of MetS identification in children and adolescents.[86] With or without associated obesity or diabetes, hypertension correlates with insulin resistance,[87] and patients with it are significantly more likely to develop diabetes and cardiovascular disease than normotensive patients.[88] Insulin resistance and hypertension are likely linked via insulin's enhanced effect on renal sodium reabsorption, stimulation of the sympathetic nervous system, inflammatory effects on blood vessels, and defective nitric-oxide generation that impairs glucose uptake and vasodilation[89]; also, there is activation of the tissue renin-angiotensin system with similar effects. Insulin resistance and the renin-angiotensin system are closely linked.[90]

Microalbuminuria, resulting from loss of circulating protein into the urine from the glomerulus, reflects a general process of widespread vascular damage that also occurs in nonrenal vessels, which are structurally and functionally similar to glomerular vessels and susceptible to the same inflammatory adversities. Microalbuminuria is another risk factor for cardiovascular disease (see Table 1) and also heralds the existence of renal damage.[91] It rises with increasing age[92] and is easy to measure.

Dysfunction in vascular endothelium, reflected in elevated endothelin 1 levels, is yet another well-established occurrence in the metabolic syndrome and, in conjunction with several other stressors (ie, dyslipidemia; disrupted nitric-oxide synthesis with, in turn, inhibited leukocyte migration, platelet aggregation, and smooth muscle cell function; hypertension; hyperglycemia), predisposes to atherogenesis and thrombosis.[93] Elevated C-peptide, another marker of inflammation, is an adverse prognostic indicator for vascular disease, and its level is regularly elevated in the metabolic syndrome,[94] correlating with insulin resistance and hyperinsulinemia, visceral obesity, and dyslipidemia.

Obstructive sleep apnea is a frequent part of insulin-resistance syndrome, particularly in those with higher BMIs. It may appear independently in nonobese persons without other features of the syndrome,[95,96] but its presence may stimulate, and not merely be a physical consequence of, the insulin-resistance syndrome. It may occur in young children, for whom there may be major benefits to obtaining lipid profiles and C-reactive protein levels after tonsillectomy.[97,98] It is 3 times more prevalent among patients with diabetes than in the general population.[99] It may be independent of BMI and is often undiagnosed.

The Ovary and PCOS (a Syndrome Within a Syndrome)

In 1935, Stein and Leventhal[100] described 7 women with a syndrome presenting with obesity, abnormal menses, reduced fertility, and hirsutism; they noted the ovaries to be polycystic. We now know that PCOS is an insulin-resistant state associated with hyperandrogenemia. It is recognized as one of the most common disorders among female subjects, affecting 5% to 10% of this population during the reproductive years.[101] The cardinal features of PCOS are noted in Table 4.[102 103] Premature pubarche or menarche may be a PCOS feature noted in the first decade of life, whereas oligomenorrhea may be a feature in adolescents.[101] Factors that increase the risk for PCOS include having a low birth weight and a positive family history for diabetes mellitus as well as early cardiovascular disorder.[104] PCOS must be distinguished from other disorders that present with irregular menses and hirsutism, including nonclassical congenital adrenal hyperplasia, virilizing neoplasm, Cushing's syndrome, use of androgenizing drugs, hyperthecosis syndrome, or normal individuals with idiopathic hirsutism. Adolescents with PCOS have a higher prevalence of MetS than the general adolescent population, and hyperandrogenemia is a risk factor for MetS that is independent of obesity and insulin resistance.[105]

The pathogenesis of PCOS is complex and results in increased levels of androgen production by the ovary. Abnormal gonadotropin-releasing hormone pulses and consequent abnormal luteinizing hormone (LH) pulses occur with augmented LH production as compared with follicle-stimulating hormone. LH stimulates androgen production by ovarian theca cells to produce androstenedione and then testosterone. Insulin, in this hyperinsulinemic state, is a costimulator, with LH, of testosterone production, a process innately more efficient in patients with PCOS than in normal females.[106] Testosterone inhibits production by the liver of sex-hormone–binding globulin, enhancing the proportion of testosterone that is circulating free, with virilizing consequences that include menstrual disorders,

Table 4
Diagnostic features of PCOS

History
Precocious puberty or premature pubarche
Menstrual irregularities
Physical diagnosis
Centripetal obesity (BMI ≥30 kg/m^2); waist/hip ratio ≥0.85
Blood pressure ≥140/90 mm Hg
Acanthosis nigricans
Hirsutism (frequently unrelated to androgen excess or PCOS; idiopathic)
Terminal hair (mustache, chin stubble/beard, chest, abdomen, back)
Persistent acne vulgaris
Alopecia
Polycystic ovaries (shown ultrasonographically)
May not develop or may develop for several years after menarche
May not be distinguishable from normal-variant ovarian cysts
Laboratory studies
Testosterone elevation (may not develop for several years after menarche)
Repeat testing indicated if initially normal
Glucose-tolerance test of hemoglobin A1c
Rule out other diagnoses with overlapping presentations

Not all features need to be present in a given individual.

acne, and hirsutism, in addition to all the other pathologies of insulin-resistance syndrome. Testosterone levels correlate with hyperinsulinemia in PCOS and vary with its different phenotypic expressions.[107] It blunts sensitivity to insulin in both liver and muscle, stimulates lipolysis, and increases in FFAs. In chronic excess, it is directly associated with observable vascular damage.[108]

Obesity is found in many, but not all, adolescent girls with PCOS. In obese individuals with PCOS, worsening obesity seems to worsen the consequences of the syndrome, and diabetes mellitus tends to appear early in life.[109] Nonobese females with PCOS, however, are also insulin resistant, with reduced adiponectin levels and other biochemical markers of insulin-resistance syndrome.[110] Nearly half of those with PCOS ultimately develop type 2 diabetes.[111] Nondiabetic women with PCOS make sufficient insulin to avoid frank diabetes, particularly in earlier years of the syndrome, but many nonetheless have subtle defects in their insulin responses to meals or to a formal glucose challenge that may become clinically important in pregnancy or other physiologically stressful situations.[112]

Those with PCOS are inclined toward development of macrovascular disease,[113] a risk that seems to be related to the common atherogenic predisposers in the insulin-resistance syndrome, augmented by additional risks unique to PCOS that demand aggressive case-finding and management. As might also be expected, obstructive sleep apnea is frequently associated with PCOS and, again, is not merely a function of obesity.[114] Disordered breathing is more strongly correlated with insulin resistance than with BMI or testosterone levels.[114]

Gynecologic cancers are thought to possibly be associated with PCOS,[115,116] although this linkage remains speculative and subject to controversy. Hyperandrogenism, obesity, and hyperinsulinemia are possible risk factors for endometrial carcinoma; however, it has not been shown that endometrial cancer is more prevalent in women with PCOS than in unaffected women.[117] PCOS seems to be an inherited, complex, multigenic disorder, a topic that is under active investigation.[118,119] The roles of eating behaviors and dietary composition are still more controversial.[120,121]

METABOLIC SYNDROME THERAPY

Managing patients with metabolic syndrome is a labor-intensive endeavor, partly because of the varied array of presentations. Presently, there is no way to deal with the syndrome as a single entity; rather, the clinician must grapple with each of the individual aspects as they reveal themselves. However, an interdisciplinary approach that emphasizes comprehensive management produces maximum benefit in reducing the prevalence of metabolic syndrome and its consequences in adolescents.[122]

Obesity

The most frequent feature of the metabolic syndrome is obesity, and obese children and adolescents may begin to have clinical and biochemical features of MetS that need early screening and management.[22,123] Even small weight loss can lead to some reduction in risk factors for diabetes and cardiovascular diseases.[32] The first line of treatment for adolescents with MetS should include efforts to engage them in regular physical exercise and healthy nutrition intake to encourage needed weight loss and weight control.[53,124–126] Diet intake should include restriction of saturated and trans fatty acids; if weight reduction is needed, carbohydrate intake needs to be restricted with emphasis on reduction of refined sugars along with intake of dietary fiber to improve insulin sensitivity.[53,127] The benefit of physical activity alone in adolescents has been noted, with recent research examining the effect of exercise on adipocytokines and mitochondrial function.[128]

However, frustration in correcting obesity is universal for both patient and clinician. It is much better understood in laboratory animals than in human subjects despite multitudes of studies that have dealt with its hormonal aspects, various dietary regimens,[129] use of appetite-suppressing drugs,[130] surgical techniques, the effects of culture and ethnicity, the benefits of physical activity, psychological cofactors, and other issues. However, it is important to note that successful weight loss is a paramount ingredient in coming to grips with the ravages of insulin resistance and is the best method of treating MetS and PCOS in overweight adolescents.

Hypertension needs to be treated aggressively to lessen insulin resistance and to minimize long-term detrimental effects on the kidney and vasculature in children and adolescents with MetS.[131] A growing pharmacopoeia is available to clinicians for managing high blood pressure in adolescents, although success may be elusive regardless of modality. Angiotensin-converting enzyme inhibitors and angiotensin-receptor blockers, which can reduce albuminuria, possess renal protective effects and should be used early in youth with diabetes mellitus.[132–134] A possible relationship between hypertension and oxidative stress has been proposed that may be responsive to ascorbic acid supplementation.[135]

Diabetes

A family history of diabetes mellitus is associated with hyperinsulinemia in children and adolescents, whereas obesity and hypertension, per se, are not.[136] More research is need to identify better biochemical markers for type 2 diabetes mellitus.[58] Research suggests that careful attention to obesity in childhood and adolescence can lower the incidence of diabetes in later life.[137] Type 2 diabetes in the context of insulin-resistance syndrome is a highly complex and arduous management problem that requires incorporating ongoing efforts against obesity, hyperglycemia, hyperlipidemia, and hypertension. Several classes of agents are now available for treating diabetes, including metformin, thiazolidinediones, starch blockers, sulfonylureas, and related compounds. Metformin lowers insulin resistance predominantly in the liver and, in our view, should be widely used in adolescents with type 2 diabetes mellitus. Thiazolidinediones lower insulin resistance predominantly in fat and muscle, whereas starch blockers hinder carbohydrate absorption from the intestine. Sulfonylureas and related compounds stimulate insulin production by remaining β cells and are used infrequently in our clinics.

Management also includes insulin, the effective use of which demands significant expertise, a diabetes education mechanism, and a motivated youth with appropriate cognitive skills.[138] Incretin-based therapies, including injectable exenetide, a glucagon-like peptide 1 (GLP-1) receptor binder, and so-called dipeptidyl peptidase-4 (DPP-4) inhibitors (sitagliptin, vildagliptin) play important roles in modulating appetite and postprandial hyperglycemia and also in lowering hemoglobin A1c levels in youth with diabetes.[139,140] These modalities are in growing use in adult patients with diabetes, and their use in children and adolescents is being investigated.[141]

Hyperlipidemia

Hyperlipidemia in the metabolic syndrome presents with the lipid abnormalities already described, and efforts against them combine diet modification, effective management of diabetes, and use of an array of pharmacotherapies for children, adolescents, and adults.[142] Pharmacotherapies include statins (which act principally to inhibit production of LDL by blocking hepatic 3-hydroxy-3-methylglutaryl coenzyme A reductase) and fibrates (which inhibit hepatic production of VLDL, partly by activation of peroxisome proliferator-activated [PPAR] receptors).[132,142] Fibrates raise HDL levels by stimulating synthesis of apolipoproteins A, particles that act to transport cholesterol out of the circulation. Statins and fibrates, used together in managing combined dyslipidemias, may uncommonly have adverse effects but are usually safe and effective in combination.[142,143] Nicotinic acid, fish oil, and other agents also find utility in managing dyslipidemias, although there are occasions when more radical methods may be required.[144]

Knowledge of postprandial values of both lipid and glucose is an essential part of management of both the metabolic syndrome and hyperlipidemia. When elevated, both are important metabolic indices of risk of cardiovascular events, mediated by oxidant stress related to increased glucose level after a meal. The accompanying rise in free radicals triggers inflammation, endothelial dysfunction, and hypercoagulability, among other adverse events.[145] Hypercoagulability and inflammation in the metabolic syndrome are risk equivalents for coronary occlusion and stroke. Oral agents commonly used to combat them include low-dose aspirin and antiplatelet agents such as clopidogrel.

Management of PCOS in the adolescent involves managing the other features of metabolic syndrome with specific attention to management of obesity and hyperandrogenism.[101,146] Those with irregular menstruation, acne, and/or hirsutism can be placed on oral contraceptives (including the patch).[101] If irregular menstruation is the main concern, oral contraceptives or a cyclical progestin regimen can be used, such as 10 mg of medroxyprogesterone acetate for 12 to 14 days each month to induce withdrawal bleeding. Regular use of oral contraceptives offers management of PCOS-induced anovulation and unopposed estrogen stimulation of the endometrium.

In addition, hirsutism may be treated through use of antiandrogens, of which spironolactone at 100 to 200 mg/day (which also has important antihypertensive effects) is often prescribed.[147] Other agents for this purpose include cyproterone acetate, finasteride, and flutamide. These antiandrogenic agents may work well in concert with a carefully chosen oral contraceptive, the most frequently used form of which is a combined estrogen/progesterone preparation. The estrogen portion of the medication suppresses LH and ovarian androgen synthesis. It also stimulates hepatic synthesis of sex-hormone–binding globulin, binding a larger fraction of circulating testosterone.

Metformin and thiazolidione agents can lower insulin resistance in PCOS and sometimes restore fertility in adolescents with PCOS.[101,132,146] Metformin (Glucophage and others) is an oral biguanide that was approved to treat type 2 diabetes mellitus in adults in 1994, and there has been limited research with regard to its use in children and adolescents.[5] Metformin use leads to a reduction in gluconeogenesis in the liver while also inducing improvement in glucose movement in fatty tissue and skeletal muscle cell membranes. It is used to reduce weight in overweight/obese individuals as well as those without obesity.[5,148,149] In 1 study of adolescent boys (aged 9–18 years) given 1 g of metformin twice per day, there was an average weight loss of 4.35 kg over 6 months.[150] Metformin can be used alone or in conjunction with oral contraceptives in the management of PCOS in adolescent girls.[101,146]

In those with PCOS, metformin improves insulin sensitivity by decreasing levels of insulin and reducing symptoms seen with hyperinsulinemia and hyperandrogenism.[146,151,152] In PCOS, metformin may lead to greater regularity of ovulation because of induced weight loss, improved menstrual cycle regularity, and reduced levels of androgens.[152] If used in adolescents metformin is usually started at a dose of 500 mg twice per day, and if used to manage diabetes mellitus 2, the dose is increased by 500 mg/week to a daily maximum of 2 g as determined by specific blood glucose levels. Adverse effects (noted in Table 5) are usually dose dependent and usually improve with time.[153] Lactic acidosis is noted in 1 in every 30 000 patients, with a 50% mortality rate, and this serious adverse effect is seen especially in those with renal insufficiency. Contraindications to metformin include congestive heart failure, liver disease, severe hypoxia,

Table 5
Adverse effects of metformin[146]

Appetite loss
Cramps
Diarrhea
Emesis
Flatulence
Lactic acidosis
Nausea
Vitamin B_{12} malabsorption

renal insufficiency, and critical illness in general. Rosiglitazone is likely superior to metformin in reducing insulin resistance and has been associated with improved insulin sensitivity, more regular menses, and decreased androgen levels.[154]

CONCLUSIONS

Insulin resistance is rampant in the industrialized world, and it has consequences that are deadly for all patients, including adolescents. Obesity and physical inactivity are becoming alarmingly more prevalent. The health consequences are already devastating and will grow worse if our weight-control efforts continue to fail. Medications may help, but prevention of obesity and maintaining physical fitness play the most important roles in avoiding the disorders cascading from the metabolic syndrome.

These are the rightful struggles of physicians and patients, schools, governments, the media, and industry. Much can be accomplished by using the knowledge clinicians have in hand, but these efforts are minimized when faced with community apathy, large numbers of unmotivated patients, cash-strapped schools with other priorities, disinterested government, and media and industry working at cross purposes. These current challenges make the prospects for preventing obesity and encouraging physical fitness not bright at this point in time.

REFERENCES

1. Sullivan PW, Ghushchyan V, Wyatt HR, Wu EQ, Hill JO. Productivity costs associated with cardiometabolic risk factor clusters in the United States. *Value Health*. 2007;10(6):443–450
2. Zimmet P, Alberti G, Kaufman F, et al. The metabolic syndrome in children and adolescents. *Lancet*. 2007;369(9579):2059–2061
3. Saland JM. Update on the metabolic syndrome in children. *Curr Opin Pediatr*. 2007;19(2): 183–191
4. Draznin MB, Kamboj M. The endocrine system. In: Greydanus DE, Feinberg AN, Patel DR, Homnick DN, eds. *The Pediatric Diagnostic Examination*. New York, NY: McGraw-Hill Medical Publishers; 2008:427
5. Rowlett J. Obesity in the adolescent. In: Greydanus DE, Patel DR, Pratt HD, eds. *Essential Adolescent Medicine*. New York, NY: McGraw-Hill Medical Publishers; 2008:656–657

6. James WP, Rigby N, Leach R. Obesity and the metabolic syndrome: the stress on society. *Ann N Y Acad Sci.* 2006;1083:1–10
7. Grundy SM. Metabolic syndrome: connecting and reconciling cardiovascular and diabetes worlds. *J Am Coll Cardiol.* 2006;47(6):1093–1100
8. Song SH, Hardisty CA. Early-onset type 2 diabetes mellitus: an increasing phenomenon of elevated cardiovascular risk. *Expert Rev Cardiovasc Ther.* 2008;6(3):315–322
9. Cali AM, Caprio S. Prediabetes and type 2 diabetes in youth: an emerging epidemic disease? *Curr Opin Endocrinol Diabetes Obes.* 2008;15(2):123–127
10. Reaven GM. Banting lecture 1988: role of insulin resistance in human disease. *Diabetes.* 1988;37(12):1595–1607
11. Lebovitz HE. Insulin resistance: a common link between type 2 diabetes and cardiovascular disease. *Diabetes Obes Metab.* 2006;8(3):237–249
12. DeFronzo RA, Ferrannini E. Insulin resistance: a multifaceted syndrome responsible for NIDDM, obesity, hypertension, dyslipidemia, and atherosclerotic cardiovascular disease. *Diabetes Care.* 1991;14(3):173–194
13. Cook S, Weitzman M, Auinger P, et al. Prevalence of a metabolic syndrome phenotype in adolescents: findings from the Third National Health and Nutrition Examination Survey, 1998–1994. *Arch Pediatr Adolesc Med.* 2003;157(8):821–827
14. Vissers D, Vanroy C, De Meulenaere A, et al. Metabolic syndrome in youth: a cross-sectional school-based survey. *Acta Paediatr.* 2007;96(12):1809–1813
15. Duncan GE, Li SM, Zhou XH. Prevalence and trends of a metabolic syndrome phenotype among U.S. adolescents, 1999–2000. *Diabetes Care.* 2004;27(10):2438–2443
16. Csábi G, Török K, Jeges S, Molnár D. Presence of metabolic cardiovascular syndrome in obese children. *Eur J Pediatr.* 2000;159(1–2):91–94
17. Boney CM, Verma A, Tucker R, Vohr BR. Metabolic syndrome in childhood: association with birth weight, maternal obesity, and gestational diabetes mellitus. *Pediatrics.* 2005;115(3). Available at: www.pediatrics.org/cgi/content/full/115/3/e290
18. Golley RK, Magarey AM, Steinbeck KS, Baur LA, Daniels LA. Comparison of metabolic syndrome prevalence using six different definitions in overweight pre-pubertal children enrolled in a weight management study. *Int J Obes (Lond).* 2006;30(5):853–660
19. de Ferranti SD, Gauvreau K, Ludwig DS, Neufeld EJ, Newburger JW, Rifai N. Prevalence of the metabolic syndrome in American adolescents: findings from the Third National Health and Nutrition Examination Survey. *Circulation.* 2004;110(16):2494–2497
20. Lambert M, Paradis G, O'Loughlin J, Delvin EE, Hanley JA, Levy E. Insulin resistance syndrome in a representative sample of children and adolescents from Quebec, Canada. *Int J Obes Relat Metab Disord.* 2004;28(7):833–841
21. Rodríguez-Morán M, Salazar-Vázquez B, Violante R, Guerrero-Romero F. Metabolic syndrome among children and adolescents aged 10–18 years. *Diabetes Care.* 2004;27(10):2516–2517
22. Weiss R, Dziura J, Burgert TS, et al. Obesity and the metabolic syndrome in children and adolescents. *N Engl J Med.* 2004;350(23):2362–2374
23. Ford ES, Li C, Zhao G, Pearson WS, Mokdad AH. Prevalence of the metabolic syndrome among U.S. adolescents using the definition from the International Diabetes Federation. *Diabetes Care.* 2008;31(3):587–589
24. Kelishadi R. Childhood overweight, obesity, and the metabolic syndrome in developing countries. *Epidemiol Rev.* 2007;29:1–26. Available at: http://epirev.oxfordjournals.org/cgi/content/full/mxm003v1. Accessed June 30, 2008
25. Ford ES, Li C. Defining the metabolic syndrome in children and adolescents: will the real definition please stand up? *J Pediatr.* 2008;152(2):160–164
26. Misra A, Khurana L, Vikram NK, Goel A, Wasir JS. Metabolic syndrome in children: current issues and South Asian perspective. *Nutrition.* 2007;23(11–12):895–910
27. Cook S, Auinger P, Li C, Ford ES. Metabolic syndrome rates in United States adolescents, from the National Health and Nutrition Examination Survey, 1999–2002. *J Pediatr.* 2008;152(2): 165–170

28. Jolliffe CJ, Janssen I. Development of age-specific adolescent metabolic syndrome criteria that are linked to the Adult Treatment Panel III and International Diabetes Federation criteria. *J Am Coll Cardiol*. 2007;49(8):891–898
29. Goodman E, Daniels SR, Meigs JB, Dolan LM. Instability in the diagnosis of metabolic syndrome in adolescents. *Circulation*. 2007;115(17):2316–2322
30. Goodman E. Metabolic syndrome and the mismeasure of risk. *J Adolesc Health*. 2008;42(6): 538–540
31. Goodman E. Pediatric metabolic syndrome: smoke and mirrors or true magic? *J Pediatr*. 2006;148(2):149–150
32. Pietrobelli A, Malavolti M, Battistini NC, Fuiano N. Metabolic syndrome: a child is not a small adult. *Int J Pediatr Obes*. 2008;3(suppl 1):67–71
33. Jones KL. The dilemma of the metabolic syndrome in children and adolescents: disease or distraction? *Pediatr Diabetes*. 2006;7(6):311–321
34. Li C, Ford ES. Is there a single underlying factor for the metabolic syndrome in adolescents? A confirmatory factor analysis. *Diabetes Care*. 2007;30(6):1556–1561
35. Gerich JE. Glucagon as a counter-regulatory hormone. In: Lefebvre PJ, ed. *Glucagon*. Vol II. Berlin, Germany: Springer; 1983:275–951
36. Baron AD, Schaeffer L, Shragg P, Kolterman OG. Role of hyperglucagonemia in maintenance of increased rates of hepatic glucose output in type II diabetes. *Diabetes*. 1987;36(3):274–283
37. Butler AE, Janson J, Bonner-Weir S, et al. Beta cell deficit and increased beta cell apoptosis in humans with type 2 diabetes. *Diabetes*. 2003;52(1):102–110
38. Umpierrez GE, Smiley D, Gosmanov A, Thomason D. Ketosis-prone type 2 diabetes: effect of hyperglycemia on beta-cell function and skeletal muscle insulin signaling. *Endocr Pract*. 2007;13(3):283–290
39. Revers RR, Fink R, Griffin J, Olefsky JM, Kolterman OG. Influence of hyperglycemia on insulin's in vivo effects in type II diabetes. *J Clin Invest*. 1984;73(3):664–672
40. Love-Osborne KA, Nadeau KJ, Sheeder J, Fenton LZ, Zeitler P. Presence of the metabolic syndrome in obese adolescents predicts impaired glucose tolerance and nonalcoholic fatty liver disease. *J Adolesc Health*. 2008;42(6):543–548
41. Abdelmalek MF, Diehl AM. Nonalcoholic fatty liver disease as a complication of insulin resistance. *Med Clin North Am*. 2007;91(6):1125–1149, ix
42. Gholam PM, Flancbaum L, Machan JT, Charney DA, Kotler DP. Nonalcoholic fatty liver disease in severely obese subjects. *Am J Gastroenterol*. 2007;102(2):399–408
43. Targher G, Bertolini L, Padovani R. Non-alcoholic fatty liver disease is associated with carotid artery wall thickness in diet-controlled type 2 diabetic patients. *J Endocrinol Invest*. 2006; 29(1):55–60
44. Toshimitsu K, Matsuura B, Ohkubo I, et al. Dietary habits and nutrient intake in non-alcoholic steatohepatitis. *Nutrition*. 2007;23(1):46–52
45. Kang H, Greenson JK, Omo JT, et al. Metabolic syndrome is associated with greater histologic severity, higher carbohydrate, and lower fat diet in patients with NAFLD. *Am J Gastroenterol*. 2006;101(10):2247–2253
46. Gerich JE. Metabolic abnormalities in impaired glucose tolerance. *Metabolism*. 1997;46(12 suppl 1):40–43
47. Amiel SA, Tamborlane WV, Simonson DC, Sherwin RS. Defective glucose counterregulation after strict glycemic control of insulin-dependent diabetes mellitus. *N Engl J Med*. 1987; 316(22):1376–1383
48. Hoffman RP. Sympathetic mechanisms of hypoglycemic counterregulation. *Curr Diabetes Rev*. 2007;3(3):185–193
49. Gerich JE. Lilly lecture 1988: glucose counterregulation and its impact on diabetes mellitus. *Diabetes*. 1988;37(12):1608–1617
50. Tschritter O, Preissl H, Hennige AM, et al. The cerebrocortical response to hyperinsulinemia is reduced in overweight humans: a magnetoencephalographic study. *Proc Natl Acad Sci U S A*. 2006;103(32):12103–12108

51. Maffeis C, Banzato C, Talamini G; Obesity Study Group of the Italian Society of Pediatric Endocrinology and Diabetology. Waist-to-height ratio, a useful index to identify high metabolic risk in overweight children. *J Pediatr.* 2008;152(2):207–213
52. Kelishadi R, Cook SR, Motlagh ME, et al. Metabolically obese normal weight and phenotypically obese metabolically normal youths: the CASPIAN study. *J Am Diet Assoc.* 2008;108(1): 82–90
53. Crespo PS, Prieto Perera JA, Lodeiro FA, Azuara LA. Metabolic syndrome in childhood. *Public Health Nutr.* 2007;10(10A):1121–1125
54. Hirschler V, Roque MI, Calcagno ML, et al. Maternal weight circumference and prediction of children's metabolic syndrome. *Arch Pediatr Adolesc Med.* 2007;161(12):1205–1210
55. Schneider HJ, Glaesmer H, Klotsche J, et al. Accuracy of anthropometric indicators of obesity to predict cardiovascular risk. *J Clin Endocrinol Metab.* 2007;92(2):589–594
56. Qi Y, Takahashi N, Hileman SM, et al. Adiponectin acts in the brain to decrease body weight [published correction appears in *Nat Med.* 2004;10(6):649]. *Nat Med.* 2004;10(5):524–529
57. Amemiya S, Dobashi K, Urakami T, Sugihara S, Ohzeki T, Tajima N. Metabolic syndrome in youths. *Pediatr Diabetes.* 2007;8(suppl 9):48–54
58. Weyer C, Funahashi T, Tanaka S, Hotta K, Matsuzawa Y, Pratley RE, Tataranni PA. Hypoadiponectinemia in obesity and type 2 diabetes: close association with insulin resistance and hyperinsulinemia. *J Clin Endocrinol Metab.* 2001;86(5):1930–1935
59. Pischon T, Girman CJ, Hotamisligil GS, Rifai N, Hu FB, Rimm EB. Plasma adiponectin levels and risk of myocardial infarction in men. *JAMA.* 2004;291(14):1730–1737
60. Guerre-Millo M. Adiponectin: an update. *Diabetes Metab.* 2008;34(1):12–18
61. Considine RV, Sinha MK, Heiman ML, et al. Serum immunoreactive-leptin concentrations in normal-weight and obese humans. *N Engl J Med.* 1996;334(5):292–295
62. Montague CT, Farooqi IS, Whitehead JP, et al. Congenital leptin deficiency is associated with severe early-onset obesity in humans. *Nature.* 1997;387(6636):903–908
63. Farooqi IS, Matarese G, Lord GM, et al. Beneficial effects of leptin on obesity, T cell hyporesponsiveness, and neuroendocrine/metabolic dysfunction of human congenital leptin deficiency. *J Clin Invest.* 2002;110(8):1093–1103
64. Heymsfield SB, Greenberg AS, Fujioka K, et al. Recombinant leptin for weight loss in obese and lean adults: a randomized, controlled, dose-escalation trial. *JAMA.* 1999;282(16):1568–1575
65. Petersen KF, Oral EA, Dufour S, et al. Leptin reverses insulin resistance and hepatic steatosis in patients with severe lipodystrophy. *J Clin Invest.* 2002;109(10):1345–1350
66. Yamauchi T, Kamon J, Waki H, et al. The fat-derived hormone adiponectin reverses insulin resistance associated with both lipoatrophy and obesity. *Nat Med.* 2001;7(8):941–946
67. Aquilante CL, Kosmiski LA, Knutsen SD, Zineh I. Relationship between plasma resistin concentrations, inflammatory chemokines, and components of the metabolic syndrome in adults. *Metabolism.* 2008;57(4):494–501
68. Hsieh CH, Pei D, Kuo SW, et al. Correlation between white blood cell count and metabolic syndrome in adolescence. *Pediatr Int.* 2007;49(6):827–832
69. Bahceci M, Gokalp D, Bahceci S, Tuzcu A, Atmaca S, Arikan S. The correlation between adiposity and adiponectin, tumor necrosis factor alpha, interleukin-6 and high sensitivity C-reactive protein levels: is adipocyte size associated with inflammation in adults? *J Endocrinol Invest.* 2007;30(3):210–214
70. Bruun JM, Lihn AS, Verdich C, Pedersen SB, et al. Regulation of adiponectin by adipose tissue-derived cytokines: in vivo and in vitro investigations in humans. *Am J Physiol Endocrinol Metab.* 2003;285(3):E527–E533
71. Greenberg AS, McDaniel ML. Identifying the links between obesity, insulin resistance and beta-cell function: potential role of adipocyte-derived cytokines in the pathogenesis of type 2 diabetes. *Eur J Clin Invest.* 2002;32(suppl 3):24–34
72. Ridker PM, Rifai N, Pfeffer M, Sacks F, Lepage S, Braunwald E. Elevation of tumor necrosis factor-alpha and increased risk of recurrent coronary events after myocardial infarction. *Circulation.* 2000;101(18):2149–2153

73. Volkova NB, Deedwania PC. The metabolic syndrome and its effects on cardiovascular risks. In: Fonseca V, ed. *Clinical Diabetes*. Philadelphia, PA: Elsevier; 2006:64–77
74. Butler AE, Janson J, Soeller WC, Butler PC. Increased beta-cell apoptosis prevents adaptive increase in beta-cell mass in mouse model of type 2 diabetes: evidence for role of islet amyloid formation rather than direct action of amyloid. *Diabetes*. 2003;52(9):2304–2314
75. DeFronzo RA, Bonadonna RC, Ferrannini E. Pathogenesis of NIDDM: a balanced overview. *Diabetes Care*. 1992;15(3):318–368
76. Brudaşcă I, Cucuianu M. Pathogenic role of abnormal fatty acids and adipokines in the portal flow. Relevance for metabolic syndrome, hepatic steatosis and steatohepatitis. *Rom J Intern Med*. 2007;45(2):149–157
77. Oprescu AI, Bikopoulos G, Naassan A, et al. Free fatty acid-induced reduction in glucose-stimulated insulin secretion: evidence for a role of oxidative stress in vitro and in vivo. *Diabetes*. 2007;56(12):2927–2937
78. Isomaa B, Almgren P, Tuomi T, et al. Cardiovascular morbidity and mortality associated with the metabolic syndrome. *Diabetes Care*. 2001;24(4):683–689
79. Beilin L, Huang RC. Childhood obesity, hypertension, the metabolic syndrome and adult cardiovascular disease. *Clin Exp Pharmacol Physiol*. 2008;35(4):409–411
80. Wilson PW, Kannel WB, Silbershatz H, D'Agostino RB. Clustering of metabolic factors and coronary heart disease. *Arch Intern Med*. 1999;159(10):1104–1109
81. Morrison JA, Friedman LA, Gray-McGuire C. Metabolic syndrome in childhood predicts adult cardiovascular disease 25 years later: the Princeton Lipid Research Clinics Follow-up Study. *Pediatrics*. 2007;120(2):340–345
82. Chapman MJ. Metabolic syndrome and type 2 diabetes: lipid and physiological consequences. *Diab Vasc Dis Res*. 2007;4(suppl 3):S5–S8
83. Eckel RH. Familial combined hyperlipidemia and insulin resistance: distant relatives linked by intra-abdominal fat? *Arterioscler Thromb Vasc Biol*. 2001;21(4):469–470
84. Mamo JC, Yu KC, Elsegood CL, et al. Is atherosclerosis exclusively a postprandial phenomenon? *Clin Exp Pharmacol Physiol*. 1997;24(3–4):288–293
85. Lee IK, Kim HS, Bae JH. Endothelial dysfunction: its relationship with acute hyperglycaemia and hyperlipidemia. *Int J Clin Pract Suppl*. 2002;129(129):59–64
86. Rappaport EB. Identifying and evaluating the metabolic syndrome in children and adolescents. *Ethn Dis*. 2007;17(3 suppl 4):S4–S16
87. Sowers JR. Insulin resistance and hypertension. *Am J Physiol Heart Circ Physiol*. 2004;286(5): H1597–H1602
88. Ferrannini E, Buzzigoli G, Bonadonna R, et al. Insulin resistance in essential hypertension. *N Engl J Med*. 1987;317(6):350–357
89. Muniyappa R, Montagnani M, Koh KK, Quon MJ. Cardiovascular actions of insulin. *Endocr Rev*. 2007;28(5):463–491
90. Katovich MJ, Pachori A. Effects of inhibition of the renin-angiotensin system on the cardiovascular actions of insulin. *Diabetes Obes Metab*. 2000;2(1):3–14
91. Naidoo DP. The link between microalbuminuria, endothelial dysfunction and cardiovascular disease in diabetes. *Cardiovasc J S Afr*. 2002;13(4):194–199
92. Agrawal B, Berger A, Wolf K, Luft FC. Microalbuminuria screening by reagent strip predicts cardiovascular risk in hypertension. *J Hypertens*. 1996;14(2):223–228
93. Yu Y, Suo L, Yu H, Wang C, Tang H. Insulin resistance and endothelial dysfunction in type 2 diabetes patients with or without microalbuminuria. *Diabetes Res Clin Pract*. 2004;65(2): 95–104
94. Forouhi MG, Sattar N, McKeigue PM. Relation of C-reactive protein to body fat distribution and features of the metabolic syndrome in Europeans and South Asians. *Int J Obes Relat Metab Disord*. 2001;25(9):1327–1331
95. Vgontzas AN, Legro RS, Bixler EO, Grayev A, Kales A, Chrousos GP. Polycystic ovary syndrome is associated with obstructive sleep apnea and daytime sleepiness: role of insulin resistance. *J Clin Endocrinol Metab*. 2001;86(2):517–520

96. Gopal M, Duntley S, Uhles M, Attarian H. The role of obesity in the increased prevalence of obstructive sleep apnea syndrome in patients with polycystic ovary syndrome. *Sleep Med.* 2002;3(5):401–404
97. Gozal D, Sans Capdevila O, Kheirandish-Gozal L. Metabolic alterations and systemic inflammation in obstructive sleep apnea among nonobese and obese prepubertal children. *Am J Respir Crit Care Med.* 2008;177(10):1142–1149
98. Tasali E, Ip MS. Obstructive sleep apnea and metabolic syndrome: alterations in glucose metabolism and inflammation. *Proc Am Thorac Soc.* 2008;5(2):207–217
99. West SD, Nicoll DJ, Stradling JR. Prevalence of obstructive sleep apnoea in men with type 2 diabetes. *Thorax.* 2006;61(11):945–950
100. Stein IF, Leventhal ML. Amenorrhea associated with bilaaterral polycystic ovaries. *Am J Obstet Gynecol.* 1935;29:181–191
101. Mastorakos G, Lambrinoudaki I, Creatsas G. Polycystic ovary syndrome in adolescents: current and future treatment options. *Paediatr Drugs.* 2006;8(5):311–318
102. Ehrmann, DA. Polycystic ovary syndrome. *N Engl J Med.* 2005;352(12):1223–1236
103. Orio F, Vuolo L, Palomba S, Lombardi G, Colao A. Metabolic and cardiovascular consequences of polycystic ovary syndrome. *Minerva Ginecol.* 2008;60(1):39–51
104. Gluckman PD, Hanson MA, Cooper C, Thornburg KL. Effect of in utero and early-life conditions on adult health and disease. *N Engl J Med.* 2008;359(1):61–72
105. Coviello AD, Legro RS, Dunaif A. Adolescent girls with polycystic ovary syndrome have an increased risk of the metabolic syndrome associated with increasing androgen levels independent of obesity and insulin resistance. *J Clin Endocrinol Metab.* 2006;91(2):492–497
106. Nelson VL, Qin KN, Rosenfield RL, et al. The biochemical basis for increased testosterone production in theca cells propagated from patients with polycystic ovary syndrome. *J Clin Endocrinol Metab.* 2001;86(12):5925–5933
107. Kauffman RP, Baker TE, Baker VM, DiMarino P, Castracane VD. Endocrine and metabolic differences among phenotypic expressions of polycystic ovary syndrome according to the 2003 Rotterdam consensus criteria. *Am J Obstet Gynecol.* 2008;198(6):670.e1–670.e7; discussion 670.e7–670.e10
108. Luque-Ramírez M, Mendieta-Azcona C, Alvarez-Blasco F, Escobar-Morreale HF. Androgen excess is associated with the increased carotid intima-media thickness observed in young women with polycystic ovary syndrome. *Hum Reprod.* 2007;22(12):3197–3203
109. Legro RS, Kunselman AR, Dodson WC, Dunaif A. Prevalence and predictors of risk for type 2 diabetes mellitus and impaired glucose tolerance in polycystic ovary syndrome: a prospective, controlled study in 254 affected women. *J Clin Endocrinol Metab.* 1999;84(1):165–169
110. Ardawi MS, Rouzi AA. Plasma adiponectin and insulin resistance in women with polycystic ovary syndrome. *Fertil Steril.* 2005;83(6):1708–1716
111. Ehrmann DA, Barnes RB, Rosenfield RL, Cavaghan MK, Imperial J. Prevalence of impaired glucose tolerance and diabetes in women with polycystic ovary syndrome. *Diabetes Care.* 1999;22(1):141–146
112. Kousta E, Cela E, Lawrence N, et al. The prevalence of polycystic ovaries in women with a history of gestational diabetes. *Clin Endocrinol (Oxf).* 2000;53(4):501–507
113. Shroff R, Kerchner A, Maifeld M, Van Beek EJ, Jagasia D, Dokras A. Young obese women with polycystic ovary syndrome have evidence of early coronary atherosclerosis. *J Clin Endocrinol Metab.* 2007;92(12):4609–4614
114. Fogel RB, Malhotra A, Pillar G, Pittman SD, Dunaif A, White DP. Increased prevalence of obstructive sleep apnea syndrome in obese women with polycystic ovary syndrome. *J Clin Endocrinol Metab.* 2001;86(3):1175–1180
115. Balen A. Polycystic ovary syndrome and cancer. *Hum Reprod Update.* 2001;7(6):522–525
116. Gadducci A, Gargini A, Palla E, Fanucchi A, Genazzani AR. Polycystic ovary syndrome and gynecological cancers: is there a link? *Gynecol Endocrinol.* 2005;20(4):200–208
117. Navaratnarajah R, Pillay OC, Hardiman P. Polycystic ovary syndrome and endometrial cancer. *Semin Reprod Med.* 2008;26(1):62–71

118. Kahsar-Miller MD, Nixon C, Boots LR, Go RC, Azziz R. Prevalence of polycystic ovary syndrome (PCOS) in first-degree relatives of patients with PCOS. *Fertil Steril.* 2001;75(1): 53–58
119. Li Z, Huang H. Epigenetic abnormality: a possible mechanism underlying the fetal origin of polycystic ovary syndrome. *Med Hypotheses.* 2008;70(3):638–642
120. Katcher HI, Kunselman AR, Dmitrovic R, et al. Comparison of hormonal and metabolic markers after a high-fat, Western meal versus a low-fat, high-fiber meal in women with polycystic ovary syndrome. *Fertil Steril.* 2008; In press
121. Pasquali R, Gambineri A, Biscotti D, et al. Effect of long-term treatment with metformin added to hypocaloric diet on body composition, fat distribution, and androgen and insulin levels in abdominally obese women with and without the polycystic ovary syndrome. *J Clin Endocrinol Metab.* 2000;85(8):2767–2774
122. Caranti DA, de Mello MT, Prado WL, et al. Short- and long-term beneficial effects of a multidisciplinary therapy for the control of metabolic syndrome in obese adolescents. *Metabolism.* 2007;56(9):1293–1300
123. Papadopoulou-Alataki E, Papadopoulou-Legbelou K, Doukas L, Karatzidou K, Pavlitou-Tsiontsi A, Pagkalos E. Clinical and biochemical manifestations of syndrome X in obese children. *Eur J Pediatr.* 2004;163(10):573–579
124. Pan Y, Pratt CA. Metabolic syndrome and its association with diet and physical activity in US adolescents. *J Am Diet Assoc.* 2008;108(2):276–286
125. Quintos JB, Castells S. Management of metabolic syndrome in morbidly obese children and adolescents. *Pediatr Endocrinol Rev.* 2006;3(suppl 4):564–570
126. Chen AK, Roberts CK, Barnard RJ. Effect of a short-term diet and exercise intervention on metabolic syndrome in overweight children. *Metabolism.* 2006;55(7):871–878
127. Kranz S, Mahood L, Wagstaff DA. Diagnostic criteria patterns of U.S. children with metabolic syndrome: NHANES 1999–2002. *Nutr J.* 2007;6:38–41
128. Eisenmann JC. Aerobic fitness, fatness and the metabolic syndrome in children and adolescents. *Acta Paediatr.* 2007;96(12):1723–1729
129. O'Keefe JH, Gheewala NM, O'Keefe JO. Dietary strategies for improving post-prandial glucose, lipids, inflammation, and cardiovascular health. *J Am Coll Cardiol.* 2008;51(3):249–255
130. Greydanus DE, Feucht C, Patel DR. Pharmacotherapy for obese adolescents. *Int J Child Health Hum Dev.* 2009;7(3):22–35
131. Puri M, Flynn JT. Management of hypertension in children and adolescents with the metabolic syndrome. *J Cardiometab Syndr.* 2006;1(4):259–268
132. Ornstein RM, Jacobson MS. Supersize teens: the metabolic syndrome. *Adolesc Med Clin.* 2006;17(3):565–587; abstract x
133. Bakris GL, Toto RD, McCullough PA, et al. Effects of different ACE inhibitor combinations on albuminuria: results of the GUARD study. *Kidney Int.* 2008;73(11):1303–1309
134. Lewis EJ, Lewis JB. Treatment of diabetic nephropathy with angiotensin II receptor antagonist. *Clin Exp Nephrol.* 2003;7(1):1–8
135. Rodrigo R, Prat H, Passalacqua W, Araya J, Guichard C, Bächler JP. Relationship between oxidative stress and essential hypertension. *Hypertens Res.* 2007;30(12):1159–1167
136. Rodríguez-Morán M, Guerrero-Romero F. Hyperinsulinemia in healthy children and adolescents with a positive family history for type 2 diabetes. *Pediatrics.* 2006;118(5). Available at: www.pediatrics.org/cgi/content/full/118/5/e1516
137. Franks PW, Hanson RL, Knowler WC, et al. Childhood predictors of young-onset type 2 diabetes. *Diabetes.* 2007;56(12):2964–2972
138. Executive Summary: Standards of Medical Care in Diabetes—2008 American Diabetes Association: clinical practice recommendations. *Diabetes Care.* 2008;31(suppl):S5–S11
139. Donekal S, Shomali ME. Effectiveness of the novel anti-diabetes medication exenatide in everyday practice: comparison with clinical trials. *Diabetes Res Clin Pract.* 2008;80(2):e4–e6

140. Klonoff DC, Buse JB, Nielsen LL, et al. Exenatide effects on diabetes, obesity, cardiovascular risk factors and hepatic biomarkers in patients with type 2 diabetes treated for at least 3 years. *Curr Med Res Opin.* 2008;24(1):275–286
141. Jeha GS, Heptulla RA. Newer therapeutic options for children with diabetes mellitus: theoretical and practical considerations. *Pediatr Diabetes.* 2006;7(2):122–138
142. Daniels SR, Greer FR; American Academy of Pediatrics, Committee on Nutrition. Lipid screening and cardiovascular health in childhood. *Pediatrics.* 2008;122(1):198–208
143. Fazio S. Management of mixed dyslipidemia in patients with or at risk for cardiovascular disease: a role for combination fibrate therapy. *Clin Ther.* 2008;30(2):294–306
144. Moriarty PM. LDL-apheresis therapy. *Curr Treat Options Cardiovasc Med.* 2006;8(4):282–288
145. O'Keefe JH, Bell DS. Postprandial hyperglycemia/hyperlipidemia (postprandial dysmetabolism) is a cardiovascular risk factor. *Am J Cardiol.* 2007;100(5):899–904
146. Greydanus DE, Omar HA, Tsitsika AK, Patel DR. Menstrual disorders in adolescent females: current concepts. *Dis Mon.* 2009;55(4):65–125
147. Spritzer PM, Lisboa KO, Mattiello S, Lhullier F. Spironolactone as a single agent for long-term therapy of hirsute patients. *Clin Endocrinol (Oxf).* 2000;52(5):587–594
148. Kasa-Vubu J. Metformin as a weight tool in "at risk" obese adolescents: a magic bullet? *J Pediatr.* 2008;152(6):750–752
149. Eneli I, Mantinan KD. Managing the overweight child. In: Davies HD, Fitzgerald HE, eds. *Obesity in Childhood and Adolescence.* Westport, CT: Praeger; 2008:214–220
150. Srinivasan S, Ambler GR, Bauer LA, et al. Randomized, controlled trial of metformin for obesity and insulin resistance in children and adolescents: improvement in body composition and fasting insulin. *J Clin Endocrinol Metabol.* 2006;91(6):2074–2080
151. Hoppin AG, Katz ES, Kaplan LM, Lauwers GY. Case records of the Massachusetts General Hospital: case 31-2006—a 15-year-old girl with severe obesity. *N Engl J Med.* 2006;355(15): 1593–1602
152. Nestler JE. Metformin for the treatment of polycystic ovary syndrome. *N Engl J Med.* 2008;358(1):47–54
153. Aubuchon M. Polycystic ovarian syndrome (PCOS). In: Hillard PJA, ed. *The 5-Minute Obstetrics-Gynecology Consult.* Philadelphia, PA: Wolters Kluwer/Lippincott Williams & Wilkins; 2008:158–159
154. Jensterle M, Janez A, Mlinar B, Marc J, Prezelj J, Pfeifer M. Impact of metformin and rosiglitazone treatment on glucose transporter 4 mRNA expression in women with polycystic ovary syndrome. *Eur J Endocrinol.* 2008;158(6):793–801
155. DeFronzo RA. Lilly lecture: the triumvirate—beta cell, muscle, liver. A collusion responsible for NIDDM. *Diabetes.* 1988;37(6):667–687
156. Felig P, Wahren J, Hendler R. Influence of maturity-onset diabetes on splanchnic glucose balance after oral glucose ingestion. *Diabetes.* 1978;27(2):121–126
157. Svedberg J, Strömblad G, Wirth A, Smith U, Björntorp P. Fatty acids in the portal vein regulate hepatic insulin clearance. *J Clin Invest.* 1991;88(6):2054–2058
158. Pittas AG, Joseph NA, Greenberg AS. Adipocytokines and insulin resistance. *J Clin Endocrinol Metab.* 2004;89(2):447–452
159. Chavez BE, Henry RH. Type 2: diabetes—insulin resistance, beta cell dysfunction, and other metabolic and hormonal abnormalities. In: Fonseca VA, ed. *Clinical Diabetes: Translating Research Into Practice.* Philadelphia, PA: Saunders Elsevier; 2006:21–34
160. Fagan TC, Deedwania PC. The cardiovascular dysmetabolic syndrome. *Am J Med.* 1998; 105(1A):77S–82S

Adolesc Med 19 (2008) 498–506

Type 2 Diabetes

Martin B. Draznin, MD, FAAP*

Departments of Pediatrics and Human Development, Michigan State University College of Human Medicine, B240 Life Sciences Building, East Lansing, MI 48824-1317, USA

Pediatric Endocrinology Subspecialty Clinics, Michigan State University Kalamazoo Center for Medical Studies, 1000 Oakland Drive, Kalamazoo, MI 49008-1284, USA

Type 2 diabetes mellitus occurs when an individual can no longer respond sufficiently to endogenous insulin to maintain blood glucose levels in the normal range. It has strong familial expression[1] with high concordance between identical twins, unlike type 1 diabetes, which is predominately autoimmune in origin.[2] The incidence of type 2 diabetes in adolescents has seemingly increased along with the increase in the prevalence of obesity, and for some ethnic groups the risk seems to be much higher than in others.[3]

Symptoms and signs of type 2 diabetes can be subtle, as in adults. However, a significant percentage of youth with newly diagnosed type 2 diabetes present with ketoacidosis,[4] causing confusion with type 1 diabetes. Some of the newer antipsychotic medications are associated with weight gain and onset of type 2 diabetes.[5] Monogenic diabetes, previously known as maturity-onset diabetes of youth (MODY), can present as a mild-seeming form of diabetes in youth that is not associated with obesity and may be confused with type 2 diabetes.[6] Finally, with the increasing rate of obesity, type 1 diabetes occurring in obese children and adolescents may be diagnosed before they have experienced significant weight loss. Laboratory assessment of circulating antibodies to islet-cell antigens and to insulin as well as measuring C peptide in the circulation can help to differentiate type 1 from type 2 diabetes, although there have been reports of antibodies at presentation in some cases of typical-seeming type 2 diabetes.[7] Interested readers can get an idea of the potential for confusion from a recent editorial.[8] The diagnosis of diabetes is made when the standard criteria have been met (Table 1). The fasting blood glucose level may be relatively insensitive compared with the postprandial level or a so-called random level. In some instances, glucose-tolerance testing may be required. Preparation for the oral glucose-tolerance test includes proper nutrition (with ≥300 g carbohydrates)

*Corresponding author.
E-mail address: draznin@kcms.msu.edu (M. B. Draznin).

 ISSN 1934-4287

Table 1
Diagnostic criteria for diabetes

1. Fasting plasma glucose level of ≥126 mg/dL (8 h with no caloric intake), or
2. Symptoms of hyperglycemia and a random plasma glucose level of ≥200 mg/dL (random is without regard to time since last meal or time of day; symptoms of hyperglycemia include polyuria, polydipsia and unexplained weight loss), or
3. 2-h plasma glucose level of ≥200 mg/dL during an oral glucose-tolerance test (the test should be performed by using 1.75 g of glucose per kg of body weight up to a maximum of 75 g)

Modified from American Diabetes Association. *Diabetes Care.* 2008;31(suppl 1):S55–S60.

based on total caloric need for size and age, eaten per day for the 3 days beforehand, to avoid a false-positive study and entails an overnight fast before the challenge with glucose solution.

So-called lifestyle modifications (improved nutrition, increased physical activity, and weight loss) have been the foundation of treatment for type 2 diabetes, because they can have a profound effect on the diabetic state, yielding a transient remission in some cases. Lifestyle changes may be difficult for some youth; if the entire family is not supportive of their efforts, and other family members do not adopt some of the changes in support of their efforts, success is hard to achieve. Control of total caloric intake, avoidance of a diet high in simple carbohydrates, and possibly low-carbohydrate diets can all lead to improved glucose tolerance by virtue of weight reduction.

Complications of type 2 diabetes include those occurring in the short-term and over the long-term (Table 2). Recurrent ketoacidosis should be much less common in youth with type 2 diabetes than in type 1 diabetes, because the initial presentation with ketoacidosis in subjects with type 2 diabetes occurs in those naive to any treatment, and they are less prone to ketoacidosis when being treated. A hyperglycemic hyperosmolar state is a serious emergency and requires

Table 2
Complications of diabetes

Short-term
- Ketoacidosis
- Hyperglycemic hyperosmolar state
- Hypoglycemia (caused by medications)

Long-term
- Retinopathy
- Nephropathy with or without hypertension
- Dyslipidemia
- Neuropathy (usually a late consequence)
- Large blood vessel disease (usually a late consequence)
- Cutaneous lesions
- Cataracts (usually a late consequence)

exquisite attention to detail in managing fluid and electrolyte balance during its treatment.[9,10] When the so-called oral hypoglycemic agents, those which increase insulin secretion, are in use or when agents leading to delayed absorption of carbohydrates from the gastrointestinal tract are used, hypoglycemia can be a significant risk. Long-term complications of diabetes are thought to be a result of the exposure to hyperglycemia over time; thus, the goal of achieving control of blood glucose levels is just as important as it is in the patient with type 1 diabetes. Nonproliferative retinopathy caused by damage to retinal capillaries with exudates, bleeding into the retina, and macular edema may be succeeded by proliferative retinopathy, in which unregulated revascularization can lead to retinal detachment. Damage to the glomerular ground substance and increased pressure of blood flow through the glomerulus is also thought to be a result of hyperglycemia and leads to initial proteinuria and hypertension with eventual renal failure. Similarly, neuropathy seems related to experiencing hyperglycemia over time. Of concern is that microalbuminuria and hypertension seem to be occurring earlier in youth with type 2 diabetes than in their counterparts with type 1 disease.[11]

Medications for type 2 diabetes (Table 3) include several types with differing properties and adverse effects. There has been insufficient study of safety and efficacy in children of most antidiabetic drugs for there to be US Food and Drug Administration (FDA) indications for their use; off-label use has been a historical inevitability in the care of children and adolescents but should never be done casually, and it ideally should have its basis in well-conducted clinical trials, although those trials are not sufficiently powered for FDA recognition. Information about the mode of action, adverse effects, and whether there is a pediatric indication for these agents was obtained from the Physician's Desk Reference for 2008. It may be reasonable, but not supported by robust evidence, to assume that

Table 3
Medications for type 2 diabetes

Agent	Class	Pediatric Indication?	Action(s)	Adverse Effects
Metformin	Biguanide	Yes	Lowerspp glucose	Gastrointestinal
Several	Oral hypoglycemic agents	No	Increase insulin secretion	Low blood glucose level
Several	Thiazolidinedione (PPAR activators)	No	Increase insulin Weight gain	
Several	α-Glucosidase inhibitors	No	Lower glucose excursion	Gastrointestinal
Exenatide	Glucagon-like peptide 1 mimic	No	Lowers glucose excursion, leads to satiety	Gastrointestinal
Pramlintide	Incretin mimic	≥15 y	Similar to exenatide	Gastrointestinal
Sitagliptin	DPP-4 inhibitor	No	Enhances incretin action	Idiosyncratic allergic

older adolescents may experience similar risk/benefit characteristics with these medications as do younger adults. Metformin, a biguanide, has long-term evidence of efficacy for type 2 diabetes and a good safety profile, especially because youth would not have experienced much risk of renal insufficiency from their diabetes at diagnosis, which makes lactic acidosis unlikely. The adverse effects may be quite unpleasant but resolve over days to weeks for all but a handful of patients. Metformin also affects weight loss, even more so in individuals who faithfully adhere to their nutrition and exercise plans. Hypoglycemia is uncommon in patients treated solely with metformin. Metformin has a pediatric indication from the FDA. The oral hypoglycemic agents, such as glipizide, are also effective in blood glucose control but present an increased risk of hypoglycemia and can add to weight gain because of their mechanism (increased release of insulin after meals). Thiazolidinedione medications, also known as peroxisome proliferator activating receptor (PPAR) agents, act on muscle, liver, and adipose tissue to increase sensitivity to insulin. In the adult literature there has been concern about fluid retention, edema, and even congestive heart failure.[12] The first-generation PPAR agent, troglitazone, was associated with hepatic failure, which was fatal in some cases; it is no longer marketed. The major drawback with these agents other than uncertainty about long-term safety and lack of FDA indication in youth is that their use is associated with weight gain. The α-glucosidase enzyme inhibitors act to slow the absorption of glucose so that the patient's endogenous insulin can act more effectively. They are occasionally associated with hypoglycemia, but the main drawbacks to their use are complaints of abdominal pain, diarrhea, and flatulence, all of which are secondary to presentation of sugars to the flora in the lower intestine, at which carbohydrates would otherwise have been absorbed earlier after being digested higher in the gastrointestinal tract. These adverse effects may be ameliorated with time. At present, however, there is not an FDA indication for their use in children.

Exenatide is an agent that mimics the activity of glucagon-like peptide 1 (GLP-1). Used in combination with metformin or oral hypoglycemic agents, it is given by injection twice daily to increase insulin secretion by the pancreatic β cells, diminish inappropriate glucagon secretion, and slow the rate of gastric emptying. These 3 actions complement the other agents. The adverse effects, abdominal pain and diarrhea, may be intolerable to some patients. For those who do tolerate exenatide, there is the added benefit of weight reduction. Exenatide does not currently have an FDA pediatric indication. Although a recent notification by the FDA of cases of fatal and nonfatal cases of pancreatitis in patients using exenatide did not specifically list children and adolescents as at risk, caution in using this agent was advised for all patients.[13] Pramlintide, another newer agent, is also injected and is indicated to be used solely as an adjunct to insulin therapy. It can be used for both type 1 and type 2 diabetes. It is an incretin analog and acts to modulate gastric emptying to delay and minimize the postprandial elevation of blood glucose. Its use also leads to a sensation of fullness. Use of pramlintide is associated with a risk for hypoglycemia and requires reduction of the insulin dose. Lowering the insulin requirement and generating a sensation of satiety may assist in weight reduction. At present, pramlintide does have a pediatric indication from the FDA; however, it is limited to those aged ≥15 years. Sitagliptin is an inhibitor of dipeptidyl peptidase 4, a proteolytic enzyme that degrades incretins regardless of whether they are endogenous or mimics taken as drugs, it is given orally, and it has not yet been given an FDA indication for use in children and youth.

Insulin therapy for type 2 diabetes (Table 4) has a long history. The original crystalline or "regular" insulin required multiple injections throughout the day. Development of the recently discontinued Lente insulin, a suspension of insulin crystals to slow the absorption of the insulin, and of neutral protamine Hagedorn (NPH) insulin, in which a buffered suspension containing insulin and protamine reduced the solubility both gave prolonged action and assisted type 2 diabetic patients with simplification of care. With the advent of molecular genetics and a better understanding of blood glucose fluctuation, development of the very rapidly acting insulin analogs (lispro, aspart, and glulisine) afforded true "prandial" insulin to more accurately cover meals eaten with less residual postprandial persistence of high insulin levels. At about the same time, insulin glargine and insulin detemir were developed to provide "basal" insulin to prevent non–meal-related blood glucose elevation. Varying strategies for insulin coverage with these new analogs have been introduced for type 2 diabetes, such as prandial insulin alone or with other agents, basal insulin alone, basal insulin with prandial insulin, continuous subcutaneous insulin infusion (insulin pumps), premixed fixed-ratio NPH with analog insulin to minimize the numbers of daily injections, etc. All forms of insulin therapy present the associated risk of hypoglycemia, and

Table 4
Insulin therapy for type 2 diabetes

Type	Use	Characteristics
Human		
Regular	Prandial	Longer acting than optimal' need to inject 45 min before eating
NPH	Basal	Has large peak at 6–8 h and does not last 24 h
Human insulin analogs		
Lispro, aspart, and glulisine	Prandial	Optimal pharmacokinetics; more expensive; glulisine does not yet have a pediatric indication
Glargine	Basal	Very nearly without significant peak, good duration stings
Detemir	Basal	May need large total dose for true 24-h coverage
Premixed	Combined	Lack of flexibility may be troublesome; easier to use
NPH and analogs		

all forms of insulin therapy can lead to an increase in weight unless nutritional therapy is carefully followed. Treatment goals in type 2 diabetes are near-normalization of blood glucose levels, weight control or reduction, normalization of lipid levels, normalization of blood pressure, and prevention or at least slowing of the onset of long-term complications. At the same time, avoidance of hypoglycemia, a hyperosmotic crisis, or diabetic ketoacidosis in some individuals must be stressed. Recommended standards of care are summarized in Table 5. Standards of care include self-monitoring of blood glucose levels. This monitoring had historically been limited to the morning fasting level, although recent studies suggest that postprandial blood glucose excursion may be an important factor that confers risk of complications (see ref 14 for a concise review of the issue). Glycohemoglobin levels assess previous average blood glucose levels over a span of up to 3 months. Assessment of weight control, blood pressure, and ophthalmologic, renal, and neurologic status must all be part of the office visit.

A structured team approach to diabetes clinic visits is valuable for assisting youth in their self-management. Diabetes self-care education should not stop with the first hospitalization or initial diagnosis. Nutrition education should also be provided in an ongoing manner to provide support and help to optimize adherence. Visits as often as every 3 months are warranted to help sustain the continued efforts by the youth and family members to get good results. The interval history should assess the self-care that is being done, how accurately the treatment plan has been followed, what the blood glucose testing has shown, what impact the diabetes has had on daily life, and what effects any intercurrent illness may have had on the diabetes care. Assessments of growth, progression in puberty, blood pressure control, retinal screening examination with a handheld ophthalmoscope

Table 5
Standards for care

- Clinic visits every 3 mo if possible
- History: Details of self-care, how accurately it is done, log book or blood glucose meter download to assess self-blood glucose monitoring; nutrition, exercise, taking of medications, symptoms related to diabetes or diabetes therapy, intercurrent illness and effect on the diabetes, how well school and/or work are going, whether there is any barrier to excellent self-care at school or work, family support, emotional well-being
- Solicit questions by patient/family about self-care or other diabetes-related matters (eg, how well expenses for supplies are being covered by insurance, any lapses in care)
- Physical examination: height and weight for growth assessment, progress through puberty or any sign of delay, BMI, blood pressure, examination of retinas (yearly slit-lamp examination through dilated pupils by expert consultant in addition to routine examination each time in clinic), signs of cardiovascular changes, assess for peripheral neuropathy annually, inspection of teeth and gums for gingival inflammation, etc, skin evaluation for specific changes such as lipohypertrophy from not rotating insulin injection site, infections
- Laboratory: hemoglobin A1c level at each visit, annual lipid panel, annual albumin/creatinine ratio, hepatic enzyme levels if using metformin
- Continuing diabetes self-care education: at each visit as needed

(with referral for an annual dilated-pupil slit-lamp examination by an expert consultant), dental evaluation with strong recommendations for twice-annual dental examination and cleaning, assessment of any adverse effects from medications or of complication from insulin injections and blood glucose monitoring, annual assessment of lipid levels, nutritional assessment and counseling, weight-management assessment and counseling, and assessment of family support for the self-care by the youth are all needed to optimize outcome.

Treatment of complications may require expert consultation and treatment from colleagues in ophthalmology, nephrology, and neurology. Psychosocial health is an important foundation for both success in "lifestyle" modification and use of medications, and at the same time it is an area in which expert consultation and treatment may be required to allow treatment goals to be met. Medications/treatments for diabetes complications (Table 6) may be administered by the diabetes physician or by a specialist consultant (eg, nephrologist, cardiologist).

Ideally, retinopathy should be prevented by tight blood glucose control. The retina specialist must be involved to provide any needed laser or other surgical treatments for macular edema or proliferative retinopathy. For hypertension and/or nephropathy, the first-line treatment would include improved control of blood glucose and weight reduction. Angiotensin-converting enzyme antagonists are highly effective but have adverse effects of dry cough and rash and a significant risk of teratogenicity when taken by a pregnant adolescent. The mechanism of action yields a renal-protective dilatation of the efferent arterioles, which lowers filtration pressure across the glomerulus; this can lessen proteinuria

Table 6
Treatment for diabetes complications

Complication	Agent/Treatment	Benefits	Risks
Retinopathy	Blood glucose control	Visual protection	Hypoglycemia?
	Ophthalmologic procedures	Halts progression	Risks of procedure
Hypertension	Angiotensin-converting enzyme inhibitors	Renal protection	Cough, rash, birth defects
	Angiotensin receptor blockers		Weight loss
Nephropathy	Angiotensin-converting enzyme inhibitors, angiotensin receptor blockers	Blood glucose control	Hypoglycemia, same as for hypertension
Dyslipidemia	Blood glucose control	Many	Hypoglycemia
	Exercise	Normalize lipids	Skeletal muscle, liver damage
	Weight loss		
	Statin class drugs		
Neuropathy	Blood glucose control	May reverse?	Hypoglycemia
	Pain-relief medicines		
	Autonomic symptom relief		

as well as lower blood pressure. Angiotensin receptor blockers have a similar effect, but although they act at a different part of the pathway, they also introduce the risk for teratogenesis. Dyslipidemia should initially be approached as a consequence of blood glucose levels and weight control, but elevation of the low-density lipoprotein cholesterol fraction above 100 mg/dL that does not respond to dietary improvement, lowering of blood glucose, and increased exercise may warrant treatment with a statin-class drug. There is little experience with these agents in children; the hepatic and skeletal muscle complications noted in the adult material in the Physician's Desk Reference suggest that careful laboratory follow-up and routine questioning about fatigue and muscle weakness or pain would be prudent in youth.

Goals for therapy in type 2 diabetes should take into account balancing the pervasive nature of diabetes-related complications and the intrusive nature of treatments as they affect a patient who is in the process of becoming who he or she will be for an entire adult life. Blood glucose levels should be brought as close to normal as can safely be achieved; the hemoglobin A1c level is usually used as the index of glycemic control, but controlling the postprandial excursion of blood glucose may, with more experience, be found to be even more important. More data are needed before applying that standard, with its increased requirement for blood glucose testing, to youthful patients. Weight should be decreased toward a BMI in the healthy range. Physical activity should be encouraged to protect cardiovascular health and improve blood glucose control. The onset of microvascular and macrovascular complications should be slowed or prevented by good blood glucose control. Kidney function should also be maintained, and damage to the peripheral and autonomous nervous system should be minimized. The adolescent with type 2 diabetes should be able to live a full and active life. Emotional health should be supported, and family involvement in the diabetes care should be appropriate in allowing autonomy without neglecting oversight.

REFERENCES

1. Pinhas-Hamiel O, Zeitler P. The global spread of type 2 diabetes in children and adolescents. *J Pediatr.* 2005;146(5):693–700
2. American Diabetes Association. Diagnosis and classification of diabetes mellitus. *Diabetes Care.* 2008;31(suppl 1):S55–S60
3. Shaw J. Epidemiology of childhood type 2 diabetes and obesity. *Pediatr Diabetes.* 2007;8(suppl 9):7–15
4. Sapru A, Gitelman SE, Bhatia S, Dubin R, Newman TB, Flori H. Prevalence and characteristics of type 2 diabetes mellitus in 9–18 year-old children with diabetic ketoacidosis. *J Pediatr Endocrinol Metab.* 2005;18(9):865–872
5. Davis V, Rosenbloom AL. Metabolic effects of antipsychotic drugs. *Pediatr Diabetes.* 2006; 7(3):176–186
6. Winter WE. Maturity-onset diabetes of youth and other genetic conditions associated with diabetes. In: Lifshitz F, ed. *Pediatric Endocrinology.* 4th ed. New York, NY: Informa Health Care; 2007:189–209
7. Umpaichitra V, Banerji MA, Castells S. Autoantibodies in children with type 2 diabetes mellitus. *J Pediatr Endocrinol Metab.* 2002;15(suppl 1):525–530

8. Rosenbloom AL. Distinguishing type 1 and type 2 diabetes at diagnosis: what is the problem? *Pediatr Diabetes*. 2007;8(2):51–52
9. Fourtner SH, Weinzimer SA, Katz LEL. Hyperglycemic hyperosmolar non-ketotic syndrome in children with type 2 diabetes. *Pediatr Diabetes*. 2005;6(3):129–135
10. Hollander AS, Olney RC, Blackett PR, Marshall BA. Fatal malignant hyperthermia-like syndrome with rhabdomyolysis complicating the presentation of diabetes mellitus in adolescent males. *Pediatrics*. 2003;111(6 pt 1):1447–1452
11. Eppens MK, Craig ME, Cusumano RN, et al. Prevalence of diabetes complications in adolescents with type 2 compared with type 1 diabetes. *Diabetes Care*. 2006;29(6):1300–1306
12. Cheng AY, Fantus IG. Thiazoladinedione-induced congestive heart failure. *Ann Pharmacother*. 2004;38(5):817–820
13. US Food and Drug Administration Center for Drug Evaluation and Research. Information for healthcare professionals exenatide (marked as Byetta). Available at: www.fda.gov/CDER/drug/InfoSheets/HCP/exenatide2008HCP.htm. Accessed October 27, 2008
14. Monnier L, Colette C. Glycemic variability: should we and can we prevent it? *Diabetes Care*. 2008;31(suppl 2):S150–S154

Adolesc Med 19 (2008) 507–520

Screening Adolescents for Lipid Disorders: What Is the Best Approach?

Brian P. Jenssen, BA[a], Marc S. Jacobson, MD*[b]

[a]*University of Rochester School of Medicine and Dentistry, 601 Elmwood Ave, Box 40, Rochester, NY 14642, USA*

[b]*Department of Pediatrics and Epidemiology, Albert Einstein College of Medicine, 833 Northern Blvd, Suite 230, Great Neck, NY 11021, USA*

Coronary artery disease is the most common cause of death in the United States and the leading cause of hospital-related health care costs. Hypercholesterolemia is a leading risk factor for cardiovascular disease (CVD), and both genetic and environmental factors affect cholesterol levels. Although the clinical symptoms and signs of elevated cholesterol levels in children do not occur until adulthood, arterial dysfunction and plaque formation begin much earlier. Thirty-six percent of US youth have a cholesterol level that is higher than normal (>170 mg/dL), with elevated low-density lipoprotein (LDL) levels associated with atherosclerotic lesions and ultimate disease.[1] Because the disease process begins in childhood and adolescence, early prevention in childhood is critically important.

A tenet of early prevention includes screening, which entails using the evidence base concerning a condition to search for precursors or preclinical signs of that condition in ostensibly healthy people. Although screening offers the benefit of preventing potential disease, morbidity, and mortality and associated health expenditures and resources, it is not without risks and costs. These include, for example, false-positive and false-negative test results, which can lead to unnecessary and potentially harmful and costly follow-up in the former group and failing to help those at risk of disease in the latter group.

This review will focus on the potential benefits and adverse effects of screening children and adolescents for lipid disorders. Particular emphasis will be placed on the evidence base and controversy surrounding the current guidelines, the potential and utility of universal, population-based screening, and other available screening options. Brief attention will be placed also on management and treatment of lipid disorders.

*Corresponding author.
E-mail address: daktah@gmail.com (M. S. Jacobson).

 ISSN 1934-4287

ATHEROSCLEROTIC PROCESS

Atherosclerosis is a pathologic process in the arterial intima-media that begins in childhood and progresses over a period of many decades. The earliest abnormality is the fatty streak, an infiltration of lipid-laden macrophages and proliferation of smooth muscle cells within the intima of arteries at susceptible locations. These initial changes can manifest in the aorta and coronary arteries of infants and progressively worsen and result in altered endothelial structure and function by the time of adolescence. The altered endothelium, known as atheromatous plaque, can cause narrowing of the arterial lumen and a nidus for thrombus. In the relatively small coronary arteries, the narrowing caused by plaque, with concomitant stiffness and risk for thrombus, is the basis for clinical coronary heart disease (CHD).

The development of atherosclerotic lesions has been studied extensively in adolescents by using pathologic autopsy data combined with premortem and postmortem risk-factor assessments and in vivo studies. Studies over the past 20 years have shown clearly that the commonly described risk factors in adults, such as elevated LDL cholesterol level, low high-density lipoprotein (HDL) cholesterol level, high triglyceride level, hypertension, obesity, diabetes, and smoking, are directly associated in a dose-response fashion with the prevalence and extent of arterial lesions in adolescents and young adults. Newer in vivo imaging studies have shown that early vascular stiffening and intimal thickening can be measured in adolescents at risk, including those with a family history of premature myocardial infarction. These studies also have shown that improvements in observed risk factors, such as elevated LDL cholesterol level and BMI, can be correlated with improved vascular reactivity. Thus, a large evidence base has identified the pediatric risk factors associated with CVD, and there is a growing body of literature in support of techniques available to ameliorate the markers of future disease.

DYSLIPIDEMIA

Abnormal cholesterol concentrations, or dyslipidemia, are disturbances of lipoprotein metabolism defined by statistically determined criteria and laboratory testing. They are highly correlated with the extent and progression of plaque. An elevated LDL cholesterol level is the most often used clinical determinant of dyslipidemia in children, whereas other markers can include elevations in total cholesterol (TC) or triglyceride level or deficiencies in HDL cholesterol. A screening program could identify abnormal cholesterol concentrations within 3 main groups of adolescents: (1) those with monogenic dyslipidemias, such as familial hypercholesterolemia (FH); (2) those with dyslipidemias secondary to diseases such as diabetes, hypothyroidism, hepatitis, or AIDS; and (3) those with multifactorial dyslipidemia, including risk factors related to environment, such as obesity or diet. The majority of children and adolescents with dyslipidemias will present with the multifactorial categorization, whereas a minority of them will present with the specific genetic variant.

Monogenic dyslipidemias are those related to genetic disorders. FH, the one disorder in this group with the highest risk of early disease, is an autosomal dominant condition that results from a loss-of-function mutation in alleles that produce hepatic cell-surface LDL receptors. The lessened receptor activity, a result of either decreased number or function, reduces clearance of LDL particles from the blood, resulting in severely elevated LDL levels and subsequent accelerated atherosclerosis and early coronary artery disease. The homozygous form of FH is rare, whereas its heterozygous form is more common, occurring in ~1 in 500 individuals in the United States. Individuals with heterozygous FH have a 20% risk of myocardial infarction in their 20s, and the risk increases to 75% by their 50s.

Unlike the genetically linked FH, multifactorial dyslipidemias include a constellation of risk factors that impart an elevated risk of CVD. Metabolic syndrome, a cluster of risk factors of unknown etiology, is the disorder most representative of this group. The lipid-profile pattern associated with this syndrome includes normal to mildly increased TC and LDL cholesterol levels, moderate-to-severe increase in triglyceride level, and reduced HDL cholesterol level. In adults, metabolic syndrome is currently diagnosed in individuals with ≥3 of the following: high triglyceride level, low HDL cholesterol level, hypertension, central adiposity, and elevated glucose level. In children, a definition is less concrete, and significant debate has yet to lead to a consensus on what exactly constitutes pediatric metabolic syndrome. Regardless, with the rise in incidence of obesity in adolescents, metabolic syndrome will most likely become the most frequent cause of lipid abnormalities seen in pediatric practice.

EVALUATION/ASSESSMENT: CURRENT GUIDELINES

Existing guidelines from the American Academy of Pediatrics (AAP), American Heart Association (AHA), and other major professional groups for screening and managing lipoprotein abnormalities in children and adolescents were based on a report published in 1992 by the National Cholesterol Education Program (NCEP) Expert Panel on Blood Cholesterol Levels in Children and Adolescents.[2] With the goal of lowering elevated cholesterol levels in children and adolescents, the panel recommended 2 strategies: a population-based approach aimed at shifting the population distribution of cholesterol levels and a targeted screening approach to identify those individuals with elevated LDL cholesterol levels in need of further monitoring and management.

For the high-risk individual approach, the panel supported selective screening in the context of regular health care, targeting children and adolescents with a family history of premature CVD or at least 1 parent with high blood cholesterol levels. Specific classifications of abnormal lipid levels were delineated (see Table 1). For children with borderline or at-risk levels, a repeat measurement, averaged with the previous one, was recommended before initiation of treatment.

Before advocating for selective screening, however, the panel considered the utility of universal screening and specifically recommended against it. Four reasons were cited. First, although high cholesterol levels in children generally predict cholesterol elevations in adulthood, "quite a few" children with cholesterol levels identified as high in childhood would not have high enough levels once they reach adulthood to meet criteria for individualized treatment. Second, universal screening could cause many children to be labeled as patients with a disease, causing undue anxiety for children and their families. Third, for most children not from high-risk families, sufficient time exists to allow delaying cholesterol-lowering therapies until they reach adulthood. Finally, insufficient evidence exists concerning the long-term safety and efficacy of drug therapy in childhood to reduce CHD morbidity and mortality in adulthood, and universal screening could lead to overuse of cholesterol-lowering drugs in childhood and adolescence. Although the NCEP guidelines, including the recommendation against universal screening, have been considered the standard of care for more than a decade, there is vigorous debate in the literature concerning updating the NCEP guidelines, including the option of promoting universal screening using blood tests.

CHALLENGES WITH EXISTING NCEP GUIDELINES

A recent scientific statement from the AHA provides a comprehensive review and summary of the challenges with the existing NCEP guidelines.[3] First, the panel seems to have underestimated the number of children who would be targeted for screening, possibly by as much 20% (see Table 2). Second, several studies have revealed that targeted screening based on family history has a relatively low efficacy. Third, limited compliance with the guidelines, both from physicians and families, may further reduce their effectiveness. Fourth, additional limitations may exist with the sensitivity and specificity of the screening cut points. The guidelines use set thresholds that apply across race, gender, and age and fail to account for the variability in TC and HDL cholesterol levels that occur throughout these groupings, thus altering the statistical accuracy of the screening method. Other effects on sensitivity and specificity include measure-

Table 1
1992 NCEP classification of lipid risk for children and adolescents

	At Risk	Borderline	Within Guidelines
TC level, mg/dL	>200	170–200	<170
LDL cholesterol level, mg/dL	>160	130–160	<130

Table 2
AHA challenges with NCEP guidelines

Challenge	Reason
Underestimation of number of children targeted for screening	Panel estimated that family history would lead to ~25% of children and adolescents being targeted for screening
	Population-based studies, including several published around the same time of the NCEP guidelines, estimated that between 36% and 46% of children and adolescents would be screened
Low efficacy of targeted screening based on family history	Only 50% of children and adolescents with an elevated LDL cholesterol level would be selected for screening when using guidelines
	Low efficacy in part related to incomplete or unavailable family history
Limited physician and family compliance	Two studies, reported 10 y apart, showed that only two thirds of pediatric health care providers self-report that they selectively screen children on the basis of family history of CVD
	Low levels of parental compliance with both cholesterol screening and intervention are also reported
Sensitivity/specificity limitations in universal set cut points	Guidelines fail to account for variability in TC and HDL cholesterol levels in race, gender, and sexual maturation (eg, girls tend to have higher TC levels than boys, increasing the sensitivity but decreasing the specificity for girls)
	Measurement error and intraindividual variation
	Only 41% of children with a TC level of >200 mg/dL had a level that high 1 y later
Focus solely on elevated LDL cholesterol levels	Fails to address other lipoprotein abnormalities, including decreased HDL cholesterol or elevated triglyceride levels
	Increasing prevalence of these disorders based on their association with obesity and metabolic syndrome

ment error and intraindividual variation in cholesterol levels. Finally, another important limitation in the screening recommended by the NCEP guidelines includes focusing only on elevated LDL cholesterol without addressing other lipoprotein abnormalities.

In addition to the challenges with the current guidelines, the AHA committee also addressed the groups of children for which the NCEP did not make specific recommendations. Overweight and obesity, which increase the risk for type 2 diabetes, hypertension, insulin resistance, and the metabolic syndrome, have increased significantly over the last 10 to 15 years. The association and impact of these various, often interrelated disorders on lipoprotein abnormalities, along with the reasons underlying their increased prevalence, will most likely require new ways of both identifying and managing those children at risk. The NCEP guidelines also did not make specific recommendations about lipid abnormalities other than elevated LDL cholesterol levels, although the AHA panelists noted that a sufficient evidence base is lacking concerning screening and management of these other disorders. Finally, specific conditions that place individuals at high risk of both lipoprotein abnormalities and CVD, such as diabetes, transplantation, or HIV infection, are without recommendations for management.

After summarizing the limitations and shortcomings of the NCEP guidelines, the AHA committee suggested 5 modifications. Two of the suggested modifications focus on screening, and 3 of them focus on drug treatment (not within the scope of this review). For screening, in addition to family history, the presence of overweight and/or obesity should trigger screening. If those children are identified as having lipid abnormalities, further screening should focus on other aspects of the metabolic syndrome, including insulin resistance and type 2 diabetes, hypertension, or central adiposity.

SHOULD ALL CHILDREN BE SCREENED?

Although the AHA committee suggested important modifications to the current guidelines, the scientific statement did not explicitly discuss the utility of universal screening of cholesterol levels. Considering the rising epidemic of obesity and overweight in children and adolescents and the associated rise in dyslipidemia, the pertinent question remains: Should all children and adolescents be screened for dyslipidemia? The US Preventive Services Task Force (USPSTF) has provided a systematic evidence review of this question and focused on screening relevant to children in primary care settings without previously identified dyslipidemias.[4]

The explicit goal of the USPSTF review was to synthesize the published evidence regarding the effectiveness of selecting, testing, and managing children and adolescents with dyslipidemia in the course of routine primary care. The review, which followed the strict methodology used by other USPSTF reviews, identified relevant studies through Medline searches from 1966 until September 2005. The answers to 7 key questions relevant to general principles of effective screening were sought (see Table 3). Their literature search identified 2507 unique citations, which included 144 articles about screening and testing for dyslipidemia, 43 about interventions and tracking lipid values over time, 6 about the adverse effects of screening, and 84 about adverse effects of treatment. The reviewers concluded that "the evidence is insufficient to recommend for or against routine screening for lipid disorders in infants, children, adolescents or young adults (up to age 20)." The conclusion was rated as a grade I statement, meaning that "the USPSTF concludes that the current evidence is insufficient to assess the balance of benefits and harms of the service. Evidence is lacking, of poor quality, or conflicting, and the balance of benefits and harms cannot be determined."[5]

The conclusions drawn from the USPSTF report are telling. Several of the key questions identified by the panel have not been addressed. Studies are lacking

Table 3
USPSTF general principles of effective screening

Question	Conclusions
Is screening children/adolescents for dyslipidemia effective in delaying the onset and/or reducing the incidence of CHD-related events?	No evidence
What is the accuracy and feasibility of screening for dyslipidemia in identifying children/adolescents at risk for CVD? (6 subquestions)	
a. What are abnormal lipid values in children/adolescents?	Discusses NCEP guidelines; noted growing body of literature that questions utility of fixed screening cut points across age, gender, and race
b. What are the appropriate tests, and how well do they identify children/adolescents with dyslipidemia?	TC, initial laboratory measurement, but use the LDL cholesterol level as the basis for initiating treatment and determining goals of therapy; ability of TC levels to detect elevated LDL cholesterol, examined with Lipid Research Clinics data and data from the Bogalusa cohort (elevated fasting TC level identified elevated LDL cholesterol in ranges of 44%–69% sensitivity and 90%–98% specificity); following recommendations for adults, discussed potential benefits in measuring both TC and HDL cholesterol levels; may help distinguish false-negative and true-negative results
What is the available information about lipid-level tracking from childhood to adulthood?	Various US and non-US cohorts have shown that ~40%–55% of children with elevated lipid levels, defined by percentile within the population distribution, will continue to have elevated lipid levels on follow-up (4–15 y)
c. What is the accuracy of family history in determining risk?	Evaluated several "good-quality" studies; variety of definitions of family history risk factors; regardless, using positive family history to select for cholesterol screening misses a large percentage of children with elevated cholesterol levels, ranging from 17% to 90% overall and 30% to 60% in most studies
What, besides family history, are other important risk factors?	Overweight or body fat composition measures, with childhood overweight, as measured with BMI, being the best independent predictor of adult dyslipidemia after LDL cholesterol level
d. What are effective screening strategies?	Current screening strategies have limited diagnostic accuracy, low adherence to guidelines by providers, and limited compliance by parents and children; no trials have compared strategies of screening in children (eg, school, pediatric clinic, or hospital)

(*Continued*)

Table 3
(Continued)

Question	Conclusions
2. What are the adverse effects of screening, including statistical errors and psychological effects?	Studies have demonstrated lack of parental compliance with screening and follow-up recommendations; studies don't seem to have addressed the issue of false-positive and false-negative results, instead focusing on issues of "labeling"; no studies have reported increased anxiety or depression among screened children or parents
3. What is the effectiveness of various therapies in reducing incidence of adult dyslipidemia and/or reducing the incidence or delaying the onset of CHD-related events?	No evidence
4. What is the effectiveness of drug, diet, exercise, and combination therapy for treating dyslipidemia in children/adolescents?	40 randomized, controlled trials included; (1) for children with probable or definite FH; drug treatment showed statins are effective for reducing TC and LDL levels; diet treatment marginally effective; exercise treatment, no studies; (2) for children with elevated lipids without FH; no studies; diet treatment marginally effective; exercise treatment, no change in lipids; combination diet and exercise, few trials, but all showed improvement in lipid levels
5. What are the adverse effects of such treatments?	Studies not of sufficient duration to determine long-term effects of either short or extended use of any therapy; information available: statins associated with elevated liver enzyme and creatine kinase levels, bile acid–binding resins with adverse gastrointestinal effects, decreased levels of serum vitamins and minerals, low-fat diets associated with growth retardation in 3 children, although most studies have shown normal growth and development in children >2 y old on monitored diets, and few adverse effects other than ephemeral elevated blood pressures noted with exercise
6. Does improving non-FH dyslipidemia in childhood reduce risk of dyslipidemia in adulthood?	No evidence

concerning 3 areas of interest: the ability of screening to delay the onset and reduce the incidence of CHD-related events, if improving dyslipidemia in children reduces risk of adult dyslipidemia, and the effectiveness of treatments in children in reducing the risks of CHD-related events in adulthood. The USPSTF panel also noted the lack of information about which specific childhood risk factors are most predictive of adult disease, information that could contribute to a risk-assessment screening tool. They also noted the limited information about drug treatments for the general pediatric population (ie, those not diagnosed with monogenic dyslipidemias such as FH). The panel concluded that the current screening strategies are ineffective. Future research should identify risk factors other than family-history lipid levels, and randomized, controlled clinical trials of various screening strategies are needed.

OTHER SCREENING OPTIONS

The current screening guidelines are ineffective, and the evidence in support of effective screening techniques for identifying (let alone managing) children and adolescents with dyslipidemia in the course of routine primary care is sorely lacking, but are other screening options available? Some have called for changing the screening settings, advocating a move from primary care office settings to the public school system. Studies from other countries have revealed a slight increased effectiveness with this approach,[6] but their relevance to our public education system is limited. US-based cholesterol screening programs have been attempted through, for example, the rural West Virginia school systems, but their low participation rates dramatically decreased the utility and cost-effectiveness of this approach.[7]

Others have called for changing the cholesterol screening technique used or changing the lipid-level cut points. A recent small study showed that a nonfasting LDL cholesterol measure was a conceptually better screen than using TC level (ie, can be drawn on first visit and does not require multiple venipunctures),[8] but this approach has not been tested on a large scale. As mentioned earlier, the screening cut points used in current NCEP guidelines do not factor in age, gender, or race in the evaluation of elevated cholesterol levels. A recent study examined the accuracy of new age- and gender-specific lipoprotein cut points developed from National Health and Nutrition Examination Survey (NHANES) data as a means of improving the predictive value of screening cut points.[9] It is interesting to note that the authors found that the NHANES cut points, compared with those of the NCEP, were more strongly predictive of only low HDL levels in adults but less predictive of high TC, LDL, and triglyceride levels in adults.

Another option could entail cascade screening, a technique used to identify those with FH by systemically screening first-degree relatives of people with FH for the presence of a monogenic dyslipidemia. Cascade screening, also known as case finding or problem-based screening, has been tested in a pilot study in the United Kingdom and found to be acceptable and feasible, and it has been used with success in the Netherlands. It has been shown to be the most cost-effective screening option for detecting cases across the whole population, as compared with universal screening, opportunistic screening in primary care, and screening of people admitted to hospital with premature myocardial infarction.[10] Although no equally effective markers of disease exist in detecting multifactorial dyslipidemias, a risk-assessment tool used in conjunction with the cascade screening for

FH might serve as a means of at least identifying those children at greatest risk of future disease. One study implemented a nurse lead genetic register to identify FH proband patients in lipid clinics and use information garnered from those patients to identify new cases of heterozygous FH in first-degree relatives. With this method, screening of only 200 relatives revealed 121 new cases of FH; it was estimated that it would have required testing 60 000 people from the general population to find the same number.[11] A second study, which used DNA testing for identifiable mutations in the LDL-receptor gene, found that extending family screening further beyond first-degree relatives of probands to the relatives of newly detected cases yielded 2000 new cases of FH in 5 years.[12] On the basis of cost-effectiveness and general efficacy, regional and/or national networks should be developed in the United States to initiate cascade screening of relatives connected to FH probands by using serum cholesterol levels.

Screening for hypercholesterolemia identifies only 1 of the risk factors associated with CVD. An approach, similar to risk-assessment tools used in the adult population, that incorporates not only lipid levels but also risk of hypertension, hyperglycemia, obesity, and smoking as a means of evaluating risk of CHD-related disease will likely prove to be a more effective tool.[13] Also, it is important to stress that although the current guidelines using family history as an entry point for screening have proven to be less than optimal, that does not mean that family history should be completely disregarded. Family history is an important marker for future CVD in children and provides an opportunity to increase the success of family-based interventions.[14,15] Thus, new guidelines should focus on various risk factors, including family history and lipid levels, to identify those children and adolescents at greater risk of CVD.

NEW TREATMENT OPTIONS

Effective screening depends on, among other factors, accuracy of the screening test for detecting the disease and, equally important, effective and acceptable treatment for the disease detected through screening. In this article we have summarized the evidence of the ineffectiveness of current screening strategies for hypercholesterolemia in children and adolescents. Although the evidence base surrounding available treatments for hypercholesterolemia in children and adolescents is slowly growing, treatment of multifactorial dyslipidemias, especially pharmacologic treatment, remains limited and controversial without clear evidence as to which children and adolescents specifically should be targeted.

Treatment should be initiated for children and adolescents at high risk of CVD, such as those with a family history of CVD or individual high cholesterol levels (as outlined in Table 1). Initial treatment for all types of hypercholesterolemia consists of diet modification, weight control, and exercise. Diet needs to be explored with a prospective diet diary, a food-frequency questionnaire, or questions in the clinical interview, with special focus on sources of saturated fat and simple sugars, especially sugar-sweetened beverages. Specific dietary modification should be based on the principles listed in the AAP position statement on cholesterol in childhood (see Table 4).[16] Exercise may be a useful adjunct to a comprehensive diet program, because it can help maintain ideal body weight and general cardiovascular and pulmonary fitness. AAP guidelines on physical activity for children and adolescents recommend limiting sedentary activity and/or screen time to <2 hours per day while promoting 1 hour of physical activity per day on most days of the week. In addition, interventions for reducing secondhand smoke exposure and/or smoking cessation should be attempted when appropriate.

Only children and adolescents with severe family histories, high levels of LDL cholesterol, and failure to respond to diet modifications require pharmacotherapy. A recent AAP report included a review of pharmacologic agents and indications for treating dyslipidemia in children and adolescents.[17] In their summary, the authors offered 3 situations in which pharmacologic intervention should be considered (see Table 5). Finally, when pharmacologic therapy is warranted, several classes of agents are available for treatment in children and adolescents (see Table 6).

RECOMMENDATIONS

The evidence regarding screening children and adolescents for lipid disorders in the primary care settings remains incomplete. Although using family history as a screening tool has been found to be no more effective than general population screening in identifying FH,[18] this method does have the advantage of identifying children and adolescents from families at high risk, giving subsequent interventions a clearer rationale. Nonetheless, screening must be used to identify children with the dyslipidemia most likely to cause morbidity and mortality (FH). If not recognized and treated, half of male and 15% of female heterozygotes of this autosomal dominant disorder will die before the age of 60 years. Thus, the World Health Organization has targeted FH for individualized intervention strategies, because this relatively small percentage of the population accounts for a disproportionately high percentage of CVD and mortality.[19] As mentioned above, recent studies have evaluated the efficacy of cascade family screening for FH and found it to be optimal for the United Kingdom in identifying cases in terms of

Table 4
Dietary recommendations for management of hypercholesterolemia

- Cholesterol intake: <300 mg/d
- Fat intake: 20%–30% of total energy intake, averaged over several days
- Saturated fat: <10% of total energy intake
- Polyunsaturated fat: <10% of total energy intake
- Monounsaturated fat: intake to make up the remainder
- Overall energy intake for adequate growth, achieved by consuming a variety of foods

Table 5
AAP Committee on Nutrition: recommended LDL concentrations for pharmacologic treatment and LDL treatment goals in children and adolescents

Patient Risk Factors	LDL Cholesterol Concentrations, mg/dL	LDL Cholesterol Treatment Goals, mg/dL
No other risk factors for CVD	Persistently >190	<160
Other risk factors present, such as cigarette smoking, obesity, hypertension, or family history of premature CVD	Persistently >160	As low as 130–100
Children with diabetes mellitus	>130	As low as 130–100

Includes children and adolescents who are ≥8 years old.

cost-effectiveness. A close second to proband-based case finding in their analysis was universal screening of adolescents, specifically screening targeted at 16-year-olds. The UK findings, however, using an approach based under a universal, socialized health care system organized as the National Health Service, are most likely not applicable to the United States, with our high rates of geographic mobility and varying health care coverage. Proband-based screening would certainly be less effective in our fragmented system compared with a national health care system. Therefore, we should adopt the universal screening of adolescents as the most likely method to cost-effectively identify individuals

Table 6
Pharmacologic therapies available for hyperlipidemia treatment of children and adolescents

Drug Class	Examples	Action	Common Adverse Effects
Statin	Atorvastatin, fluvastatin[a], lovastatin, pravastatin, rosuvastatin[a], simvastatin	HMG-CoA reductase inhibitors, inhibiting hepatic cholesterol synthesis	Myalgia, myositis, elevated AST and ALT levels
Niacin	Extended-release niacin	Lowers VLDL synthesis	Flushing, raised AST and ALT levels
Fibrate	Gemfibrozil[a], fenofibrate[a]	Lowers VLDL synthesis	Dyspepsia, constipation, myositis, anemia
Bile acid sequestrants	Cholestyramine, colesevelam[a]	Binds intestinal bile acids, interrupts enterohepatic recirculation	Flatulence, bloating, constipation, cramps
Cholesterol-absorption inhibitor	Ezetimibe[a]	Inhibits cholesterol absorption from small intestine	Flatulence, bloating, constipation

HMG-CoA indicates 3-hydroxy-3-methylglutaryl coenzyme A; AST, aspartate aminotransferase; ALT, alanine aminotransferase; VLDL, very low density lipoprotein.
[a] Not FDA approved under age 18.

with FH who need intensive and early preventative care. An additional benefit of universal adolescent screening is the identification of secondary and multifactorial dyslipidemias early in their course, when preventative measures are most likely to be beneficial.

Finally, we should remember that practice-based screening and treatments for childhood hypercholesterolemia and obesity are individual efforts to combat a problem that is an interaction of genetic propensity with the lifestyle environment. Efforts should be made to change social factors that promote dyslipidemia and obesity, including unhealthy eating habits at school and at home, general lack of exercise, and, more controversially, food marketing that targets children who are too young to distinguish advertising from truth.[20] Without broad changes in our society, health care efforts will continue to struggle against the effects of dyslipidemia and obesity without ever addressing the underlying causes.

REFERENCES

1. Green RF. Summary of workgroup meeting on use of family history information in pediatric primary care and public health. *Pediatrics.* 2007;120(suppl 2):S87–S100
2. American Academy of Pediatrics. National Cholesterol Education Program: report of the Expert Panel on Blood Cholesterol Levels in Children and Adolescents. *Pediatrics.* 1992;89(3 pt 2):525–584
3. McCrindle BW, Urbina EM, Dennison BA, et al. Drug therapy of high-risk lipid abnormalities in children and adolescents: a scientific statement from the American Heart Association Atherosclerosis, Hypertension, and Obesity in Youth Committee, Council of Cardiovascular Disease in the Young, with the Council on Cardiovascular Nursing. *Circulation.* 2007;115(14):1948–1967
4. Haney EM, Huffman LH, Bougatsos C, Freeman M, Steiner RD, Nelson HD. Screening and treatment for lipid disorders in children and adolescents: systematic evidence review for the US Preventive Services Task Force. *Pediatrics.* 2007;120(1). Available at: www.pediatrics.org/cgi/content/full/120/1/e189
5. US Preventive Services Task Force, Agency for Healthcare Research and Quality. Screening for lipid disorders in children, topic page. July 2007. Available at: www.ahrq.gov/clinic/uspstf/uspschlip.htm. Accessed November 10, 2008
6. Derinoz O, Tumer L, Hasanoglu A, Pasaoglu H, Aksakal FN, Ceyhan MN. Cholesterol screening in school children: is family history reliable to choose the ones to screen? *Acta Paediatr.* 2007;96(12):1794–1798
7. Deskins S, Harris CV, Bradlyn AS, et al. Preventive care in Appalachia: use of the theory of planned behavior to identify barriers to participation in cholesterol screenings among West Virginians. *J Rural Health.* 2006;22(4):367–374
8. de Ferranti S, Shapiro D, Markowitz R, Neufeld E, Rifai N, Bernstein H. Nonfasting low-density lipoprotein testing: utility for cholesterol screening in pediatric primary care. *Clin Pediatr (Phila).* 2007;46(5):441–445
9. Magnussen CG, Raitakari OT, Thomson R, et al. Utility of currently recommended pediatric dyslipidemia classifications in predicting dyslipidemia in adulthood: evidence from the Childhood Determinants of Adult Health (CDAH) study, Cardiovascular Risk in Young Finns Study, and Bogalusa Heart Study. *Circulation.* 20081;117(1):32–42
10. Marks D, Wonderling D, Thorogood M, Lambert H, Humphries SE, Neil HA. Cost effectiveness analysis of different approaches of screening for familial hypercholesterolaemia. *BMJ.* 2002; 324(7349):1303

11. Bhatnagar D, Morgan J, Siddiq S, Mackness MI, Miller JP, Durrington PN. Outcome of case finding among relatives of patients with known heterozygous familial hypercholesterolaemia. *BMJ*. 2000;321(7275):1497–1500
12. Umans-Eckenhausen MA, Defesche JC, Sijbrands EJ, Scheerder RL, Kastelein JJ. Review of first 5 years of screening for familial hypercholesterolaemia in the Netherlands. *Lancet*. 2001; 357(9251):165–168
13. McGill HC Jr, McMahan CA, Gidding SS. Preventing heart disease in the 21st century: implications of the Pathobiological Determinants of Atherosclerosis in Youth (PDAY) study. *Circulation*. 2008;117(9):1216–1227
14. Reis EC, Kip KE, Marroquin OC, et al. Screening children to identify families at increased risk for cardiovascular disease. *Pediatrics*. 2006;118(6). Available at: www.pediatrics.org/cgi/content/full/118/6/e1789
15. Valdez R, Greenlund KJ, Khoury MJ, Yoon PW. Is family history a useful tool for detecting children at risk for diabetes and cardiovascular diseases? A public health perspective. *Pediatrics*. 2007;120(suppl 2):S78–S86
16. American Academy of Pediatrics, Committee on Nutrition. Cholesterol in childhood. *Pediatrics*. 1998;101(1 pt 1):141–147
17. Daniels SR, Greer FR; American Academy of Pediatrics, Committee on Nutrition. Lipid screening and cardiovascular health in childhood. *Pediatrics*. 2008;122(1):198–208
18. Friedman LA, Morrison JA, Daniels SR, McCarthy WF, Sprecher DL. Sensitivity and specificity of pediatric lipid determinations for adult lipid status: findings from the Princeton Lipid Research Clinics Prevalence Program Follow-up Study. *Pediatrics*. 2006;118(1):165–172
19. World Health Organization. Familial hypercholesterolaemia (FH): report of a WHO consultation. Available at: http://whqlibdoc.who.int/hq/1998/WHO_hgn_fh_CONS_98.7.pdf. Accessed July 13, 2008
20. Nestle M. Food marketing and childhood obesity: a matter of policy. *N Engl J Med*. 2006; 354(24):2527–2529

Adolesc Med 19 (2008) 521–546

Body Image, Eating Disorders, and the Media

Marjorie J. Hogan, MD[a,b], Victor C. Strasburger, MD, FAAP*[c]

[a]*Department of Pediatrics, University of Minnesota School of Medicine, 420 Delaware Street SE, Minneapolis, MN 55455, USA*

[b]*Department of Pediatrics, Hennepin County Medical Center, 701 Park Avenue, Minneapolis, MN 55415, USA*

[c]*Departments of Pediatrics and Family and Community Medicine and Division of Adolescent Medicine, Department of Pediatrics, University of New Mexico School of Medicine, MSC10 5590, Albuquerque, NM 87131, USA*

Adolescence is a time of tremendous change in physical appearance as both boys and girls move through puberty and become accustomed (or not) to their new body shape and size. Thus, body image is a major concern of teenagers. "Adolescents' development of their closely linked body image and self-concept can be particularly challenging because of the diverse, rapid, and significant changes that are heightened during this period."[1] Conventional wisdom maintains that dissatisfaction with body image seems to increase among female adolescents and decrease among males through the teen years,[2] but recent community surveys suggested that almost half (46%) of teen girls and even a startling 26% of boys are unhappy with their body shape and size; only 12% and 17%, respectively, reported liking their appearance.[3,4] Obviously, this is alarming, because "body dissatisfaction is associated with high levels of subjective distress, unhealthy weight control behaviors and extreme methods of altering appearance, such as cosmetic surgery and steroid use."[5]

WHAT IS BODY IMAGE, AND HOW IS IT CONSTRUCTED?

Body image is a merging of one's outer appearance with perceptions derived from personal and cultural factors[1]; body image is a "multidimensional construct that is influenced by biological, psychologic, and social factors."[1] Thus, an adolescent constructs her or his body image in many ways, incorporating input from family, peers, and media.[6] Pressure to emulate the Western body ideal, ultra thin for women and muscular for men, comes from parents, friends, and the media (see Fig 1).

Family influences play a major role in adolescent weight concerns. A prospective cohort study of 6770 girls and 5287 boys aged 9 to 14 years revealed that parents

*Corresponding author.
E-mail address: vstrasburger@salud.unm.edu (V. C. Strasburger).

 ISSN 1934-4287

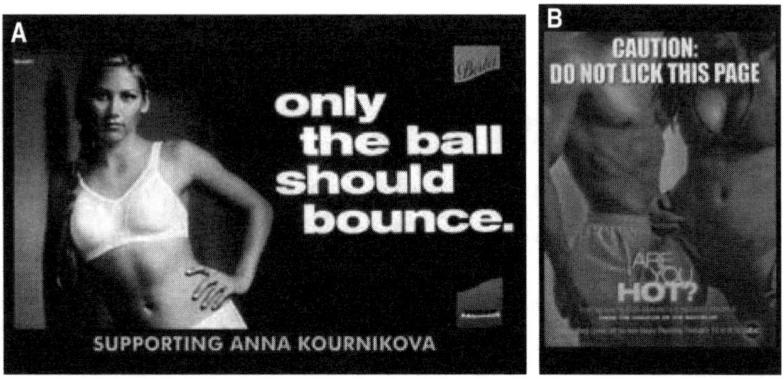
A
only the ball should bounce.
SUPPORTING ANNA KOURNIKOVA
B
CAUTION:
DO NOT LICK THIS PAGE
ARE YOU HOT?

Fig 1. A, Anna Kournikova ad for sports bras. A former tennis star, Anna Kournikova never won a major tennis tournament in her career yet outearned the Williams sisters because of her status as a sex symbol. B, "Are You Hot?" Men are frequently featured in the media for their muscular development.

influenced the development of concerns about weight and the initiation of weight-control practices.[6] An Internet-based eating disorder prevention program conducted with 455 college women found that parental negative comments about weight or shape was associated with lower self-esteem.[7] Overweight teenagers are teased more often and are at greater risk of dissatisfaction with their bodies.[7–9] Whatever the source of the comments, negative or teasing statements about weight "contribute to the development of excessive weight and body shape concerns, which is a risk factor for the development of eating disorders."[7] Teenagers believing that weight status is important to their mothers were more likely to think frequently about being thinner and about dieting in a large cross-sectional study of 11- to 18-year-old girls and boys.[10] Overt messages from parents encouraging their daughters to lose weight predict an increased drive for thinness and higher likelihood of body dissatisfaction; direct messages were more influential than parental modeling of dieting behaviors.[11]

In adolescence, the primacy of peers is notable as teenagers move from a more family-centered sphere to one dominated by friends. Peers have shown influence on body image in some studies,[1,12,13] but in others have shown negligible impact.[6] In a large prospective study of almost 7000 girls aged 9 to 14 years, Field et al[14] found peers to be highly influential on a teenager's desire to lose weight; if a peer placed emphasis on thinness, purging or using laxatives to lose weight was more likely. Another study concluded that peer practices were predictive of an adolescent developing an eating disorder.[15] For teenagers, acceptance by the peer group is important, and one study found weight-control practices to be related to those of peers, as well as being influenced by their mothers' dieting behaviors.[16] Shroff and Thompson[17] found peer and media influences to exceed parental influence in terms of body image. One study revealed that friends and family give messages to boys to increase musculature and to girls to encourage weight loss. However, messages to boys decrease over time, whereas those to girls increase.[18]

The media (discussed in more detail later) clearly exert influence on body image (see Fig 2). Perhaps media, functioning as a "superpeer,"[19] define the look and body shape to attain via images available to all teenagers in many venues, whether magazines, television programs, or film. "Hey, kids, this is the way we all should look!" Teenagers today face a growing discrepancy between their bodies and mediated role models.

Obesity in all age groups is increasing at alarming rates; 17% of American adolescents are now overweight or obese (see Fig 3).[20] Models used to weigh 8% less than the average woman; they now weigh 23% less.[21]

Borzekowski and Bayer introduced the concept of "goodness of fit' between self-evaluation of one's body, one's expectations for the physical self, and the

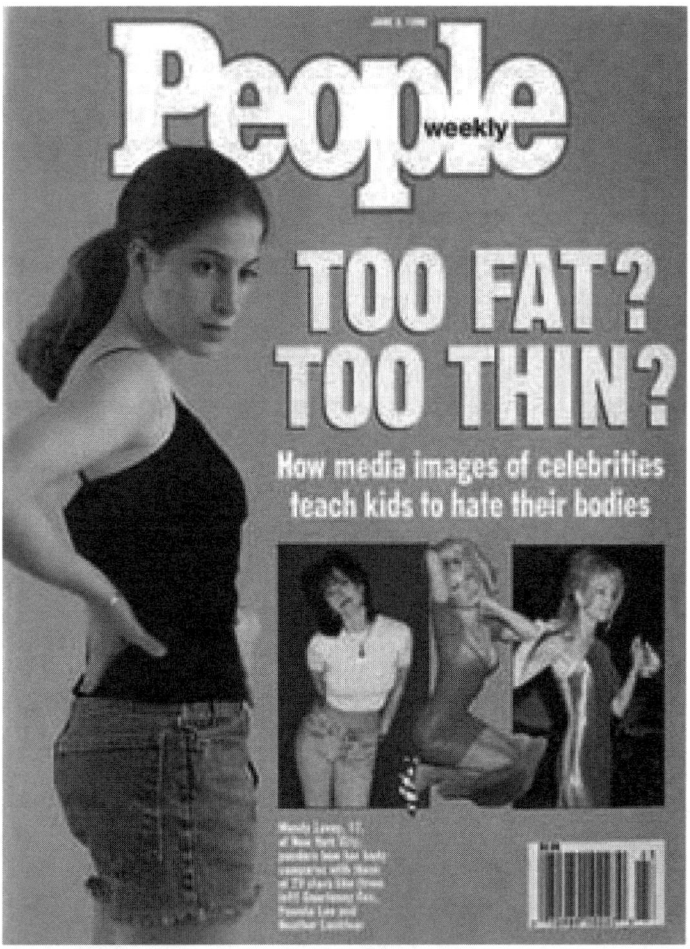
People
weekly
TOO FAT?
TOO THIN?
How media images of celebrities
teach kids to hate their bodies

Fig 2. *People* magazine.

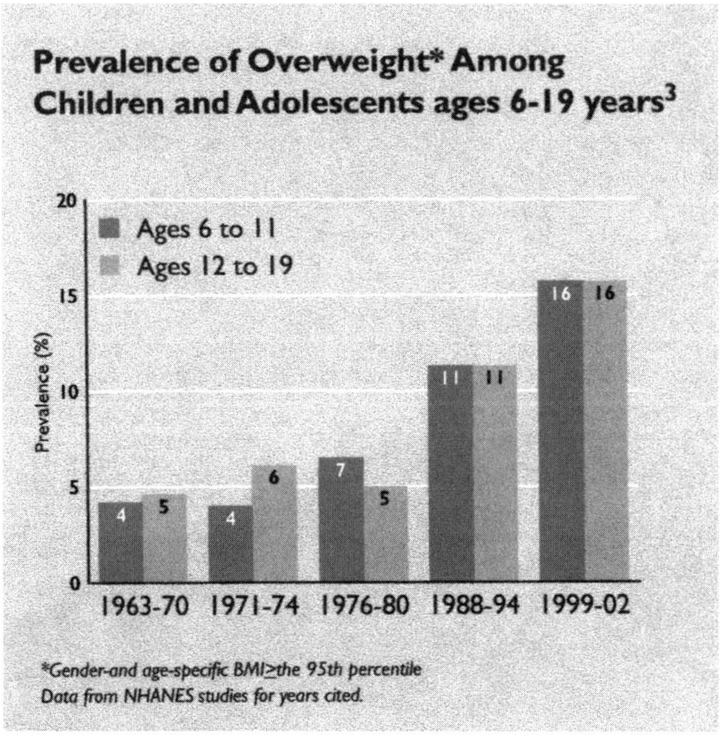

Fig 3. The prevalence of obesity continues to increase in the United States. Among adults, more are overweight or obese than normal weight.[9]

perceived evaluations of others."[1] Teen girls face a discrepancy between the realities of their own bodies and those they see in the media or reflected in the expectations of friends and family members. By the "tween" or early-adolescent years, fully 20% to 50% of girls feel too fat and 40% consider themselves overweight, yet many of these girls are normal by medical standards.[1,22,23]

WHY IS BODY IMAGE IMPORTANT?

Adults, including parents, pediatricians, and other adults, want adolescents to have a healthy body image. Eating disorders, including anorexia and bulimia, and obesity seem to be associated with a disordered body image in adolescents. All are on the rise.[20,24] Less prevalent but also alarming is the increase of those seeking cosmetic surgery to correct perceived flaws.[5,25] A cross-sectional study of >6200 girls and >4200 boys revealed use of potentially harmful supplements and anabolic steroids as other dangerous complications of disordered body image.[26] In a study of 16 862 children and young teenagers, contemplation of smoking initiation was positively related to concerns about weight: "Adolescents are susceptible to society's emphasis on slenderness and may initiate smoking as a weight control measure."[27]

Adolescents confront daunting tasks as they move through puberty toward adulthood. Establishing a healthy, positive view of one's body is key to a successful transition. Researchers have found a wide array of harmful emotional outcomes associated with negative body image, including depression and poor self-esteem.[28,29]

HOW DO TEENAGERS USE MEDIA?

Today's adolescents live in a world surrounded and defined by media.[30] They are heavy users of media (see Fig 4),[31,32] many of which proffer unhealthy and unrealistic body images for adolescent viewers. Television, Internet, music videos, magazines, and movies all feature unrealistic, unattainable icons of beauty and desirability.[21]

Traditional media, specifically television, occupies less time in teenagers' lives today, supplanted largely by video games and the computer. Interactive sites such as Facebook and MySpace and the entertaining, often scintillating YouTube draw teen eyes and compete for leisure hours. Interactive sites allow teenagers to define themselves in a comfortable, positive fashion and communicate with friends. Interestingly, by posting photographs of themselves, adolescents put their desired look, face and body, on their Facebook page, so defining their chosen image.

Magazines aimed at female teenagers are extremely popular and have increased in number and availability. An estimated 33 million adolescents spend more than $175 million annually on these magazines; content heavily emphasizes clothing and fashion, appearance, and dating.[33] Teen-oriented magazines draw readers into articles and photographs, and some believe that the ultra-thin, ideal images in magazines are more accessible and believable to teenagers than those in other media, including television (see Fig 5).[30]

DO THE MEDIA AFFECT BODY IMAGE?

The research says "yes."[34] Media images and messages offer powerful cues about how we need to look, what we need to eat, and what we must buy. Whether on the television, movie screen, or the front page of teen-focused magazines or *People*, we see graphically which bodies are beautiful, which shapes are "hot," and who is successful or not (see Fig 6). We suffer through headlines about which young star is admitted to an eating-disorders program and who looks best in a bikini this season. For adolescents grappling with emerging pubertal changes, comparing themselves to the stars of stage and screen is unavoidable.

One of the most important developments in communications research over the past decade has been interest in examining the role that media play in the health of women, specifically body image and eating disorders. The British Medical Association issued a landmark report on this subject (see Fig 7),[35] and other experts have contributed to knowledge in this area.[6,26,34,36,37]

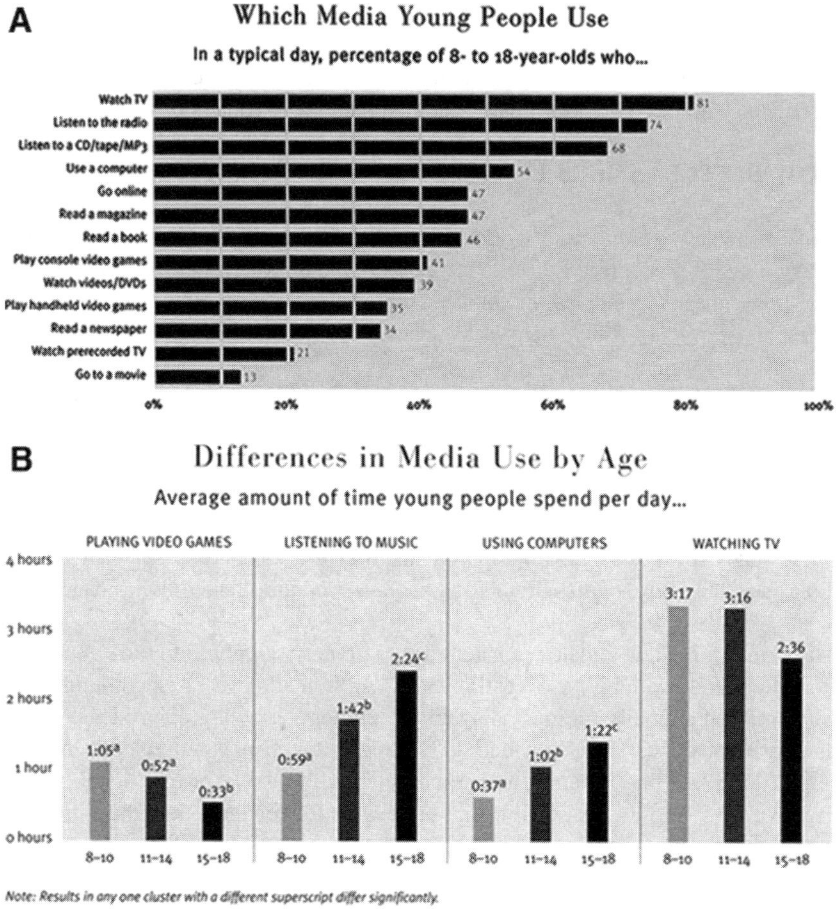

Fig 4. A, In a typical day, percentage of 8- to 18-year-olds who spend more than 1 hour watching television, listening to music, etc. B, Which media young people use.

Almost 30 years ago, Kaufman[38] examined eating behavior on prime-time television. In a content analysis, she determined that television characters were not happy in the presence of food. Food was rarely used to satisfy hunger but, rather, to bribe others or facilitate social interactions. Her conclusion was that television is obsessed with thinness: 88% of all television characters had a thin or average body build; obesity was confined to middle or old age; and being overweight routinely provided comic ammunition.[38,39] More-recent researchers have found that shows appealing to adolescents feature characters below average in weight 94% of the time.[40]

Certainly, the combination of ubiquitous commercials for foods (mostly unhealthy) and advertising and programming emphasis on female beauty and thinness predictably lead to confusion and dissatisfaction for young viewers.[34,41–44]

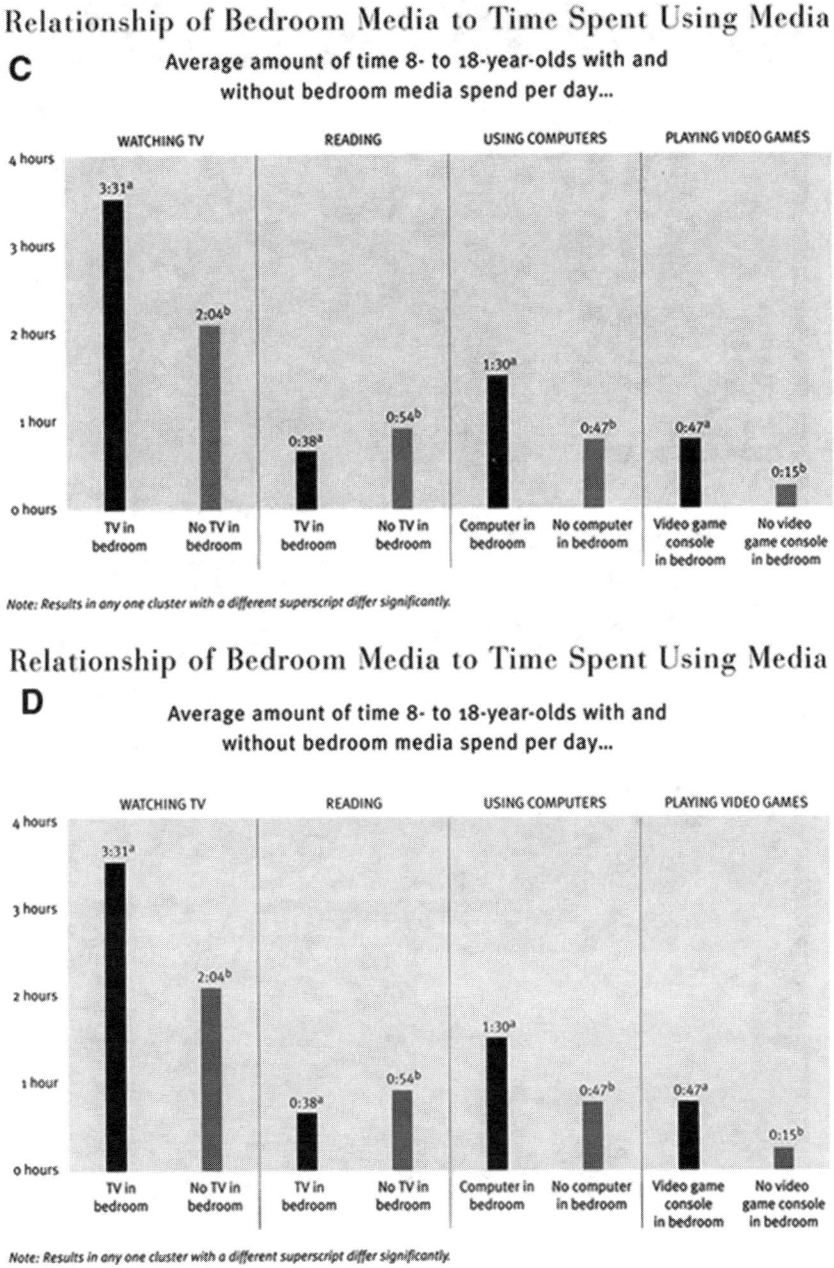

Fig 4 (continued). C, Differences in media use according to age. D, Relationship of bedroom media to time spent using media: a snapshot of preteens' and teens' media use. Teenagers spend more time with media than in any other leisure-time activity except for sleeping. (Copyright Kaiser Family Foundation. Used with permission.)

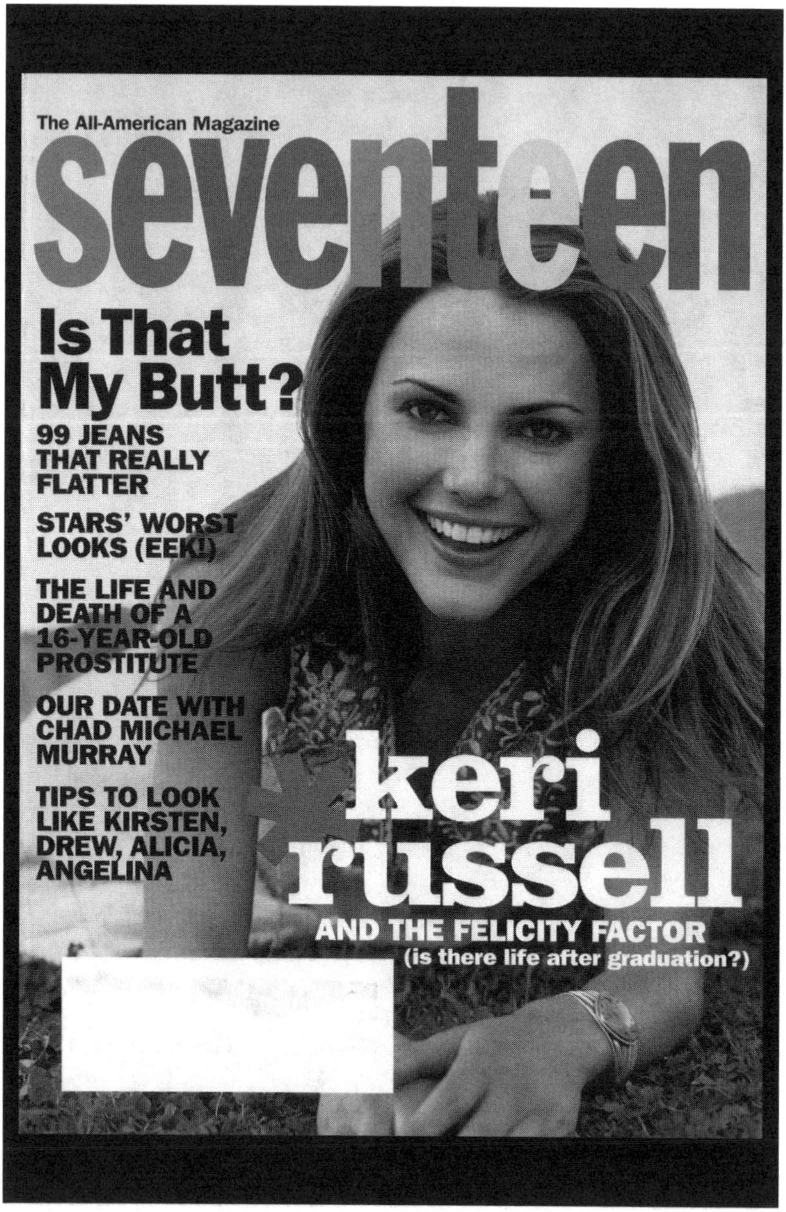

Fig 5. Cover of *Seventeen* magazine.

Others have suggested that situation comedies add to this dilemma, because thin female characters receive significantly more positive verbal comments from male characters than do heavier characters.[45,46] A 1999 study reinforced the primacy of the thin-ideal female in television programs that are popular with young

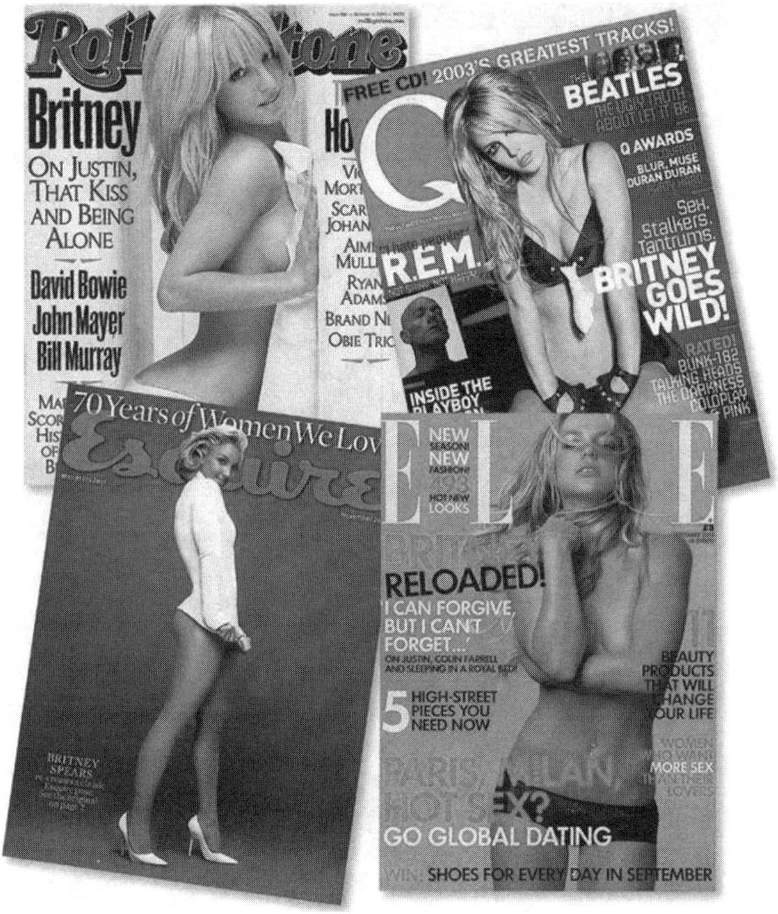

Fig 6. Four covers of mainstream magazines.

viewers. The thin females won positive comments from male characters; but the more female characters were dieting, the more they made negative comments about other women's bodies and weight, consistent with low self-esteem.[47]

Historically, there has been an association between advertising and disordered body image and disordered eating. Interestingly, as advertisements for diet-food products increased on television between 1973 and 1991, a rise in eating disorders occurred as well.[48] Similarly, studies have revealed that the increase in thin models and actresses from 1910 to 1930 and 1950 to 1980 was accompanied by an increase in disordered eating.[49] Kilbourne[21] wrote that the American diet industry tripled in the 1990s, from $10 to $36 billion per year. During the same decade, women's magazines featured a dramatic increase in articles about dieting and exercise, far more than in men's magazines.[50,51] During this time, magazines

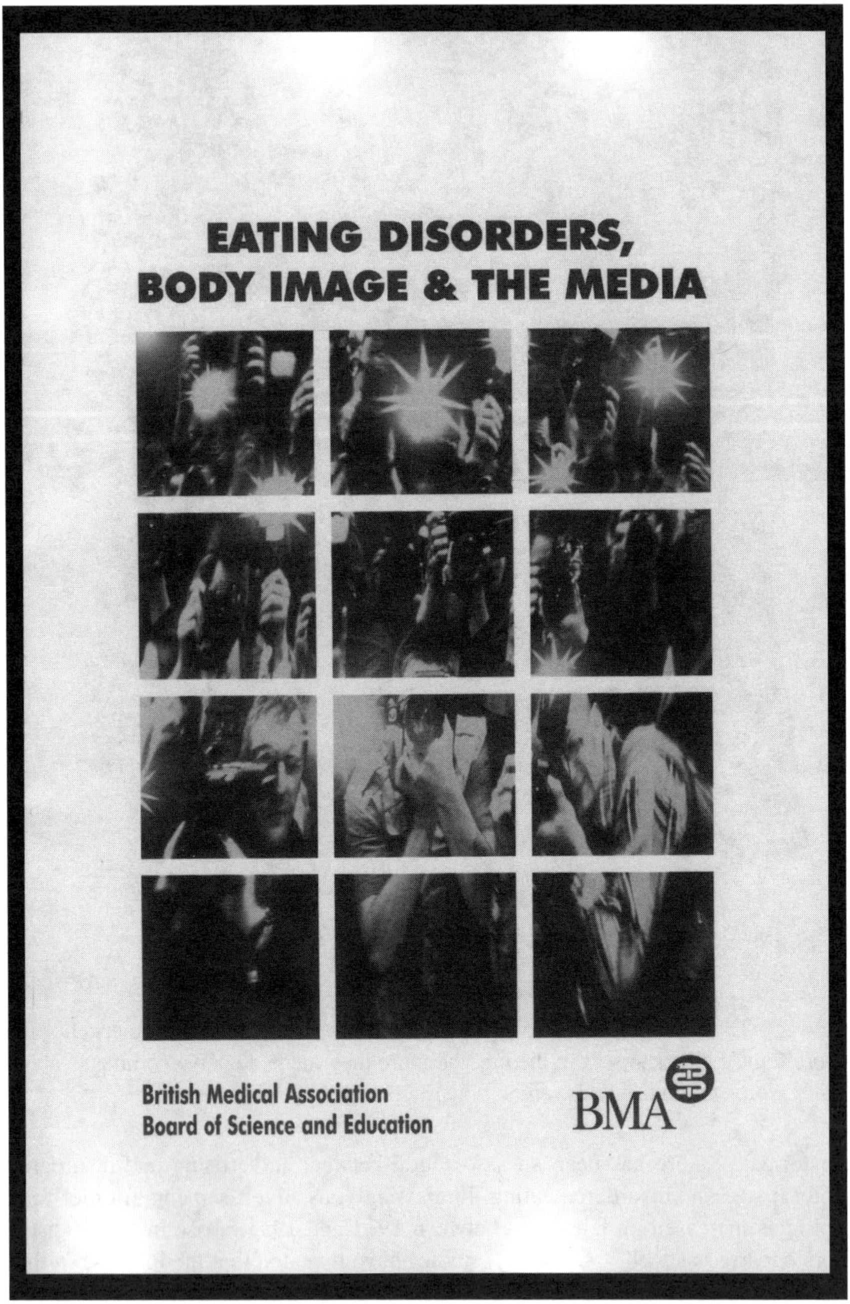

Fig 7. Cover of a British Medical Association report.

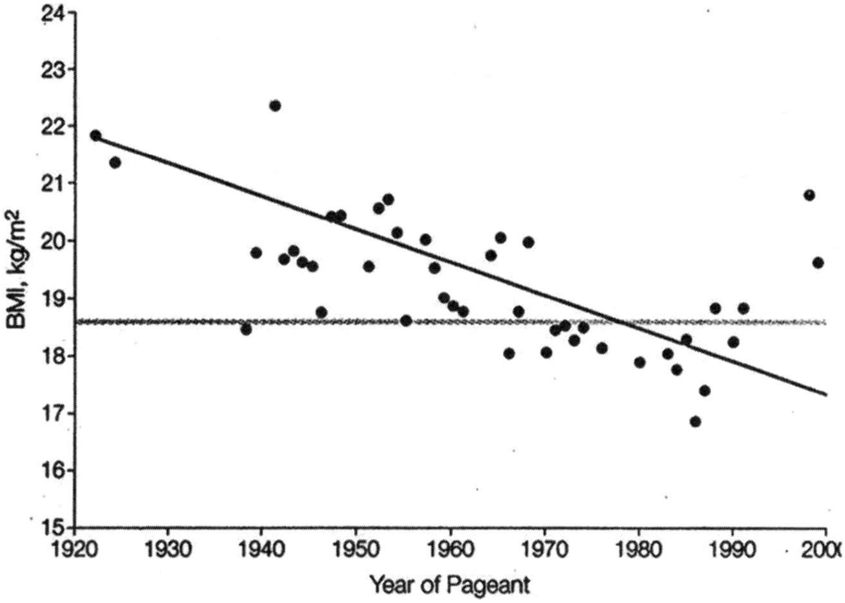

Fig 8. Trend in BMI of Miss America Pageant winners, 1922–1999. The gray horizontal line represents the World Health Organization's BMI cutoff point for undernutrition (18.5). (Reproduced with permission from Rubinstein S, Caballero B. *JAMA*. 2000;283:1569; copyright © American Medical Association.)

aimed at adolescent girls more than tripled, and a majority of 15- to 18-year-old girls reported reading these magazines daily.[52] Studies have shown that girls reading these fashion magazines compare themselves to models in the ads and articles and have more negative feelings about their own appearances.[26,53,54]

"Whether this is cause and effect or simply correlational is arguable."[34] The connection between the diet industry and the real world is complicated. Kilbourne illustrated this with the example of a WeightWatchers ad showing a piece of pie with the caption: "Feel free to act on impulse." Why would WeightWatchers encourage indulgence in Boston cream pie? It is "[b]ecause it is in their best business interest to fatten people up and then want them to diet or fail to lose weight so that their revenues will continue to grow."[21] A quick perusal of popular women's magazines at the grocery store check-out counter gives testament to the dilemma: a cover boasts a story about the latest fad diet in big letters, while just beneath is a story about the 10 best, decadent chocolate desserts of the year, followed by a sure-fire way to tighten your abs and glutes in preparation for the summer season at the beach. The irony cannot be missed.

The ideal of female beauty in America continues to shrink steadily. Researchers studied Playboy centerfolds and Miss America contestants over a 10-year period and found that the body weight of these women was 13% to 19% below average.[50,55] The BMI of aspiring Miss America contestants has declined from 22 in 1922 to <18 in 1999, the latter BMI indicating undernutrition.[56] Almost 20 years ago, adolescent girls described their "ideal girl" as an almost impossible 5 feet 7 inches tall, weighing 100 lb, and with long blond hair and blue eyes[57] (see Fig 8).

"Evidence is increasing that there are tremendous pressures on today's girls and young women to try to attain body shapes that are unhealthy, unnatural, and dictated by media norms."[35] Many scholars believe that this "internalization of the thin-ideal body image" has resulted in females in America being increasingly dissatisfied with their bodies, possibly leading to eating disorders.[6,34,36,37,58–60]

A 2004 study revealed that even movies aimed at a young audience, *Cinderella* or *The Little Mermaid*, for example, contain body-image–related themes.[61] A disturbing study in Australia revealed that of 128 children aged 5 to 8 years, many wanted to be thinner by 6 years of age.[62] In 2007, Australian researchers tested 265 primary school girls to determine if the importance of appearance relates to body dissatisfaction. They found that exposure to media and peer influence were negatively related to body esteem.[63]

Is There Solid Research That This Actually Occurs?

A growing body of literature indicates an association between media portrayals of the ideal female body and disordered body image in viewers. As many as half of normal-weight adolescent girls consider themselves overweight and have tried to lose weight.[64,65] All media subtypes (television, film, magazines, music videos) portray female characters with impossibly thin bodies, which puts pressure on adolescents to conform or be dissatisfied with their own looks[6,26,37,44,54] (see Fig 2).

Popular television comedies, including *Ally McBeal* and *Friends*, soap operas (popular with adolescent girls), music videos, and films aimed at teenagers may expose viewers to potential role models who actually suffer from eating disorders themselves.[34,37] In a critical twist, overweight female characters tend to be criticized by male characters, whereas overweight male characters may make fun of themselves but do not engender negative comments from others.[47] A study of 837 ninth-grade girls found that the number of hours watching music videos was associated with their feelings about the importance of appearance and their weight concerns.[66] Similarly, girls watching a music video that emphasized appearance had more body dissatisfaction than those watching a neutral video.[67] Clay et al[53] found that exposing young girls to thin or average-sized models in magazines lowered self-esteem and body satisfaction. The authors of 3 meta-analyses[68–70] examined the association between media exposure and body dissatisfaction; only one study revealed no association.[70]

In What Ways Might Sociocultural Factors, Including Media Exposure, Play an Important Role in Body Image?

There are 4 key components to the theory that media images and messages do influence the body image of young viewers.[71]

1. Although the "ideal" woman has gotten increasingly thinner over the past 2 decades, the real woman has actually gotten heavier.[40,56]

2. Thinness has become associated with social, personal, and professional success.[72,73]

3. Especially for teen girls, the thin look has become normative,[35,73,74] which could relate to the superpeer concept.[19]

4. Adolescent girls and grown women have been led to believe that thinness can actually be attained easily.[35,74]

In 1997, Signorelli[73] conducted a content analysis of girls in the media and made several relevant observations. Teen-oriented shows featured advertisements using beauty as a product appeal in 56% of ads targeting females and 3% of ads targeting male viewers. Fully 56% of female characters in movies had their looks remarked on, and 70% of girls wanted to look like a television character (compared with 40% of boys). Half of those girls did something to change their appearance as a result. Women are often caught up in the trap of living in a culture in which they are expected to be the objects of the male gaze, but then feel the need to compare favorably with ultra-thin role models.[75,76]

Similarly, 2 literature reviews[37,77] concluded that female viewers exposed to ultra-thin characters in the media are prone to idealize and internalize these models and, thus, become dissatisfied with their own bodies: this is "thin internalization."[77] Levine and Harrison[37] built on the social-comparison theory,[78] whereby media exposure leads to dissatisfaction with a viewer's body, a drive to be thin, and, ultimately, down a pathway to disordered eating. This review revealed small but positive associations between media exposure and impact on body image. The social-comparison theory asserts that individuals tend to evaluate themselves through comparisons with others, maybe either upward (comparing to those considered superior or, possibly, thinner) or downward (the other is perceived as being inferior).[30] In the case of media, with ultra-thin and glamorous characters, comparisons for the average viewer would be upward: the models and celebrities in the media are quite different from the viewers' self-appraisal, which leads to feelings of dissatisfaction and lower self-esteem.[79] "Our upward social comparisons could compel us to eat in a disordered fashion and strive to be thin."[30]

In a recent review, Cohen[30] reviewed the current literature and examined the social-comparison theory[78] but also introduced the relevance of Gerbner's cultivation theory[80] in the context of body dissatisfaction. The cultivation theory simply "predicts that people who are more exposed to greater degrees of television will have attitudes that are more reflective of media realities, and less reflective of real-world social realities."[30] The author gave the apt example of an ultra-thin woman on television consuming junk food and not exercising; "incomplete information about the link between diet and fitness are communicated with the viewer."[30] She concluded, "Media exposure does seem to have an impact on body dissatisfaction, disordered eating, and drive for thinness."[30] The relationship is stronger for magazines than for television, both of which are "thin-depicting" media, but the former is a more engaging pastime.[30]

One study of college women showed that those who were concerned about their body shape judged thin celebrities as thinner than they were; however, those comfortable with their body shape judged the celebrities accurately.[81] Field et al[74] conducted a series of studies using a large database of 6770 adolescent girls aged 9 to 14 years. Girls wanting to look like characters on television, in movies, or in magazines were twice as likely to be concerned about weight, become constant dieters, or engage in purging behaviors.[6,14,74] A longitudinal study revealed that television viewing predicted thinner ideal body shapes and disordered eating 1 year later among 257 preteen girls,[82] and a recent study of 11 000 adolescents, both male and female, found a concerning correlation between wanting to look like media role models and being more likely to use anabolic steroids or unproven protein supplements.[26]

A decade ago, *Seventeen*, *Teen*, and *YM* enjoyed readerships of >6 million young females[52]; subsequently, the teen-magazine market exploded, and *Teen People*, *Elle Girl*, *Teen Vogue*, and others appeared. All of these magazines define the look that is desirable, dictating that thin is good, thin with large breasts and small hips being best. One adolescent stated: "Everybody feels like they are not good enough, not pretty enough, not skinny enough . . .. Every time you open a magazine you always see beautiful people . . . you have to look good to be a good person."[83] Several studies have found a robust association between reading teen-oriented magazines and weight concerns and/or symptoms of eating disorders in girls.[54,74,75,84,85] In a study of 548 middle and high school girls, Field et al[74] found most of them to be dissatisfied with their body shape; 69% believed that their ideal body shape was influenced by magazines or other media images. The more frequently girls read fashion magazines, the higher the likelihood they had been on diets or started an exercise program to lose weight. The study authors concluded that "print media could serve a public health role by refraining from relying on models who are severely underweight and printing more articles on the benefits of physical activity."[74]

An innovative study of college women found association between reading fashion magazines and symptoms of body dissatisfaction. Young women in a waiting room were provided either 4 fashion or 4 news magazines before answering a survey about their body image and dieting practices. Those who chose a fashion magazine reported more dissatisfaction with their weight, guilt associated with eating, and greater fear of getting fat.[86] An ongoing meta-analysis of >20 experimental studies indicated that exposure to images of thin models causes an increase in a young woman's negative feelings about her own body.[87]

Surveys have revealed, despite the participants' actual body weight, exaggerated fears of obesity among adolescents.[88,89] Viewers trust media, especially television,[90] but media portrayals of the ideal woman are distorted, especially with today's rising rates of overweight and obesity. With few exceptions, notably Rosanne Barr years ago and Queen Latifah more recently, there is a dearth of successful, charismatic overweight female media role models.[34]

In 1985, the BBC banned televising beauty pageants, labeling them "an anachronism."[91] In the world of high fashion, the use of ultraskinny models is being scrutinized, and in some situations models have been banned from the fashion runway.[92] American media seem obsessed by the ups and downs the weight of popular film and television stars and models; "whether this degree of publicity about actresses' (and models') body weights is healthy or harmful remains to be tested."[34] Everyone follows Oprah's struggles with weight vicariously.

Is Everyone Susceptible?

Body image and dissatisfaction with one's body vary across ethnic and racial groups in America.[1,79] Specifically, black female adolescents are "more tolerant of adiposity," and Asian American college-age adolescents are less so.[93,94] However, black young women who are dissatisfied with their body image may be at increased risk for unintended pregnancies and sexually transmitted infections.[95] One study revealed that ethnic identity did not mitigate the relationship between depression and body dissatisfaction for females,[29] and a 2006 study suggested little difference in body dissatisfaction among women self-identifying as black, Asian American, or Hispanic.[96]

There has been little research on factors of personal characteristics that may enhance body satisfaction. Some studies have suggested that positive relationships with parents or feeling supported by surrounding social network are likely buffers.[97–99] Presnell et al speculated that "theoretically, cognitive factors such as attributional style or perceived control, which have been linked to depression and anxiety, may be associated with body dissatisfaction."[97] More research on resilience and protective factors for positive body image is needed.

Similar to other harmful effects of media, including violence, heavy viewers and users of the plethora of media types may be at greater risk for body dissatisfaction simply because they see more images. More research is needed on vulnerability: which children and teenagers are at greater risk of internalizing media images and messages?

Is It Just Girls, or Boys, Too?

Although the bulk of research has involved females, males are clearly not immune to mediated images and messages. More research on male children and teenagers is needed.[3,4,6,87] One study of boys' action figures (often featured on television shows) between 1964 and 1998 found that the characters all had smaller waist sizes with ballooning chests and biceps.[100] Boys are more interested in bulking up, not weight loss.[44,75] In a study of >10 000 adolescents, Field et al[26] found that 8% of girls and 10% of boys reported using substances to enhance muscle mass, appearance, or strength. Boys used the substances to bulk up muscle, but girls also reported a desire to lose weight. Both genders were more likely to use substances if influenced by the appearance of models in the media: "concern with muscle definition and media images may lead young people to use unhealthful products to achieve a more desired physique."[26] Boys seemingly possess sociocultural ideas that are different from young women. However, the increasing epidemic of overweight and obesity in all age groups and both genders may change these observations. The heavily publicized use of anabolic steroids in baseball and other sports venues may influence adolescents, particularly young men. A 1999 review revealed that young males are often dissatisfied with their bodies, not because they are not thin enough but because they want to be both lean and muscular at the same time. Some boys are concerned about weight loss; "there is evidence that boys are divided between those who desire to lose weight and those who wish to gain weight and musculature."[101] Girls uniquely strive for thinness, but "there may be 2 pathways to body dissatisfaction among boys—weight concerns and muscularity concerns."[101] However, both genders aim toward a media-dictated body-image ideal.

DO THE MEDIA PLAY A ROLE IN EATING DISORDERS?

As startling as the research discussed above seems, the existing studies do not yield a simplistic "yes" or "no" answer to the question of whether media exposure causes eating disorders. "Probably the most conservative view is that there is now considerable evidence that the media influence body image and self-dissatisfaction among young girls and women"[34] (see Fig 9). At the same time, several cross-sectional studies have revealed an apparent link between the

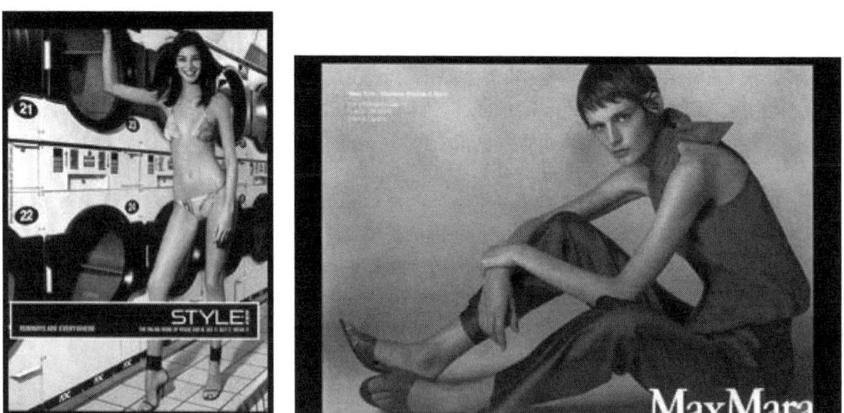

Fig 9. Thin models in *Style* and *Max Mara*.

level (and type) of media exposure and the likelihood of having an eating disorder or symptoms of disordered eating.[14,71,102–106]

The authors of a meta-analysis of 66 studies concluded that distorted, negative body image plays a key role in the development of an eating disorder.[107] As discussed above, body-image development comes from many sources, including family and peers but also media exposure. Looking from a different perspective, young women with diagnosed eating disorders have reported being influenced by magazines and newspapers.[105] In experimental studies, this group of young women overestimates body sizes.[108,109]

- A large survey of 11 000 adolescents revealed that those wanting to emulate the looks of media role models were more likely to be concerned about weight than their peers. As well, this study yielded a greater likelihood of purging by those teenagers endorsing a "media ideal" of beauty.[6]
- A prospective cohort study of almost 7000 girls (aged 9–14 years) revealed both peer and media influences on purging: girls purging or using laxatives at least monthly to control weight (~1% of the sample) cited the importance of thinness to peers and trying to look like models on television, in movies, or in magazines. Girls wanting to look like their media role models had twice the risk of purging monthly.[14]
- A recent longitudinal study of >2500 girls from middle through high school revealed that those who were heavy readers of magazines with dieting and weight-loss articles were twice as likely to engage in unhealthy behaviors of purging and laxative use after 5 years.[110]
- Even young girls in elementary and middle school who read fashion magazines were dissatisfied with their bodies and had more eating-disorder symptoms; their own bodies suffered in comparison to the models in magazines.[71,104]
- In 1 study, college women who "internalized" the cultural bias toward thinness scored higher on tests of body dissatisfaction and bulimia.[111]
- A cohort of college women exposed to "thin-ideal television" among 40 prime-time programs was a significant predictor of disordered eating for women of all races. In the same study, women exposed to sports media did not report disordered eating.[112]
- In an interesting approach, girls who decreased their reading of fashion magazines had fewer eating-disorder symptoms.[113]

The Internet, often a valuable learning tool, is also a minefield of dangerous information for the weight- and body-image–conscious teenager. A recent study identified at least 20 proanorexia Web sites that offer encouragement for disordered eating behaviors.[114] "The general attitude of the pro-ana (anorexia) and pro-mia (bulimia) sites is one of superiority, empowerment, and pride, where young women encourage one another to demonstrate self-control and reject weak societal values."[115] These unmonitored sites clearly represent a danger to vulnerable, possibly seriously ill young people; typical visitors on these sites are overweight young women and others who have eating disorders or other mental health problems.[1]

A naturalistic study reinforced concerns about the connection between media exposure and eating disorders. Three years after the introduction of American television to the island of Fiji, 15% of girls reported vomiting to control weight. Before the introduction of American television shows, only 3% were dissatisfied with their weight or appearance. The number of Fijian teenagers who scored high on a test for disordered eating doubled, and 75% of the girls reported feeling "too big or fat" after mainstream American shows such as *Beverly Hills 90210* came to their country. Those girls watching television >3 nights per week were 50% more likely to have negative body image and 30% more likely to diet.[116] Similarly, a recent longitudinal study of 3000 Spanish adolescents over 19 months found that those who read fashion magazines were 2 times more likely to develop an eating disorder.[117] The very young are not immune either. Harrison[103] studied 300 children aged 6 to 8 years at 2 schools in the Midwest and found a correlation between television viewing and eating-disorder symptoms.

Not all researchers have found an association between exposure to certain media images and eating disorders.[118–122] Some studies have revealed one media subtype to correlate with abnormal eating habits but not others (eg, fashion magazines, music videos, and soap operas but not television in general).[119,123] These findings could relate to sometimes unreliable self-reporting of media exposure by subjects or to the "third person effect" (teenagers are known to be susceptible to the belief that "media affects everyone but me").[124]

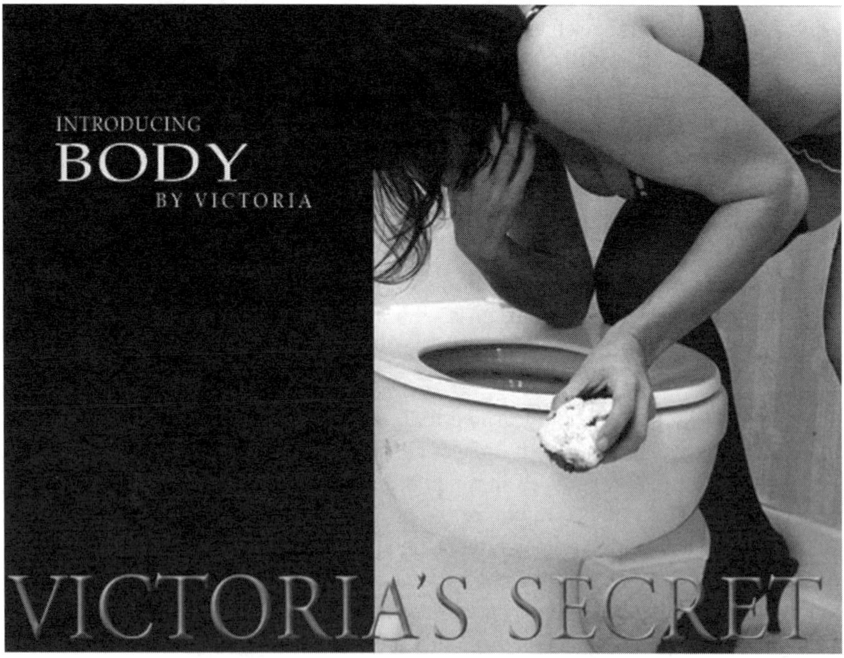

Fig 10. Spoof of a Victoria's Secret ad by Adbusters.org.

WHAT CAN BE DONE TO MAKE THE MEDIA HEALTHIER FOR KIDS, VIS-A-VIS BODY SELF-IMAGE?

The media could certainly play a role as a catalyst or intermediate influence, rather than a direct and complete cause of eating problems, perhaps only by certain subgroups of young women.[125] It is highly likely that media images and messages contribute to the construction of a young women's body image, often negative.[35] In turn, a negative body image occurring during early adolescence may make disordered eating more likely.[126] Until these associations are examined further, adults must make media healthier for young viewers and users of the increasing array of media today.

Media education presents the best opportunity to counter the harmful messages and images on large and small screens and in the print media. Media education involves teaching young people to be savvy, wise consumers of all media. Media-educated teenagers learn several lessons[127,128]:

- Media have political, social, and economic implications.
- All media are constructed for a reason.
- Media contain ideological and value messages.
- Media construct our culture.
- Each form of media uses its own language and techniques.
- No two people experience media the same way.

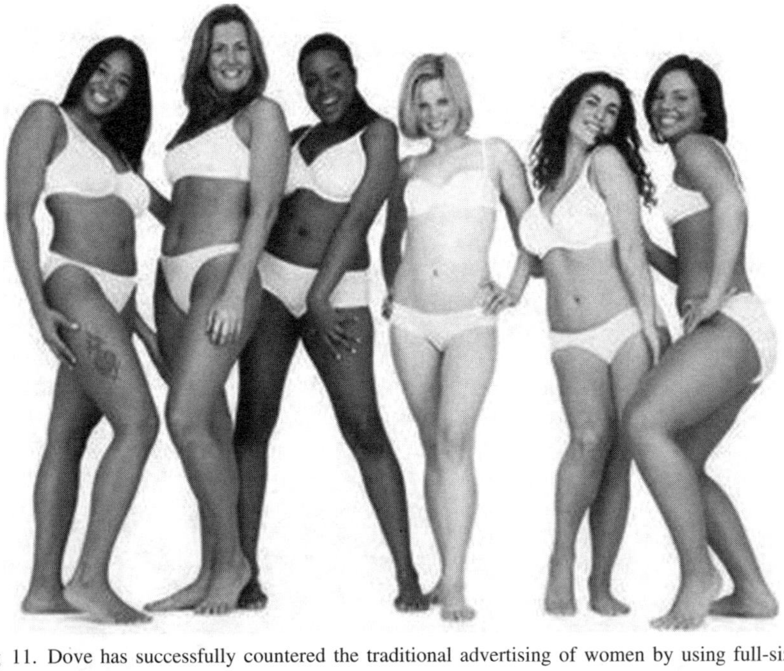

Fig 11. Dove has successfully countered the traditional advertising of women by using full-sized models in their ads.

Adolescents can practice media education at home if involved, concerned parents co-view media and encourage critical thinking and deconstruction of images and messages. Young people also need access to healthy media; a new magazine for girls, *New Moon*, emphasizes robust health and activity and engenders pride in caring for the body you have. Although schools are already burdened to provide more than the 3 R's, they should incorporate media education into relevant health units. Youth can also be steered to create their own media products, possibly countering the dangerous body-image models so prevalent in media now. The National Institute on Media and the Family created an innovative program to help families, educators, and communities become "MediaWise."[129]

As daunting as the prospect seems, engaging the media to provide healthier messages about body images must be a key component of improving media for young people.

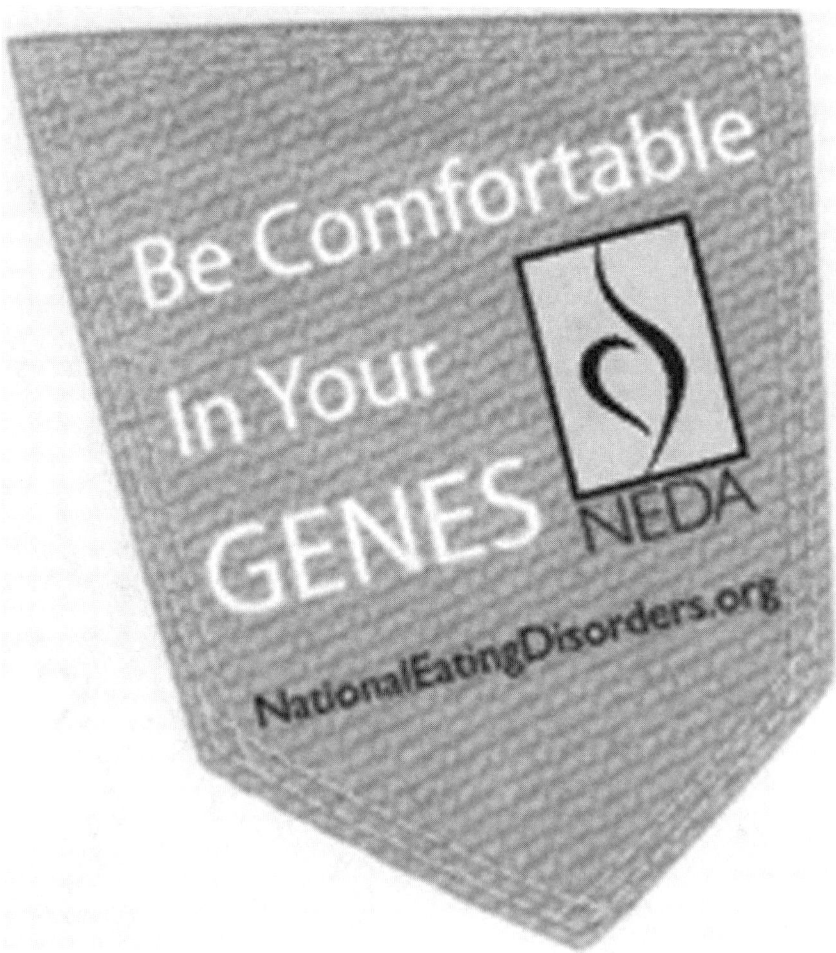

Fig 12.

Ads that feature normal teenagers and shows that feature normal teenagers of all shapes and sizes could go a long way in reorienting body image toward normalcy (see Fig 10). Consumer complaints about magazine ads and articles and television programs should be encouraged. Not surprisingly, other countries are more attuned to the media's role in body-image formation (eg, Great Britain).[35] Ideally, shows, articles, and advertisements would depict healthy nutritional choices and exercise as the hallmarks of good health. Occasionally, examples of positive, believable, non-skinny media characters do appear: the 2002 movie *Real Women Have Curves* depicted an overweight Hispanic teenager played by America Ferrera, who is also featured in the teen movie *The Sisterhood of the Traveling Pants* and the television hit *Ugly Betty*.

Pediatricians and public health leaders must continue to recognize, prevent, and treat obesity and eating disorders. Many professionals are viewing the epidemic of obesity as one of the primary health concerns facing children and youth. Acknowledging the role of media in influencing the escalating rates of these problems is key. The new American Academy of Pediatrics guidelines for preventing obesity and its complications in childhood and adolescence recommend limited media use daily as part of a comprehensive management plan.[130] In addition to healthy dietary choices (emphasizing fruits and vegetables) and 60 minutes of vigorous exercise daily, media use is clearly recognized as a contributor to the obesity epidemic. In a staged approach for children with a BMI between the 85th and 94th percentiles, screen time should be <2 hours daily as a preventive measure. For children and adolescents requiring a structured weight-management protocol, the total screen-time recommendation is <1 hour daily.[130]

CONCLUSIONS

Body image in adolescence is constructed from several factors: individual, familial, peer, and cultural. "Interventions that reduce sociocultural pressures to be thin and educate adolescents to more critically evaluate messages from the media hold promise in reducing body dissatisfaction,"[97] ultimately encouraging positive body image and self-esteem and reducing the risk of harmful outcomes, both physical and emotional (Fig 11).

REFERENCES

1. Borzekowski DL, Bayer AM. Body image and media use among adolescents. *Adolesc Med Clin*. 2005;16(2):289–313
2. Bearman SK, Martinez E, Stice E. The skinny on body dissatisfaction: a longitudinal study of adolescent girls and boys. *J Youth Adolesc*. 2006;35(2):217–229
3. Neumark-Sztainer D, Story M, Hannan PJ, Perry CL, Irving LM. Weight-related concerns and behaviors among overweight and nonoverweight adolescents: implications for preventing weight-related disorders. *Arch Pediatr Adolesc Med*. 2002;156(2):171–178
4. Ricciardelli LA, McCabe MP. Dietary restraint and negative affect as mediators of body dissatisfaction and bulimic behavior in adolescent girls and boys. *Behav Res Ther*. 2001;39(11):1317–1328
5. Neumark-Sztainer D, Paxton SJ, Hannan PJ, Haines J, Story M. Does body satisfaction matter? Five-year longitudinal associations between body satisfaction and health behaviors in adolescent females and males. *J Adolesc Health*. 2006;39(2):244–251

6. Field AE, Camargo CA Jr, Taylor CB, Berkey CS, Roberts SB, Colditz GA. Peer, parent, and media influences on the development of weight concerns and frequent dieting among preadolescent and adolescent girls and boys. *Pediatrics*. 2001;107(1):54–60
7. Taylor CB, Bryson S, Celio Doyle AA, et al. The adverse effect of negative comments about weight and shape from family and siblings on women at high risk for eating disorders. *Pediatrics*. 2006;118(2):731–738
8. Stice E. Risk and maintenance factors for eating pathology: a meta-analytic review. *Psychol Bull*. 2002;128(5):825–848
9. McKnight Investigators. Risk factors for the onset of eating disorders in adolescent girls: results of the McKnight Longitudinal Risk Factor Study. *Am J Psychiatry*. 2003;160(2):248–254
10. Field AE, Austin B, Striegel-Moore R, et al. Weight concerns and weight control behaviors of adolescents and their mothers. *Arch Pediatr Adolesc Med*. 2005;159(12):1121–1126
11. Wertheim EH, Martin G, Prior M, Sanson A, Smart D. Parent influences in the transmission of eating and weight-related values and behaviors. *Eat Disord*. 2002;10(4):321–334
12. Lieberman M, Gauvin L, Bukowski WM, White DR. Interpersonal influence and disordered eating behaviors in adolescent girls: the role of peer modeling, social reinforcement, and body-related teasing. *Eat Behav*. 2001;2(3):215–236
13. Paxton SJ, Schultz HK, Wertheim EH, Muir SL. Friendship clique and peer influences on body image concerns, dietary restraint, extreme weight-loss behaviors, and binge eating in adolescent girls. *J Abnorm Psychol*. 1999;108(2):255–266
14. Field AE, Camargo CA Jr, Taylor CB, Berkey CS, Colditz GA. Relation of peer and media influences to the development of purging behavior among preadolescent and adolescent girls. *Arch Pediatr Adolesc Med*. 1999;153(11):1184–1189
15. Stice E. Modeling of eating pathology and social reinforcement of the thin-ideal predict onset of bulimic symptoms. *Behav Res Ther*. 1998;36(10):931–944
16. Levine MP, Smolak L, Moodey AF, Shuman MD, Hessen LD. Normative developmental challenges and dieting and eating disturbances in middle school girls. *Int J Eat Disord*. 1994;15(1):11–20
17. Shroff H, Thompson JK. The tripartite influence model of body image and eating disturbance: a replication with adolescent girls. *Body Image*. 2006;3(1):17–23
18. McCabe MP, Ricciardelli LA. A prospective study of pressures from parents, peers, and the media on extreme weight change behaviors among adolescent boys and girls. *Behav Res Ther*. 2005;43(5):653–668
19. Strasburger VC, Wilson BJ, Jordan A, eds. *Children, Adolescents, and the Media*. 2nd ed. Thousand Oaks, CA: Sage; 2009
20. Centers for Disease Control and Prevention. NHANES 2003–2004: overweight and obesity. Available at: www.cdc.gov/nccdphp/dnpa/obesity/childhood/prevalence.htm. Accessed May 27, 2008
21. Kilbourne J. *Deadly Persuasion: Why Women and Girls Must Fight the Addictive Power of Advertising*. New York, NY: Free Press; 1999
22. Koff E, Rierdan J. Perceptions of weight and attitudes toward eating in early adolescent girls. *J Adolesc Health*. 1991;12(4):307–312
23. Smolak L, Levine MP. Toward an empirical basis for primary prevention of eating problems with elementary school children. *Eat Disord*. 1994;2(4):293–307
24. Eating Disorders Coalition. Statistics & study findings. Available at: www.eatingdisorderscoalition.org/reports/statistics.html. Accessed May 25, 2008
25. Zuckerman D. Body image: teenagers and cosmetic surgery. Available at: www.ourbodiesourselves.org/book/companion.asp?id=1&compID=102. Accessed May 27, 2008
26. Field AE, Austin SB, Camargo CA, et al. Exposure to the mass media, body shape concerns, and use of supplements to improve weight and shape among male and female adolescents. *Pediatrics*. 2005;116(2). Available at: www.pediatrics.org/cgi/content/full/116/2/e214
27. Tomeo CA, Field AE, Berkey CS, Colditz GA, Frazier AL. Weight concerns, weight control behaviors, and smoking initiation. *Pediatrics*. 1999;104(4 pt 1):918–924
28. Paxton SJ, Neumark-Sztainer D, Hannan PJ, Eisenberg ME. Body dissatisfaction prospectively predicts depressed mood and low self-esteem in adolescents girls and boys. *J Clin Child Adolesc Psychol*. 2006;35(4):539–549

29. Siegel JM. Body image change and adolescent depressive symptoms. *J Adolesc Res*. 2002; 17(1):27–41
30. Cohen SB. Media exposure and the subsequent effects on body dissatisfaction, disordered eating, and drive for thinness: a review of the current research. *Mind Matters Wesleyan J Psychol*. 2006;1:57–71
31. Kaiser Family Foundation. Generation M: media in the lives of 8–18 year-olds—report. Available at: www.kff.org/entmedia/7251.cfm. Accessed May 27, 2008
32. National Institute on Media and the Family. Fact sheet: media use. Available at: www.mediafamily.org/facts/facts_mediause.shtml. Accessed May 27, 2008
33. Kaiser Family Foundation. Tweens, teens, and magazines: fact sheet. Available at: www.kff.org/entmedia/upload/Tweens-Teens-and-Magazines-Fact-Sheet.pdf. Accessed May 27, 2008
34. Eating and eating disorders. In: Strasburger VC, Wilson BJ, Jordan AB, eds. *Children, Adolescents, and the Media*. 2nd ed. Thousand Oaks, CA: Sage; 2009:375–434
35. British Medical Association. *Eating Disorders, Body Image and the Media*. London, United Kingdom: BMA Publications; 2000
36. Kilbourne J. *Can't Buy My Love: How Advertising Changes the Way We Think and Feel*. New York, NY: Touchstone; 1999
37. Levine MP, Harrison K. The role of the mass media in the perpetuation and prevention of negative body image and disordered eating. In: Thompson JK, ed. *Handbook of Eating Disorders and Obesity*. New York, NY: Wiley; 2003:695–717
38. Kaufman L. Prime-time nutrition. *J Commun*. 1980;30(3):37–46
39. Silverstein B, Perdue L, Peterson B, Kelly E. The role of the mass media in promoting a thin standard of bodily attractiveness for women. *Sex Roles*. 1986;14(9–10):519–532
40. Levine MP, Smolak L. Media as a context for the development of disordered eating. In: Smolak L, Levine MP, Striegel-Moore R, eds. *The Developmental Psychopathology of Eating Disorders*. Mahwah, NJ: Lawrence Erlbaum; 1996:235–257
41. Botta RA. Television images and adolescent girls' body image disturbances. *J Commun*. 1999;49(2):22–41
42. Lavine H, Sweeney D, Wagner SH. Depicting women as sex objects in television advertising: effects on body dissatisfaction. *Pers Soc Psychol Bull*. 1999;25(8):1049–1058
43. Ogletree SM, Williams SW, Raffeld P, Mason B, Fricke K. Female attractiveness and eating disorders: do children's television commercials play a role? *Sex Roles*. 1990;22(11–12):791–797
44. Tiggemann M. Television and adolescent body image: the role of program content and viewing motivation. *J Soc Clin Psychol*. 2005;24(3):361–381
45. Bell R, Berger C, Townsend M. *Portrayals of Nutritional Practices and Exercise Behavior in Popular American Films, 1991–2000*. Davis, CA: Center for Advanced Studies of Nutrition and Social Marketing, University of California; 2003
46. Greenberg BS, Eastin M, Hofschire L, Lachlan K, Brownwell KD. Portrayals of overweight and obese individuals on commercial television. *Am J Public Health*. 2003;93(8):1342–1348
47. Fouts G, Burggraf K. Television situation comedies: female weight, male negative comments, and audience reactions. *Sex Roles*. 2000;42(9–10):925–932
48. Wiseman CV, Gunning FM, Gray JJ. Increasing pressure to be thin: 19 years of diet products in television commercials. *Eat Disord*. 1992;1(1):52–61
49. Silverstein B, Perlick D. *The Cost of Competence: Why Inequality Causes Depression, Eating Disorders and Illness in Women*. New York, NY: Oxford University Press; 1995
50. Wiseman CV, Gray JJ, Mosimann JE, Ahrens AH. Cultural expectations of thinness in women: an update. *Int J Eat Disord*. 1992;11(1):85–89
51. Nemeroff CJ, Stein RI, Diehl NS, Smilack KM. From the Cleavers to the Clintons: role choices and body orientation as reflected in magazine and article content. *Int J Eat Disord*. 1994;16(2):167–176
52. Roberts DF, Foehr UG, Rideout VG. Kids and media @ the new millennium. Available at: www.kff.org/entmedia/1535-index.cfm. Accessed September 26, 2008
53. Clay D, Vignoles VL, Dittmar H. Body image and self-esteem among adolescent girls: testing the influence of sociocultural factors. *J Res Adolesc*. 2005;15(4):451–477

54. Hofschire LJ, Greenberg BS. Media's impact on adolescents' body dissatisfaction. In: Brown JD, Steele JR, Walsh-Childers K, eds. *Sexual Teens, Sexual Media*. Mahwah, NJ: Lawrence Erlbaum; 2001:125–149
55. Garner D, Garfinkel PE, Schwartz D, Thompson M. Cultural expectations of thinness in women. *Psychol Rep*. 1980;47(2):483–491
56. Rubinstein S, Caballero B. Is Miss America an under-nourished role model? *JAMA*. 2000; 283(12):1569
57. Nichter M, Nichter M. Hype and weight. *Med Anthropol*. 1991;13(3):249–284
58. Nishna A, Ammon NY, Bellmore AD, Graham S. Body dissatisfaction and physical development among ethnic minority adolescents. *J Youth Adolesc*. 2006;35(2):175–191
59. Stice E, Whitenton K. Risk factors for body dissatisfaction in adolescent girls: a longitudinal investigation. *Dev Psychol*. 2002;38(5):669–678
60. Thompson JK, ed. *Handbook of Eating Disorders and Obesity*. New York, NY: Wiley; 2003
61. Herbozo S, Tantleff-Dunn S, Gokee-Larose J, Thompson J. Beauty and thinness messages in children's media: a content analysis. *Eat Disord*. 2004;12(1):21–34
62. Dohnt HK, Tiggemann M. Body image concerns in young girls: the role of peers and media prior to adolescence. *J Youth Adolesc*. 2006;35(2):135–145
63. Clark L, Tiggemann M. Sociocultural influences and body image in 9- to 12-year-old girls: the role of appearance schemas. *J Clin Child Adolesc Psychol*. 2007;36(1):76–86
64. Krowchuk DP, Kreiter SR, Woods CR, Sinal SH, DuRant RH. Problem dieting behaviors among young adolescents. *Arch Pediatr Adolesc Med*. 1998;152(9):884–888
65. Strauss RS. Self-reported weight status and dieting in a cross-sectional sample of young adolescents. *Arch Pediatr Adolesc Med*. 1999;153(7):741–747
66. Borzekowski DL, Robinson TN, Killen JD. Does the camera add ten pounds? Media use, perceived importance of appearance, and weight concerns among teenage girls. *J Adolesc Health*. 2000;26(1):36–41
67. Tiggemann M, SlaterA. Thin ideals in music television: a source of social comparison and body dissatisfaction. *Int J Eat Disord*. 2004;35(1):48–58
68. Cafri G, Yamamiya Y, Brannick M, Thompson JK. The influence of sociocultural factors on body image: a meta-analysis. *Clin Psychol Sci Pract*. 2005;12(4):421–433
69. Groesz LM, Levine MP, Murnen SK. The effect of experimental presentation of thin media images on body satisfaction: a meta-analytic review. *Int J Eat Disord*. 2002;31(1):1–16
70. Holmstrom AJ. The effects of media on body image: a meta-analysis. *J Broadcast Electronic Media*. 2004;48(2):196–217
71. Levine MP, Smolak L, Hayden H. The relation of sociocultural factors to eating attitudes and behaviors among middle school girls. *J Early Adolesc*. 1994;14(4):471–490
72. Guillen EO, Barr SI. Nutrition, dieting, and fitness messages in a magazine for adolescent women. *J Adolesc Health*. 1994;15(6):464–472
73. Signorelli N. *A Content Analysis: A Reflection of Girls in the Media*. Menlo Park, CA: Kaiser Family Foundation; 1997. Available at: www.kff.org/entmedia/1260-index.cfm. Accessed September 29, 2008
74. Field AE, Cheung L, Wolf AM, Herzog DB, Gortmaker SL, Colditz GA. Exposure to the mass media and weight concerns among girls. *Pediatrics*. 1999;103(3). Available at: www.pediatrics.org/cgi/content/full/103/3/e36
75. Jones DC, Vigfusdottir TH, Lee Y. Body image and appearance culture among adolescent girls and boys. *J Adolesc Res*. 2004;19(3):323–339
76. Martin MC, Gentry JW. Stuck in the model trap: the effects of beautiful models in ads on female pre-adolescents and adolescents. *J Advert*. 1997;26(2):19–33
77. Thompson JK, Heinberg LJ. The media's influence on body image disturbance and eating disorders: we've reviled them, now can we rehabilitate them? *J Soc Issues*. 1999;55(2):339–353
78. Festinger L. A theory of social comparison processes. *Hum Relat*. 1954;7:117–140
79. Botta RA. The mirror of television: a comparison of black and white adolescents' body image. *J Commun*. 2000;50(3):144–159
80. Gerbner G. Toward "cultural indicators": the analysis of mass mediated message systems. *AV Commun Rev*. 1969;17(2):137–148

81. King N, Touyz S, Charles M. The effect of body dissatisfaction on women's perceptions of female celebrities. *Int J Eat Disord.* 2000;27(3):341–347
82. Harrison K, Hefner V. Media exposure, current and future body ideals, and disordered eating among preadolescent girls. *J Youth Adolesc.* 2006;35(2):146–156
83. Wertheim EH, Paxton SJ, Schutz HK, Muir SL. Why do adolescent girls watch their weight? An interview study examining pressures to be thin. *J Psychosom Res.* 1997;42(4):345–355
84. Stice E, Shaw HE. Adverse effects of the media portrayed thin-ideal on women and linkages to bulimic symptomatology. *J Soc Clin Psychol.* 1994;13(3):288–308
85. Taylor CB, Sharpe T, Shisslak C, et al. Factors associated with weight concerns in adolescent girls. *Int J Eat Disord.* 1998;24(1):31–42
86. Turner SL, Hamilton H, Jacobs M, Angood LM, Dwyer DH. The influence of fashion magazines on the body image satisfaction of college women: an exploratory analysis. *Adolescence.* 1997;32(127):603–614
87. Levine MP. Mass media and body image: a brief review of the research. *Health Weight J.* 2000;14(6):84–85, 95
88. Rome ES, Ammerman S, Rosen DS, et al. Children and adolescents with eating disorders: the state of the art. *Pediatrics.* 2003;111(1). Available at: www.pediatrics.org/cgi/content/full/111/1/e98
89. Story M, Neumark-Sztainer D. Promoting healthy eating and physical activity in adolescents. *Adolesc Med State Art Rev.* 1999;10(1):109–123, vi
90. Horgen KB, Choate M, Brownell KD. Television food advertising. In: Singer DG, Singer JL, eds. *Handbook of Children and the Media.* Thousand Oaks, CA: Sage; 2001:447–461
91. BBC bans beauty contest. *Parade Magazine.* June 30, 1985
92. Trebay G. Looking beyond the runway for answers on underweight models. *New York Times.* February 6, 2007. Available at: www.nytimes.com/2007/02/06/fashion/shows/06DIARY.html. Accessed September 29, 2008
93. Padgett J, Biro FM. Different shapes in different cultures: body dissatisfaction, overweight, and obesity in African American and Caucasian females. *J Pediatr Adolesc Gynecol.* 2003;16(6):349–354
94. Haudek C, Rorty M, Henker B. The role of ethnicity and parent bonding in the eating and weight concerns of Asian-American college women. *Int J Eat Disord.* 1999;25(4):425–433
95. Wingood GM, DiClemente RJ, Harrington K, Davies SL. Body image and African American females' sexual health. *J Womens Health Gend Based Med.* 2002;11(5):433–439
96. Grabe S, Hyde JS. Ethnicity and body dissatisfaction among women in the United States: a meta-analysis. *Psychol Bull.* 2006;132(4):622–640
97. Presnell K, Bearman SK, Madelley MC. Body dissatisfaction in adolescent females and males: risk and resilience. *Prev Res.* 2007;14(3):3–6
98. Barker ET, Galambos NL. Body dissatisfaction of adolescent girls and boys: risk and resource factors. *J Early Adolesc.* 2003;23(2):141–165
99. Swarr AE, Richards MH. Longitudinal effects of adolescent girls' pubertal development, perceptions of pubertal timing, and parental relations on eating problems. *Dev Psychol.* 1996;32(4):636–646
100. Pope H. Toy muscles linked to harmful images of male body. *Harvard Med Alumni Bull.* 1999:13
101. Neumark-Sztainer D, Story M, Falkner NH, Beuhring T, Resnick MD. Sociodemographic and personal characteristics of adolescents engaged in weight loss and weight/muscle gain behaviors: who is doing what? *Prev Med.* 1999;28(1):40–50
102. Harrison K. The body electric: thin-ideal media and eating disorders in adolescents. *J Commun.* 2000;50(3):119–143
103. Harrison K. Television viewing, fat stereotyping, body shape standards, and eating disorder symptomatology in grade school children. *Commun Res.* 2000;27:617–640
104. Martin MC, Kennedy PF. Social comparison and the beauty of advertising models: the role of motives for comparison. In: Allen CT, Roedder JD, eds. *Advances in Consumer Research.* Vol 21. Provo, UT: Association for Consumer Research; 1994:365–371
105. Murray SH, Touyz SW, Beumont PJV. Awareness and perceived influence of body ideals in the media: a comparison of eating disorder patients and the general community. *Eating Disorders.* 1996;4(1):33–46
106. Stice E, Schupak-Neuberg E, Shaw HE, Stein RI. Relation of media exposure to eating disorder symptomatology: an examination of mediating mechanisms. *J Abnorm Psychol.* 1994;103(4):836–840

107. Cash TF, Deagle EA 3rd. The nature and extent of body image disturbances in anorexia nervosa and bulimia nervosa: a meta-analysis. *Int J Eat Disord.* 1997;22(2):107–125
108. Verri AP, Verticale MS, Vallero E, Bellone S, Nespoli L. Television and eating disorders: study of adolescent eating behavior [in Italian]. *Minerva Pediatr.* 1997;49(6):235–243
109. Waller G, Shaw J, Hamilton K, Baldwin G, Harding T, Summer A. Beauty is in the eye of the beholder: media influences on the psychopathology of eating problems. *Appetite.* 1994;23(3):287
110. van den Berg P, Neumark-Sztainer D, Hannan PJ, Haines J. Is dieting advice from magazines helpful or harmful? Associations with weight-control behaviors and psychological outcomes in adolescents. *Pediatrics.* 2007;119(1). Available at: www.pediatrics.org/cgi/content/full/119/1/e30
111. Thompson JK, Heinberg LJ, Altabe M, Tantleff-Dunn S. *Exacting Beauty: Theory, Assessment, and Treatment of Body Image Disturbance.* Washington DC: American Psychological Association; 1999
112. Bissell KL, Zhou P. Must-see TV or ESPN: entertainment and sports media exposure and body-image distortion in college women. *J Commun.* 2004;54(1):5–21
113. Vaughan KK, Fouts GT. Changes in television and magazine exposure and eating disorder symptomatology. *Sex Roles.* 2003;49(7–8):313–320
114. Norris ML, Boydell KM, Pinhas L, Katzman DK. Ana and the Internet: a review of pro-anorexia Web sites. *Int J Eat Disord.* 2006;39(6):443–447
115. Taylor E. *Totally in Control: The Rise of Pro-ana/Pro-mia Websites.* Oxford, United Kingdom: Social Issues Research Center; 2002
116. Becker AE, Burwell RA, Gilman SE, Herzog DB, Hamburg P. Eating behaviors and attitudes following prolonged esposure to television among ethnic Fijian adolescent girls. *Br J Psychiatry.* 2002;180:509–514
117. Martínez-González MA, Gual P, Lahortiga F, Alonso Y, Irala-Estévez J, Cervera S. Parental factors, mass media influences, and the onset of eating disorders in a prospective population-based cohort. *Pediatrics.* 2003;111(2):315–320
118. Cusumano DL, Thompson JK. Body image and body shape ideals in magazines: exposure, awareness, and internalization. *Sex Roles.* 1997;37(9–10):701–721
119. Harrison K, Cantor J. The relationship between media consumption and eating disorders. *J Commun.* 1997;47(1):40–67
120. Barrett RT. Making our own meanings: a critical review of media effects research in relation to the causation of aggression and social skills difficulties in children and anorexia nervosa in young women. *J Psychiatr Ment Health Nurs.* 1997;4(3):179–183
121. Cash TF, Ancis JR, Strachan MD. Gender attitudes, feminist identity, and body images among young college women. *Sex Roles.* 1997;36(7–8):433–447
122. Champion H, Furnham A. The effect of the media on body satisfaction in adolescent girls. *Eur Eat Disord Rev.* 1999;7(3):213–228
123. Tiggemann M, Pickering AS. Role of television in adolescent women's body dissatisfaction and drive for thinness. *Int J Eat Disord.* 1996;20(2):199–203
124. Eveland WP Jr, Nathanson AI, Detenber BH, McLeod DM. Rethinking the social distance corollary: perceived likelihood of exposure and the third-person perception. *Commun Res.* 1999;26(3):275–302
125. Harrison K. The role of self-discrepancies in the relationship between media exposure and eating disorders. *Diss Abstr Int A Humanit Soc Sci.* 1998;59(3-A):0648
126. Dietz WH. Health consequences of obesity of youth: childhood predictors of adult disease. *Pediatrics.* 1998;101(3 pt 2):518–525
127. Hogan MJ. Parent and other adults: models and monitors of healthy media habits. In: Singer DG, Singer JL, eds. *Handbook of Children and the Media.* Thousand Oaks, CA: Sage; 2001
128. McCannon R. Adolescents and media literacy. *Adolesc Med Clin.* 2005;16(2):463–480, xi
129. National Institute on Media and the Family. *MediaWise.* Minneapolis, MN: National Institute on Media and the Family; 2005
130. Barlow SE; American Academy of Pediatrics, Expert Committee. Expert committee recommendations regarding the prevention, assessment, and treatment of child and adolescent overweight and obesity: summary report. *Pediatrics.* 2007;120(suppl 4):S164–S192

Adolesc Med 19 (2008) 547–572

Eating Disorders

Eric Sigel, MD*

Department of Pediatrics, University of Colorado Denver Health Science Center, Children's Hospital, 13123 East 16th Avenue, Aurora, CO 80045, USA

Adolescents frequently engage in disordered eating behavior at an alarming rate,[1] with many developing partial or full-blown eating disorders (EDs). The spectrum of EDs includes anorexia nervosa (AN), bulimia nervosa (BN), eating disorders not otherwise specified (EDNOS), and binge-eating disorder (BED). In this article we provide the practitioner with an update on the current state-of-the-art regarding etiology and treatment of EDs and address certain clinical controversies that practitioners face on a daily basis.

EPIDEMIOLOGY

Generally, studies have supported the fact that 1% to 2% of teenagers develop AN, and 2% to 4% develop BN. Although clinical samples suggest that males comprise ~10% of the patients with EDs, larger population studies have shown that prevalence of full or partial-syndrome BN is 1.1% in males and 3.2% in females[2] (1:2.9 male/female ratio) and that prevalence of full or partial-syndrome AN is 0.9% in males and 1.8% in females (1:2 ratio), implying that males have a much higher rate of EDs than is typically seen clinically. A study from Finland[3] showed double the prevalence of AN in adolescents on the basis of a community sample at 2.2%, and a study from Australia[4] showed a lifetime prevalence of strict *Diagnostic and Statistical Manual of Mental Disorders, Fourth Edition* (DSM-IV) AN of 1.9%, with an additional 2.4% (total = 4.3%) having partial AN (menses present).

More concerning is what teenagers self-report: prevalence of ED behavior is much higher than the official incidence of AN or BN. In the most recent Youth Risk Behavior Survey of US teenagers[1] (2007), 60% of girls and 30% of boys had attempted to lose weight during the preceding 30 days. Twelve percent had fasted for >24 hours to lose weight, and 5.9% had used diet pills, powders, or liquids to lose weight (7.5% of girls and 4.2% of boys). Self-induced vomiting or laxative use was common; 6.4% of the girls and 2.2% of the boys had used 1

---

*Corresponding author.
E-mail address: sigel.eric@tchden.org (E. Sigel).

 ISSN 1934-4287

or the other. Forty-six percent of girls and 30% of boys reported at least 1 bingeing episode during their lifetime.[5] Although the number of youth with full-spectrum EDs is low, it is alarming that so many youth experiment with unhealthy weight-control habits. These signs may be precursors to the development of EDs, and clinicians should explore these practices with all of their adolescent patients.

Incidence is increasing among younger children. Often, prepubertal patients have significant associated psychiatric diagnoses.[6] Recent literature on preadolescents with EDs suggested that patients younger than 13 years are more likely to be male and more likely to have EDNOS. Younger patients are less likely to engage in behaviors characteristic of BN. They present with more rapid weight loss and lower-percentile body weight than adolescents.

ETIOLOGY

More evidence exists today than ever before that indicates genetic susceptibility to developing EDs. Twin studies[7] have supported that genetics plays a strong role for a while: the incidence of AN is 7% in first-degree relatives of anorexic patients compared with 1% to 2% in the general population. The concordance rate in monozygotic twins is 55%, compared with 7% in dizygotic twins. Twin studies have estimated the heritability of AN as 33% to 84% and BN as 28% to 83%.[8] First-degree female relatives of males with AN have a 20-fold relative risk of AN. Most studies have found a higher incidence of EDs among first-degree relatives of bulimic patients as well. Genomic regions on chromosome 1 (for AN) and chromosome 10 (for BN) seem to harbor susceptibility genes. The family of neurotrophin proteins has been shown to be involved in the regulation of eating behavior and energy metabolism and has been intensively studied to examine its potential role in genetic susceptibility to EDs. In a study of European families with EDs, Mercader et al[9] found a strong association between rs7180942, a protein located in the *NTRK3* gene, and the presence of EDs, with an undertransmission of this heterozygous genotype and an overtransmission of the homozygous genotype associated with increased phenotypic expression of EDs.

Neurotransmitter and Endocrine Aberrations

Generally, EDs do not begin intentionally. Youth may be concerned with body weight or overall health and fitness. They decide to be healthier, improve their diets, and exercise a bit more. Within a short time, they begin to lose weight and rapidly develop a distorted body image, feeling too big, with a drive to continue to restrict and lose weight. We recognize that there are multiple abnormalities in neurotransmitters and hormones that may contribute to the development of EDs, or may be the result of nutritional deficits, secondary to ED behavior.

Abnormalities of leptin,[10] a hormone secreted by adipocytes that regulates energy homeostasis and satiety signaling, do not seem to cause AN primarily but may mediate energy changes that affect the hypothalamic-pituitary axis and play a role in perpetuating AN. Leptin physiology is deranged in patients with AN. Leptin levels increase to excessive levels as individuals regain weight. The idiosyncratic higher levels of leptin may contribute to the difficulty that patients with AN have when trying to regain weight, because higher leptin levels signal the body to decrease energy intake. Leptin also plays a significant role in some of the sequelae of AN, with low levels signaling the hypothalamus to inhibit reproductive hormone production.

There is evidence of persistently altered serotonergic and dopaminergic function in AN.[11] Other alterations in neuropeptides and gut peptides are found both in AN and BN. Adiponectin[12] seems elevated in AN, although it is unclear whether these levels are caused by the malnourished state or elevated independently of malnutrition. Cholecystokinin is decreased in BN, perhaps contributing to the lack of postingestion satiety that perpetuates a binge. An alteration in dopamine has also been recognized, although its significance is not clear. Ghrelin, a gut peptide, is elevated in patients with AN[13] and does not decrease in a normal fashion after a meal in these patients.

Despite significant research into the neurobiology of EDs, it remains unclear whether alterations contribute to the development of EDs or are present as a consequence of the physiologic changes associated with the disorders. Patients with BN or BED seem to have a blunted serotonin response to eating and satiety. With a decreased satiety response, patients continue to eat, which leads to a binge. Treatment with selective serotonin-reuptake inhibitors (SSRIs) tends to equilibrate satiety regulation. More research is needed to determine which factors are causative and which are results of the ED.

New Hypothesis to Consider

Some experts have hypothesized that the intrauterine hormonal milieu may explain the differences between the prevalence of ED between females and males. Procopio and Marriott[14] have studied same-gender and opposite-gender twin pairs and the risk of developing AN in the second twin if 1 twin develops AN. There was an approximate eightfold risk of developing AN in males who had a female twin with AN compared with the risk of developing AN in males who had a male twin with AN. Although the study could not separate environmental influences, Procopio and Marriott presented evidence from animal models that supports the idea that increased exposure to estrogen and/or decreased exposure to androgens influence brain development and may play a role in determining which individuals may be at risk for developing AN.

Traditional psychological theory has suggested many environmental factors that might promote the development of EDs. Enmeshment of mother with daughter to the point that the teenager cannot develop her own identity (a key developmental marker of adolescence) may be a predisposing factor. The teenager may cope by asserting control over food, as she senses her lack of control in the developmental realm. A second theory involves father-daughter distancing. As puberty progresses and a girl's sexuality blossoms, a father may experience difficulty in dealing with his daughter as a sexual being and may respond by withdrawing both emotionally and physically. The teenaged girl may intuitively recognize this and subconsciously decrease her food intake to become prepubertal again. A third theory is related to puberty itself: some teenagers may fear or dislike their changing bodies. By restricting food intake, they lose weight, stop menstruating, and effectively reverse pubertal development.

Society has provided the message that being thin or muscular is necessary for attractiveness and success. The ease of access to diet products (foods and diet pills) and Internet instructions (proanorexia sites) make it simple for adolescents to embark on a quest for thinness or muscularity.

Together, genetic predisposition, psychological factors, and environmental factors combine to create a milieu that promotes adolescent EDs.

DIAGNOSTIC CATEGORIES

There are at least 4 types of EDs[15]: AN, BN, EDNOS, and BED (see Table 1). Distinguishing between them to this point has been important for assessment of medical risk as well as treatment interventions, although categorizing EDs has received scrutiny. Increasingly, teenagers are diagnosed with EDNOS, because teenagers may not exhibit all of the DSM-IV criteria for either AN or BN. In fact, Eddy et al[16] reported that 59% of the adolescents evaluated in an ED program had a diagnosis of EDNOS, compared with 20% for both AN and BN. Fluidity between subtypes of AN has been recognized, because the majority of adults with AN,[17] either the restricting or binge/purge type, cross over to the other disorder. Other studies have indicated that 23% of adults with BN have a history of AN.[18] These concepts raise several concerns, specifically in regard to treatment interventions. To date, most studies have used strict criteria for AN or BN to evaluate treatment outcomes, and there are sparse data from treatment studies of EDNOS. Because the majority of those with ED now seem to be falling into the EDNOS category, clinicians and researchers may not have a solid scientific basis for treatment interventions. This has also led to controversy regarding DSM-V criteria for EDs. Some experts have argued for relaxing the criteria, specifically eliminating amenorrhea as a criteria for AN, whereas others have argued for making the categories more specific. Regardless of the outcome of these debates, the clinician needs to make a diagnosis on the basis of available criteria and, more importantly, treat the medical and mental health aspects of whichever behavior in which a youth may be engaging.

Table 1
Diagnostic criteria for EDs

AN

- A. Refusal to maintain body weight at or above a minimally normal weight for age and height (eg, weight loss leading to maintenance of body weight <85% of that expected or failure to make expected weight gain during period of growth, leading to body weight <85% of that expected)
- B. Intense fear of gaining weight or becoming fat, even though underweight
- C. Disturbance in the way in which one's body weight or shape is experienced, undue influence of body weight or shape on self-evaluation, or denial of the seriousness of the current low body weight
- D. In postmenarcheal females, amenorrhea (ie, the absence of at least 3 menstrual cycles)

BN

- A. Recurrent episodes of binge eating; an episode of binge eating is characterized by both of the following
    1. Eating, in a discrete period of time (eg, within any 2-h period), an amount of food that is definitely larger than most people would eat during a similar period of time and under similar circumstances
    2. A sense of lack of control over eating during the episodes (eg, a feeling that one cannot stop eating or control what or how much one is eating)
- B. Recurrent inappropriate compensatory behavior to prevent weight gain, such as self-induction of vomiting; misuse of laxatives, diuretics, enemas, or other medications; fasting or excessive exercise
- C. The binge eating and inappropriate compensatory behaviors both occur, on average, at least twice per week for 3 mo
- D. Self-evaluation is unduly influenced by body shape and weight
- E. The disturbance does not occur exclusively during episodes of AN

EDNOS

The EDNOS category is for disorders of eating that do not meet the criteria for any specific ED; examples include the following

1. For females, all of the criteria for AN are met except that the individual has regular menses
2. All of the criteria for AN are met except that, despite significant weight loss, the individual's current weight is in the normal range
3. All of the criteria for BN are met except that the binge eating and inappropriate compensatory mechanisms occur at a frequency of less that twice per week or for duration of <3 mo
4. The regular use of inappropriate compensatory behavior by an individual of normal body weight after eating small amounts of food (eg, self-induced vomiting after the consumption of 2 cookies)
5. Repeatedly chewing and spitting out, but not swallowing, large amounts of food

BED

- A. Recurrent episodes of binge eating; an episode of binge eating is characterized by both of the following
    1. Eating, in a discrete period of time (eg, within any 2-h period), an amount of food that is definitely larger than most people would eat in a similar period of time under similar circumstances
    2. Sense of lack of control over eating during the episode (eg, a feeling that one cannot stop eating or control what or how much one is eating)

(Continued)

Table 1
(Continued)

B. The binge-eating episodes are associated with ≥3 of the following
 1. Eating much more rapidly than normal
 2. Eating until feeling uncomfortably full
 3. Eating large amounts of food when not feeling physically hungry
 4. Eating alone because of being embarrassed by how much one is eating
 5. Feeling disgusted with oneself, depressed, or very guilty after overeating
C. Marked distress regarding binge-eating at present
D. The binge eating occurs, on average, at least 2 d/wk for 6 mo
E. The binge eating is not associated with regular use of inappropriate compensatory behaviors (eg, purging, fasting, excessive exercise) and does not occur exclusively during the course of AN or BN

Adapted from the DSM-IV-TR.

RISK FACTORS

In the past, the typical anorexic patient was described as a high-achieving, athletic, straight-A student from a middle-class family. Demographics have changed, and EDs now occur across all racial and ethnic groups. Although some studies have shown a much higher prevalence of EDs in white adolescents, Shaw et al[19] found no difference between black, Asian, Hispanic, and white people in the frequency of ED symptoms or ED risk factors. Children involved in gymnastics, figure skating, and ballet (activities that emphasize [and in which coaches often require] thin bodies) are at higher risk for anorexia than are children involved in sports that do not emphasize body image. Adolescents who believe that being thin represents the ideal frame for a female, those who are dissatisfied with their bodies, and those with a history of dieting are at increased risk for EDs. Sudden changes in dietary habits, such as becoming vegetarian, may be a first sign of anorexia, especially if the change is abrupt and without good reason.

The typical bulimic patient is more impulsive, tending to engage in risk-taking behavior such as alcohol use, drug use, and sexual experimentation more frequently than youth with AN.[20] Bulimic patients are often an appropriate weight for height or slightly overweight. They have average academic performance. Youth with diabetes have an increased risk of BN. In males, wrestling predisposes to BN, and homosexual orientation is associated with binge eating.[21] Meta-analysis of 53 studies revealed an association between childhood sexual abuse and an increased likelihood of developing an ED.[22]

A recent study[23] of males who had sexual intercourse in the previous year showed that 39% of those who had sex with only females and 55% who had sex with males had some type of disordered eating. The most common disordered eating behaviors included fasting (18.4%), smoking to control weight (14.8%), and binge eating (21.2%), followed by diet-pill use (5.8%), vomiting (4%), and laxative use (3.9%). Regardless of sexual orientation, those with ≥3 sex partners had a higher risk of disordered eating than those with <3 partners.

Another risk group identified recently is girls with attention-deficit/hyperactivity disorder (ADHD), combined type. Mikami et al[24] found in a 5-year follow-up study of girls diagnosed with ADHD that there was a significant increase in symptoms of bulimia and pathologic eating compared with controls.

RECOGNIZING EDS IN THE CLINIC SETTING

All teenagers should be screened at least annually during their well-adolescent visits for the presence of EDs. Initially, clinicians should ask about self-perception: Are teenagers happy with their body size and shape? If not, what would they change? Have they tried to change their body size and shape? If so, what have they done? For teenagers who indicate that they feel too big, ask specifically if they have tried to diet or get rid of food in any way. The clinician should assess adolescents for binge eating, as well as any type of purging behavior. An entire article devoted to interviewing teenagers with an ED can be found in the April 2008 issue of *Adolescent Medicine Clinics: State of the Art Reviews*.[25] Parental history is important as well; often, teenagers are secretive about their illness. Asking parents about any concerns they have with their children's eating or dieting patterns may provide a clue for the clinician about the presence of an ED. Any reported change in food consumption, reduction in fat or carbohydrate content, acute increase in exercise patterns, or an overall decision to "get healthy" may also be initial signs of an evolving ED.

Anorexia Nervosa

There are 2 forms of AN (see Table 1). In the restricting type, patients do not regularly engage in binge eating or purging. In the purging type, classic AN is combined with binge eating, purging behavior, or both. Distinguishing between the 2 forms is important, because they carry different implications for prognosis and treatment. Although patients may not demonstrate all features of AN, they may still exhibit the deleterious symptoms associated with AN.

Clinical Signs: AN/Weight-Losing EDs

Weight loss from a baseline of normal body weight is an obvious red flag and should raise clinical suspicion for the presence of an ED. In addition, weight loss in an overweight individual may also be a sign of an ED; although praiseworthy if done in a healthy way, teenagers often lose weight in an "ED fashion." If so, intervention may keep those overweight individuals from developing full-blown EDs. BMI is an essential vital sign; a significant drop over major percentile lines, and any BMI at <25th percentile (which indicates risk for malnutrition), may be the first clue a clinician has in raising the suspicion for an ED. A BMI at <5th percentile, representing frank malnutrition, deserves evaluation. Healthy body weight (HBW) for height should be calculated by using the 50th percentile of BMI for age. A weight of <85% healthy body weight is one of the diagnostic criteria for AN. In addition, AN should be considered in any girl with secondary amenorrhea with weight loss.

Physical symptoms are usually secondary to weight loss and proportional to the degree of malnutrition.[26] The body effectively goes into hibernation, becoming functionally hypothyroid (euthyroid sick) to save energy. Body temperature decreases, and patients report being colder than normal. Patients become bradycardic, especially in the supine position. Dizziness, lightheadedness, and syncope may occur as a result of orthostasis and hypotension secondary to impaired cardiac function. Left ventricular mass[27] is decreased (as is the mass of all striated muscle), stroke volume is compromised, and peripheral resistance is increased, contributing to left ventricular systolic dysfunction. Patients can develop prolonged QTc syndrome and increased QT dispersion, putting them at risk for cardiac arrhythmias. Peripheral circulation is reduced. Hands and feet may be blue and cool. Hair thins, nails become brittle, and skin becomes dry. Lanugo develops as a primitive response to starvation. The gastrointestinal[28] tract may be affected. Inability to take in normal quantities of food, early satiety, and gastroesophageal reflux can develop as the body adapts to reduced intake. The normal gastrocolic reflex may be lost as a result of lack of stimulation by food, causing bloating and constipation. Delayed gastric emptying is present in restricting-type and purging-type AN. Long-term physical rehabilitation improves gastric emptying and dyspeptic symptoms in AN restricting type but may not in the binge/purge type.

Neurologically, patients may experience decreased cognition,[29] inability to concentrate, increased irritability, and depression, which may be related to structural brain changes and decreased cerebral blood flow.

A combination of malnutrition and stress causes hypothalamic hypogonadism. The hypothalamic-pituitary-gonadal axis shuts down as the body struggles to survive, directing finite energy resources to vital functions. This may be mediated by the effect of a low serum leptin level on the hypothalamic-pituitary axis. Both boys and girls experience decreased libido and interruption of pubertal development, depending on the timing of the illness. Skeletal growth may be interrupted also.

A hallmark physical sign of girls with AN is amenorrhea, which occurs for 2 reasons. The hypothalamic-pituitary-ovarian axis shuts down under stress, causing hypothalamic amenorrhea. In addition, adipose tissue is needed to convert estrogen to its activated form. When weight loss is significant, adipose tissue is lost, and there is not enough substrate to activate estrogen. Resumption of normal menses occurs only when both body weight and body fat increase. An adolescent girl needs ~17% body fat to restart menses and 22% body fat if she has primary amenorrhea. Golden et al[30] showed that ~73% of postmenarcheal girls will resume menstruating if they reach 90% of their HBW. Golden et al[31] repeated an evaluation of return to menses and estimated that the mean percentile BMI needed to achieve return to menses was 27.1%.

Table 2
Laboratory abnormalities and complications from AN and BN

Cardiovascular • Bradycardia • Postural hypotension • Arrhythmia, sudden death • Congestive heart failure (during refeeding) • Pericardial effusion • Mitral valve prolapse • Electrocardiographic abnormalities (prolonged QT, low voltage, T-wave abnormalities, conduction defects)	Hematologic • Leukopenia • Anemia • Thrombocytopenia • Decreased erythrocyte sedimentation rate • Impaired cell-mediated immunity
Endocrine • Decreased luteinizing hormone, follicle-stimulating hormone • Decreased triiodothyronine, increased reverse triiodothyronine, and decreased thyroxine, thyrotropin • Irregular menses • Amenorrhea • Hypercortisolism • Growth retardation • Delayed puberty	Metabolic • Dehydration • Acidosis • Hypokalemia • Hyponatremia • Hypochloremia • Hypochloremic alkalosis • Hypocalcemia • Hypophosphatemia • Hypomagnesemia • Hypercarotenemia
Gastrointestinal • Dental erosion • Parotid swelling • Esophagitis, esophageal tears • Delayed gastric emptying • Gastric dilatation (rarely rupture) • Pancreatitis • Constipation • Diarrhea (laxative abuse) • Superior mesenteric artery syndrome • Hypercholesterolemia • Elevated levels on liver function tests (fatty infiltration of the liver)	Neurologic • Cortical atrophy • Peripheral neuropathy • Seizures • Thermoregulatory abnormalities • Decreased rapid-eye-movement and slow-wave sleep
Skeletal • Osteopenia • Fractures	Renal • Hematuria • Proteinuria • Decreased renal concentrating ability

Laboratory Findings

Most organ systems can suffer some degree of damage in the anorexic patient, related both to severity and duration of illness (see Table 2). Initial screening should include complete blood count with differential; obtaining serum levels of electrolytes, serum urea nitrogen, creatinine, phosphorus, calcium, magnesium, and thyrotropin; liver function tests; and urinalysis. An electrocardiogram should be performed, because significant electrocardiographic abnormalities may be present, most importantly prolonged QT syndrome. Bone densitometry should be performed if amenorrhea has persisted for 6 months, because patients begin to accumulate risk for osteoporosis.

Differential Diagnosis

If the diagnosis is unclear (ie, the patient has lost a significant amount of weight but does not have typical body-image distortion or fat phobia), then the clinician must consider the differential diagnosis for weight loss in adolescents. This includes inflammatory bowel disease, diabetes, hyperthyroidism, malignancy, and depression. Less common diagnoses include adrenal insufficiency and malabsorption syndromes such as celiac disease. The history and physical examination should direct specific laboratory and radiologic evaluation.

Issues During Initial Treatment

Early Satiety

Patients may have significant difficulty tolerating even modest quantities of food as their bodies adapt to increased caloric intake. Gastric emptying is poor. Pancreatic and biliary secretion is diminished. Patients may benefit from a gastric-emptying agent such as metoclopramide. This complication usually resolves after a patient has become used to larger meals.

Constipation

Patients may have prolonged constipation, often not having a bowel movement for a week or longer. Two mechanisms contribute to the condition: loss of the gastrocolic reflex and loss of colonic muscle tone. Typically, stool softeners are not effective because the colon has decreased peristaltic amplitude. Agents that induce peristalsis (eg, bisacodyl) and osmotic agents (such as polyethylene glycol-electrolyte solution [MiraLAX]) are helpful. Constipation can persist for up to 6 to 8 weeks after refeeding. Occasionally, enemas are required.

Long-term Complications

Osteoporosis

Perhaps the most concerning long-term sequelae of AN is osteopenia and osteoporosis. Studies have indicated that up to 90% of adult women with AN have reduced bone mass at ≥1 site, and adolescents with AN demonstrate bone loss as well. Misra et al[32] reported that 41% of the girls in their study had a *z* score of <1.0 (osteopenia), and 11% had a *z* score of <2.0. Castro et al[33] reported that 35% of the boys with AN in their study had reduced bone mineral density (BMD) as well. More than 50% of adult women with a history of AN have a BMD below the fracture threshold and a two- to sevenfold risk of fractures compared with healthy controls.[34,35]

The causes of osteopenia and osteoporosis are multiple.[30] Bone turnover is reduced in teenagers with AN compared with controls at a time when teenagers should be accruing 40% of their bone mineral. Estrogen and testosterone are essential for potentiating bone development. Both demonstrate high antiresorptive effects, which contributes to bone accrual in the healthy individual. In the presence of AN, gonadal hormone activity is suppressed, thus leading to more bone resorption. There is a strong correlation between length of amenorrhea and associated risk of bone loss. A higher ghrelin level is an independent predicator of bone density in healthy adolescents; however, it does not seem to contribute to bone loss in patients with AN. Low body weight is most predictive of bone loss. Amenorrhea, an indicator of estrogen deficiency and hypothalamic amenorrhea, is highly correlated with osteoporosis. Studies have shown that as few as 6 months of amenorrhea can lead to osteopenia or osteoporosis.[32]

There is strong correlation between undernutrition and BMD, including BMI, fat mass, lean body mass, and insulin-like growth factor 1 (IGF-1).[36] A decrease in lean body mass lessens the force placed on bone that leads to bone formation. IGF-1 is suppressed in the malnourished state. IGF-1 is a bone trophic factor, and its absence reduces function and correlates with both the malnourished state and decreased bone formation.

Ghrelin may play a role as well. Ghrelin stimulates growth hormone and corticotropin and suppresses luteinizing hormone, which can lead to a decrease in sex steroids. Ghrelin is elevated in AN and has been found to predict decreased BMD at the spine and the hip. A more recently discovered gut peptide, PYY, is also elevated in AN and has also been found to predict low levels of bone formation.

An interesting finding that needs additional evaluation is that the presence of depression in adolescent girls with AN contributes to higher risk of osteoporosis compared with those with AN alone.[37]

Bone Loss: Evaluation and Treatment

Evaluating for osteopenia/osteoporosis remains controversial among the experts. As discussed, bone loss may be rapid and is common in those teenagers with AN. However, the dilemma resides in what to do with the results. At this point, there are no proven, clinically acceptable treatment interventions (see discussion below). Some feel that concretely pointing out the presence of bone loss may motivate a patient to get better. Conversely, a patient may be falsely reassured if bone loss is not detected. Following bone densities yearly can provide more data and information to patients and families, specifically if the illness is chronic. Clinicians need to decide what makes sense for them depending on the clinical situation.

Bone Loss: Current State of Intervention

Returning to healthy body weight, as well as resuming menses (indicating a return to normal hormonal milieu), is the most promising intervention. Long-term studies of adolescents have not been conducted. It was demonstrated in a 2-year follow-up study[38] that return to normal weight usually stabilizes BMD, compared with persistent low body weight, which leads to continued bone loss. Bone-formation markers return to normal with weight restoration, leading to the hypothesis that, eventually, BMD may increase, although that also depends on the timing of onset of AN in relation to pubertal development. Worrisome, however, are studies of adults that have shown the presence of osteopenia and osteoporosis long after weight recovery. A study by Zipfel et al[39] showed that the presence of osteopenia decreased from 35% to 13% and osteoporosis from 54% to 21% in weight-recovered adults, which translates to 34% with persistent low bone mass after recovery.

Controversy remains regarding the issue of estrogen replacement for those with AN. Most studies have not supported use of hormone-replacement therapy to improve bone recovery; however, some evidence indicates that use of hormone-replacement therapy may stop further bone loss and may be of particular benefit for patients with extremely low body weight (<70% IBW). There is additional evidence that bone-turnover markers are improved with the use of estrogen replacement, without an associated improvement in BMD. Perhaps longer-term studies may reveal some improvement in BMD with the use of hormone replacement, although the evidence does not currently exist. Bisphosphonates used to treat postmenopausal osteoporosis are currently being studied in adolescents. Two small randomized, controlled trials[40] have shown small positive effects on bone density with the use of alendronate and risedronate,[41] although clinical effectiveness has not yet been determined. Grinspoon et al[42] demonstrated that the use of recombinant IGF-1 (subcutaneous injections twice per day for 9 months) combined with oral contraceptives increases bone-formation markers and improves BMD, although the cost and practicality of such an intervention has limited its usefulness.

Summary Recommendations for Osteopenia and Osteoporosis

As discussed, controversy remains on this subject, although studies are being performed that should further our understanding of this important issue. Currently, it seems logical to obtain a BMD reading of females if they have been amenorrheic for ≥6 months and of males who have a ≥6-month history of being malnourished in relation to AN. It also seems appropriate to treat those who are at <70% healthy body weight and demonstrate bone loss with estrogen replacement until they return to healthy body weight. Ensuring adequate calcium and vitamin D intake is logical, because they are needed for bone formation, although without weight recovery, treatment with calcium and vitamin D do not seem to make a difference.

General Growth Issues

For those who have not achieved final adult height, skeletal growth can be impacted depending on the timing, extent, and duration of the malnutrition. The longer an individual stays malnourished, the more impact there will be on height growth. Puberty can be delayed in relation to the degree of malnourishment and should be assessed initially. Careful documentation of height periodically, at least every 3 months, can provide insight into the changes on height velocity. Depending on how rapid the recovery is, final adult height may be less than predicted. This information should be conveyed to the patient and his or her family to alert them to the impact the ED may have on achieving final height.

Brain Changes

As malnutrition becomes more pronounced, brain tissue (both white and gray matter) is lost, and a concomitant increase in cerebrospinal fluid occurs in the sulci and ventricles.[29] Follow-up studies of weight-recovered anorexic patients have shown a persistent loss of gray matter, although white matter returns to normal. A specific area of gray matter, the anterior cingulate cortex, has been shown to have a persistent 5% loss in anorexic patients who have been weight-recovered for 5 years.[43] Degree of malnutrition (lowest BMI) was the most significant factor contributing to this persistence. Functionally, there does not seem to be a specific relationship between cognition and brain-tissue loss, although studies have shown a decrease in cognitive ability, as well as decreased cerebral blood flow in the more severely malnourished states. Communicating to the patient and the family that brain tissue can be lost can have a significant effect on the perception of the seriousness of this disorder.

Treatment

General Approach

Factors that determine treatment interventions[44] are severity of illness, duration of illness, specific manifestations of disease, previous treatment approaches and outcomes, program availability, financial resources, and insurance coverage. Treatment options include outpatient management, day-treatment hospitalization, and inpatient medical or psychiatric hospitalization. Residential treatment is used most often when outpatient management or short-term hospitalization fails and the ED becomes chronic. Residential treatment usually lasts 2 to 6 months. Day-treatment programs are a good intervention for patients who do not yet need inpatient care but who are not improving with outpatient management. Treatment is costly. Many patients do not have insurance benefits that adequately cover the cost of treatment, which leaves parents and practitioners with profound dilemmas as to how to best provide treatment in the face of financial constraints.

Regardless of the treatment program, a multidisciplinary approach is most effective and should include medical monitoring, nutrition therapy, and individual and family psychotherapy by experienced practitioners. Family therapy is especially helpful with younger teenagers, whereas older teenagers tend to benefit more from individual therapy. Family therapy is an important means of helping families understand the development of the disease and addressing issues that may be barriers to recovery. Both types of therapy are encouraged in most treatment programs, and recovery without psychotherapy is unusual. The average length of therapy is ~6 to 9 months, although some individuals continue therapy for extended periods. Adjunctive modalities include art and horticulture therapy, therapeutic recreation, and massage therapy.

A newer family therapy approach, manualized family therapy, developed in Britain by Maudsley and adapted by Le Grange et al,[45] has shifted the therapeutic approach to adolescents with AN. Traditional therapy allowed the adolescent to control his or her eating and the parents to remain uninvolved with the food portion of recovery. The manualized approach gives power and control back to parents. Treatment is prescribed for 20 weekly sessions. The first 10 weeks are devoted to empowering parents, putting them in control of their child's nutrition and exercise. Parents are educated about the dangers of malnutrition and are instructed to supervise each meal. The next phase (sessions 11–16) returns control over eating to the adolescent once he or she accepts the demands of the parents. The last phase of treatment (sessions 17–20) occurs when the patient is maintaining a healthy weight and shifts the focus away from the ED, examining instead the affect that the ED has had on establishing a healthy adolescent identity. This approach is reported to result in good or intermediate outcomes in 90% of treated adolescents.

Lock et al[46] evaluated manualized family therapy further, comparing shorter-term treatment of 10 sessions over 6 months with 20 sessions over 1 year. Initial age at enrollment was 15.2 years, with follow-up occurring ~4 years later. There were no differences in outcomes between the short-term and long-term treatment group: groups had similar scores on the Eating Disorder Examination, similar BMIs (20.6–20.7), with 90% demonstrating a return of menses. A shorter course of treatment seemed to be just as effective. However, on a cautionary note, it should be recognized that 90% of those enrolled in the study had previous treatment for their ED; therefore, the results may not be generalizable to the average patient presenting for care.

Inpatient Treatment

The key to determining level of intervention is the degree of malnutrition, the rapidity of weight loss, the degree of medical compromise, and the presence of life-threatening electrolyte abnormalities. No absolute criteria determine level of intervention. The practitioner must examine the degree of medical compromise and consider immediate risks and the potential for an individual to reverse the situation on his or her own. Table 3 lists the criteria for hospital admission generally used in the medical community. It is usually quite difficult for a patient who is losing weight rapidly (>2 lb/wk) to reverse the weight loss, because the body is in a catabolic state.

Goals of hospitalization[44] include arresting weight loss and stabilizing hemodynamics. Nutrition is the most vital inpatient medicine. Clinicians can safely begin with a meal plan containing ~1050 kJ(~250 kcal) more than the patient has been routinely eating, which can usually be accomplished orally. Ideally, with the help of a nutritionist, patients should start with a well-balanced meal plan, with appropriate proportions of carbohydrate, protein, and fat. Patients usually tolerate oral meals. If the patient resists, nasogastric or intravenous alimentation can be used for a short time. Aside from caloric needs, the clinician needs to consider the patient's hydration and include the appropriate amount of fluid with the meal plan. Dehydration should be corrected slowly. The oral route is usually adequate. Aggressive intravenous fluid administration should be avoided, because left

Table 3
Criteria for inpatient treatment of AN

- Body weight <75% of IBW
- Supine heart rate <45 beats per min
- Symptomatic hypotension or syncope
- Hypokalemia ($K^+ < 2.5$ mEq/L)
- Rapid weight loss that cannot be interrupted during outpatient treatment
- Failure of outpatient management
- Acute food refusal

ventricular mass is compromised and a rapid increase in volume may not be tolerated. Regulating fluid intake is important, because water intoxication can contribute to abnormal electrolyte levels and falsified weights.

During the initial introduction of food, the clinician should monitor the patient for refeeding syndrome, a phenomenon that occurs if caloric intake is increased too rapidly. Signs of refeeding syndrome are decreased serum phosphorus (as the body resumes synthesis of adenosine triphosphate), decreased serum potassium (as increased insulin causes K^+ to shift from extracellular fluid into K^+-depleted cells), and, rarely, edema related to fluid shifts or congestive heart failure. Although specific guidelines do not exist, many practitioners begin phosphorus supplementation if patients are severely malnourished (<70% healthy body weight) or their intake has been consistently <2100 kJ/day (<500 kcal/day). Caloric intake can be increased 1050 kJ/day (250 kcal/day) as long as refeeding syndrome does not occur. Weight goals vary depending on the programmatic approach. Typically, intake is adjusted to reach a goal of 0.1 to 0.25 kg/day weight gain.

Overnight monitoring for bradycardia is helpful in assessing degree of metabolic compromise. Usually, the more rapid and severe the weight loss is, the worse the bradycardia. Improving bradycardia correlates with weight recovery. Orthostatic hypotension is most severe around hospital day 4, improving steadily and correcting by the third week of nutritional rehabilitation. An electrocardiogram should be obtained, because the patient is at risk for prolonged QT syndrome and junctional arrhythmias related to the severity of bradycardia.

It usually takes 1 to 2 weeks to reach the initial goals of hospitalization: steady weight gain, toleration of oral diet without signs of refeeding syndrome, corrected bradycardia (heart rate >45 beats per minute for 3 consecutive nights), and correction of orthostasis. Specific weight criteria are used by many programs when considering discharge; this depends partly on admission weight. Ideally, a patient gains at least 5% of his or her IBW. Some programs set discharge at 80%, 85%, or 90% HBW. Patient outcomes are improved with discharge at a higher body weight. One study has shown that patients do better if discharged at 95% IBW. Frequently, insurance companies do not pay for hospital stays beyond strict medical stabilization (normal vital signs and electrolyte levels). In many practitioners' experience, the relapse rate is high if patients are discharged at <75% HBW.

Pharmacotherapy

Use of psychotropic medications is common in treatment of AN despite lack of proof of efficacy. The most promising class of medication is atypical antipsychotic drugs. Several open-label trials support the use of atypical antipsychotic medications[47,48] (risperidone olanzapine, quetiapine), which target specifically the body-image distortion of these patients. One review found that olanzapine

(2.5–15.0 mg/day) was associated with improved body weight, decreased delusional thinking, improvement in body image, and decreased agitation and premeal anxiety. The first randomized, controlled trial of olanzapine versus placebo, the result of which were published in 2007, showed a modest decrease of specific psychological symptoms associated with AN. All adolescents in this study received 3 months of cognitive behavioral therapy and either placebo or olanzapine. Those receiving olanzapine showed a statistically significant improvement in depressive symptoms, compulsivity, and persistence compared with those in the placebo group. There were no change in BMI differences between the treatment and placebo groups; however, more detailed analysis showed that those receiving olanzapine who had binge/purge-type AN had significant improvement in BMI compared with those who had restrictive-type AN.

Use of SSRIs[49] has repeatedly been shown to not be helpful in the initial therapy of AN. A study by Kaye et al[50] (n = 35) had suggested that fluoxetine may be helpful for relapse prevention; however, a larger randomized, controlled trial by Walsh et al[51] (n = 93) did not find any difference in outcomes for patients receiving fluoxetine versus placebo after initial weight restoration. Neither of these studies included just adolescents; however, at this point in time, there truly is no indication for using SSRIs to treat AN. One research question that has not been addressed in this area is the effectiveness of using SSRIs to treat depression and other comorbid diagnoses in the presence of having low body weight.

Zinc deficiency is common with AN, and several studies support its use as a supplement during the initial phases of treatment.[52] Because zinc deficiency adversely affects neurotransmitters, administering zinc helps restore neurotransmitter action to baseline. In addition, zinc may restore appetite and improve depressive mood. Zinc should be administered for ~2 months from the beginning of therapy, with at least 14 mg of elemental zinc daily.

Because of global nutritional deficits, a multivitamin with iron is also recommended daily. Symptomatic treatment for disturbances in the gastrointestinal system should be used appropriately until symptoms resolve.

Outpatient Treatment

Certainly not all patients with AN need inpatient treatment, especially if parents and clinicians recognize the warning signs early. These patients can receive treatment as outpatients with the same multidisciplinary team approach. Manualized family-based treatment, described earlier under “General Approach,” is ideal for the outpatient setting if a trained therapist is available. Appropriate nutrition counseling is vital in guiding a patient and his or her family through the initial stages of recovery. As the nutrition therapist is working at increasing the patient’s caloric intake, a practitioner needs to monitor the patient’s weight and vital signs. The activity level often needs to be decreased to help reverse the catabolic state. A reasonable weight gain goal may be 0.2 to 0.5 kg/week. If weight loss persists, careful monitoring of vital signs, including supine heart rate, is important in determining whether an increased level of care is needed. Concomitantly, the patient should be referred to a psychotherapist and, if indicated, assessed by a psychiatrist.

Outcomes

Outcome in EDs, especially AN,[53] has been studied extensively. Unfortunately, most studies have focused on specific inpatient treatment programs, and few have evaluated the less-ill patients who do not need hospitalization. Generally, studies have suggested that ~40% to 50% of patients receiving treatment recover; 20% to 30% have intermittent relapses; and 20% have chronic, unremitting illness. A population-based study from Sweden[3] showed a 5-year clinical recovery rate (defined as restoration of body weight, return of menses, and absence of bingeing and purging for 1 year) of ~67%. The longer the course of illness, the recovery rate decreases and mortality rates associated with AN increase. The course of AN often includes significant weight fluctuations over time, and it may be a matter of years until recovery is achieved. Up to 50% of anorexic patients may develop bulimia, as well as major psychological complications including depression, anxiety, and substance abuse disorders. It is unclear whether age at onset affects outcome, but shorter length of time between symptom onset and therapy tends to improve outcome. Various treatment modalities can be equally effective. Favorable outcomes have been found with brief medical hospitalization and long psychiatric or residential hospitalization. Higher discharge weight seems to improve the initial outcome.

Mortality

Patients with EDs are at a higher risk of death than the general population, with death being the result of suicide, abnormal electrolyte levels, and cardiac arrhythmias. Meta-analysis has shown that the risk of dying related to AN is 5.9% over a lifetime,[54] translating into the risk of dying to be 0.56% per year. Mortality estimates vary between 0% and 18%, depending on the patient population and the duration of follow-up. A study from Sweden[55] has shown that the risk of dying has decreased significantly from 4.4% in patients hospitalized between 1977 and 1981 compared with 1.3% in patients hospitalized 1 decade later; this decrease is hypothesized to be related to improved recognition and treatment of medical issues associated with complications from AN.

Bulimia Nervosa

Table 1 lists the diagnostic criteria for BN.[15] Binge eating is either eating excessive amounts of food during a normal mealtime or having a meal (or other eating episode) last longer than usual, consuming food throughout. Bulimic individuals feel out of control while eating, and they are unable or unwilling to recognize satiety signals. Any type of food may be included in a binge, although it is typically either carbohydrates or junk food. Extreme guilt is often associated with the episode. At some point, either before or during a binge, bulimic individuals often decide to purge. The amount of food consumed feels overwhelming, and they do not want to gain weight. The most common ways to purge are self-induced vomiting, exercise, and laxative use. Some individuals will vomit multiple times during a purge episode after using large amounts of water to cleanse their system. This can induce significant electrolyte abnormalities such as decreased Na^+ and K^+, which may put the patient at acute risk for arrhythmia or seizure. Other methods of purging include diuretics, diet pills, cathartics, and nutritional supplements.

Evaluation and Diagnosis

Diagnosing BN[56] can be difficult unless the teenager is forthcoming or parents or caregivers can supply direct observations. Bulimic patients are often average or slightly above average in body weight without any physical signs of illness. Screening all teenagers for body-image concerns is essential. If the teenager expresses concern about being overweight, then the clinician needs to screen the patient about dieting methods. Asking whether patients have binge-eaten, feel out of control while eating, or whether they cannot stop eating can clarify the diagnosis. Parents may report that significant amounts of food are missing or disappearing more quickly than normal. If the physician is suspicious, direct questioning about all the ways one can purge should follow. By indicating first that the behavior in question is not unusual can make the questioning less threatening and more likely to elicit a truthful response. For example, the clinician might ask, "Some teenagers who try to lose weight make themselves vomit after eating. Have you ever considered or done that yourself ?"

Clinical Presentation

Symptoms[20,55] seen clinically are related to the mechanism of purging. Gastrointestinal problems are most prominent, with abdominal pain being a frequent complaint. This pain can be a result of gastroesophageal reflux as the lower esophageal sphincter is compromised because of repetitive vomiting. Frequent vomiting may result in esophagitis or gastritis, because the mucosa is irritated from increased exposure to acid. Early satiety, involuntary vomiting, and complaints of food "coming up" on its own are frequent. Less common but more serious complaints are of hematemesis or esophageal rupture. Patients may report bowel problems (diarrhea or constipation) if laxatives have been used. Sialadenosis (parotid pain and enlargement) may occur secondary to frequent vomiting. Erosion of dental enamel may result from increased exposure to acidity during vomiting. Because comorbid depression is common with BN, patients may report trouble sleeping and decreased energy. Lightheadedness or syncope may develop secondary to dehydration. It has been recognized that patients who vomit more than once per week[57] are 3 times more likely to have irregular menses compared with those who do not vomit to control their weight.

On physical examination, bulimic patients may be dehydrated and have orthostatic hypotension. Sialadenosis, tooth enamel loss, dental caries, and abdominal tenderness are the most common findings. Abrasion of the proximal interphalangeal joints may occur secondary to scraping the fingers against teeth while inducing vomiting. An irreversible cardiomyopathy can develop secondary to ipecac use. Tachycardia and hypertension may occur secondary to caffeine and diet-pill use.

Laboratory Findings

Electrolyte disturbances are characteristic of bulimic patients (Table 2). The method of purging results in specific laboratory abnormalities. Vomiting causes metabolic alkalosis, hypokalemia, and hypochloremia. If laxatives are used, then a metabolic acidosis can develop with hypokalemia and hypochloremia. Amylase levels may be increased secondary to chronic parotid stimulation.

Management and Treatment

Treatment of BN depends on the frequency of bingeing and purging, the severity of biochemical and psychiatric derangement, and the chronicity of illness. Similar levels of care described in the AN section are available to patients with BN. Outpatient management is usually the first intervention (with a multidisciplinary team). Medical hospitalization is indicated for significant electrolyte disturbance, most commonly related to hypokalemia, with a K^+ level of <3.0 mEq/L indicating a need for inpatient treatment. The binge/purge cycle is addictive and can be difficult for patients to interrupt on their own. If outpatient management fails, then hospitalization can offer a forced break from the cycle, allowing patients to normalize their eating, interrupt the addictive behavior, and regain the ability to recognize satiety signals. Medical monitoring consists of checking electrolytes periodically for patients who are purging and monitoring weight trends. Observing for weight loss and the symptoms associated with it are important, as is monitoring for other psychiatric comorbidities. The common symptoms that medical practitioners encounter are as follows.

Hypokalemia

Aside from being able to treat hypokalemia with supplementation, admitting patients to an inpatient setting allows close monitoring of self-induced vomiting. Cessation of vomiting alone goes a long way to correcting hypokalemia and alkalosis. If the K^+ level is <3.0 mEq/L, then inpatient medical admission is warranted. General treatment guidelines for hypokalemia are as follows: if the K^+ level is <2.5 mEq/L, then intravenous therapy is recommended; and if the

K^+ level is 2.5 to 2.9 mEq/L, oral supplementation is suggested. Typically, extracellular K^+ is spared at the expense of intracellular K^+ so that a patient may become hypokalemic several days after the serum K^+ concentration seems to be corrected. Supplementation can be stopped once K^+ levels are >3.5 mEq/L. Once the serum K^+ level is corrected and remains normal 2 days after supplements are stopped, the clinician can be confident that total body K^+ level has returned to normal. A patient with a K^+ level between 3.0 and 3.5 can be treated as an outpatient; a short course of potassium supplementation is reasonable to pursue. Many ED specialists will not treat adolescents with chronic potassium supplementation, because it allows teenagers to treat the medical problem while continuing to purge.

Fluid Accumulation

Many patients who abuse laxatives or vomit frequently may become chronically dehydrated. The renin-angiotensin-aldosterone axis, as well as the antidiuretic hormone level, may be elevated to compensate. These systems do not shut down automatically when laxatives are stopped, and fluid retention of up to 10 kg/week may result, which puts patients at risk for congestive heart failure and can scare them as their weight increases dramatically. Diuresis often occurs after ~7 to 10 days. Parents and patients should be advised of this possible complication of initial therapy to help maintain their confidence in the care plan.

Constipation

Constipation may be seen in chronic laxative abusers, because the natural regulation of their gastrointestinal system has been lost. Practitioners need to determine if a patient truly has constipation or is attempting to convince the practitioner to continue to purge. The physical examination and radiographs can be helpful in determining the need for treatment. Practitioners need to be judicious when treating laxative abusers and should inform parents as to what they are prescribing.

Sialadenosis and Dental Caries

The pain and swelling of enlarged parotid glands can be helped by sucking on tart candy and by the application of heat. Occasionally, parotid glands enlarge after self-induced vomiting has stopped. Development of caries and tooth enamel loss is related to the frequency and duration of self-induced vomiting. The most common teeth to show signs of enamel loss are the upper molars. Referral to a dentist to evaluate the extent of damage is important.

Psychotherapy

Cognitive-behavioral therapy is the most common psychotherapeutic approach used to help bulimic patients understand their disease and to offer suggestions for decreasing bingeing and purging. Dialectic behavior therapy also may be used to teach specific skills to patients confronted by certain stressors. Family therapy is important to help empower the family in a limited setting and to help address any family dynamic that may have contributed to development of the ED.

Nutrition Therapy

Nutrition therapy guides patients in ways to regulate eating patterns so that they can avoid the impulse to binge. Frequently, those with BN feel guilty about the previous day's binge, so they restrict eating the following day, until the impulse to binge eat appears again. Regular eating with 3 meals and 2 snacks per day, including breakfast, is important to help break the binge/purge pattern. Encouraging some satiety (fat) in their meal plan will also help regulate appetite.

Medications

SSRIs[58] are generally quite helpful in treating the binge/purge cycle. Fluoxetine has been studied most extensively; a dose of 60 mg/day is most effective in teenagers. Other SSRIs are thought to work similarly and are worth trying if the patient experiences adverse effects while taking fluoxetine. Course of medication should continue until the patient is symptom free for at least 3 to 4 months.

Outcomes

With appropriate intervention, patients with BN tend to recover more rapidly than those with AN.[59] However, relapse is common, and patients should be monitored for extended periods. The mortality rate in bulimic patients is similar to that in anorexic patients. Death usually results from suicide or electrolyte derangements. Bulimic patients also develop similar psychological illnesses as those with AN, including depression and anxiety, but they rarely develop AN.

Binge-Eating Disorder

The diagnostic category of BED was created in the DSM-IV[15] (Table 1). Officially, it is still considered a research diagnosis, although it seems to be a distinct entity that is perhaps more chronic than AN or BN, with the illness lasting an average of 14.4 years.[60] Studies have shown that most adults who have BED[61] (a prevalence of 2%–4%) developed symptoms during adolescence. A remarkable number of adolescents engage in binge eating, as demonstrated by the Youth Risk Behavior Survey.

Clinical Signs

BED occurs most often in overweight or obese individuals. Eighteen percent of such patients report bingeing at least once in the past year. Patients with BED have an increased incidence of depression and substance abuse. Using the DSM-IV diagnostic criteria as a guide for evaluation, the possibility of BED should be raised for any significantly overweight patient. Specific questionnaires are available for evaluating patients suspected of having BED. The clinician should assess causes and complications of obesity, and laboratory evaluation should include thyroid function tests and measurement of cholesterol and triglyceride levels.

Treatment

A combination of cognitive-behavioral therapy and antidepressant medication has been helpful in treating BED in adults. Use of SSRIs for BED in adolescents has not been studied, but in adults, fluoxetine and citalopram[62] help decrease binge episodes, improve depressive symptoms, and possibly decrease appetite. This evidence suggests that SSRIs in adolescents with BED may be helpful as well. BED has been recognized only recently, and outcomes have not been studied. Intervention with an SSRI seems to help the bingeing, but little is known regarding long-term prognosis.

REFERENCES

1. Eaton DK, Kann L, Kinchen S, et al. Youth Risk Behavior Surveillance: United States 2007. *MMWR Surveill Summ.* 2008;57(4):1–131. Available at: www.cdc.gov/HealthyYouth/yrbs/pdf/yrbss07_mmwr.pdf. Accessed September 18, 2008
2. Woodside DB, Garfinkel PE, Lin E, et al. Comparisons of men with full or partial eating disorders, men without eating disorders, and women with eating disorders in the community. *Am J Psychiatry.* 2001;158(4):570–574
3. Keski Rahkonen A, Hoek HW, Susser ES, et al. Epidemiology and course of anorexia in the community. *Am J Psychiatry.* 2007;164(8):1259–1265
4. Wade TD, Bergin JL, Tiggemann M, Bulik CM, Fairburn CG. Prevalence and long-term course of lifetime eating disorders in an adult Australian twin cohort. *Aust N Z J Psychiatry.* 2006; 40(2):121–128
5. Eaton DK, Kann L, Kinchen S, et al. Youth Risk Behavior Surveillance: United States 2005. *MMWR Surveill Summ.* 2006;55(5):1–108. Available at: www.cdc.gov/mmwr/preview/mmwrhtml/ss5505a1.htm. Accessed September 18, 2008
6. Peebles R, Wilson JL, Lock JD. How do children with eating disorders differ from adolescents with eating disorders at initial evaluation? *J Adolesc Health.* 2006;39(6):800–805
7. Strober M, Freeman R, Lampert C, Diamond J, Kaye W. Males with anorexia nervosa: a controlled study of eating disorders in first-degree relatives. *Int J Eat Disord.* 2001;29(3):263–269
8. Bulik CM, Tozzi F. Genetics in eating disorders: state of the science. *CNS Spectr.* 2004;9(7): 511–515
9. Mercader JM, Saus E, Agüera Z, et al. Association of *NTRK3* and its interaction with NGF suggest an altered cross-regulation of the neurotrophin signaling pathway in eating disorders. *Hum Mol Genet.* 2008;17(9):1234–1244
10. Chan JL, Manzoros CS. Role of leptin in energy deprived states: normal human physiology and clinical implications for hypothalamic amenorrhea and anorexia nervosa. *Lancet.* 2005; 366(9479):74–85
11. Bosanac P, Norman T, Burrows G, Beumont P. Serotonergic and dopaminergic systems in anorexia nervosa: a role for atypical antipsychotics? *Aust N Z J Psychiatry.* 2005;39(3):146–153

12. Modan-Moses D, Stein D, Pariente C. Modulation of adiponectin and leptin during refeeding of female anorexia nervosa patients. *J Clin Endocrinol Metab.* 2007;92(5):1843–1847
13. Tolle V, Kadem M, Bluet-Pajot MT, et al. Balance in ghrelin and leptin plasma levels in anorexia nervosa patients and constitutionally thin women. *J Clin Endocrinol Metab.* 2003;88(1):109–116
14. Procopio M, Marriott P. Intrauterine hormonal environment and risk of developing anorexia nervosa [retraction appears in *Arch Gen Psychiatry.* 2008;65(9):1052]. *Arch Gen Psychiatry.* 2007;64(12):1402–1407
15. American Psychiatric Association. *Diagnostic and Statistical Manual of Mental Disorders.* 4th ed. Text rev. Washington, DC: American Psychiatric Association; 2000
16. Eddy KT, Celio Doyle A, Hoste RR, Herzog DB, le Grange D. Eating disorder not otherwise specified in adolescents. *J Am Acad Child Adolesc Psychiatry.* 2008;47(2):156–164
17. Eddy KT, Dorer DJ, Franko DL, Tahilani K, Thompson-Brenner K, Herzog DB. Diagnostic crossover in anorexia nervosa and bulimia nervosa: implications for DSM-V. *Am J Psychiatry.* 2008;165(2):245–250
18. Naessén S, Carlström K, Glant R, Hoscobsson, H, Hrirschberg AL. Bone mineral density in bulimic women: influence of endocrine factors and previous anorexia. *Eur J Endocrinol.* 2006;155(2):245–251
19. Shaw H, Ramirez L, Trost A, Randall P, Stice E. Body image and eating disturbances across ethnic groups: more similarities than differences. *Psychol Addict Behav.* 2004;18(1):12–18
20. Mehler P. Bulimia nervosa. *N Engl J Med.* 2003;349(9):875–881
21. Austin SB, Ziyaheh N, Kahn JA, Camargo CA Jr, Colditz GA, Field AE. Sexual orientation, weight concerns, and eating-disordered behaviors in adolescent girls and boys. *J Am Acad Child Adolsec Psychiatry.* 2004;43(9):1115–1123
22. Smolak L, Murnen SK. A meta-analytic examination of the relationship between child sexual abuse and eating disorders. *Int J Eat Disord.* 2002;31(2):136–150
23. Ackard DM, Fedio G, Neumark-Sztainer D, Britt HR. Factors associated with disordered eating among sexually active adolescent males: gender and number of sexual partners. *Psychosom Med.* 2008;70(2):232–238
24. Mikami AY, Hinshaw SP, Patterson KA, Lee JC. Eating pathology among adolescent girls with attention-deficit/hyperactivity disorder. *J Abnorm Psychol.* 2008;117(1):225–235
25. Steinegger C, Katzman DK. Interviewing the adolescent with an eating disorder. *Adolesc Med State Art Rev.* 2008;19(1):18–40
26. Yager J, Anderson AE. Clinical practice: anorexia nervosa. *N Engl J Med.* 2005;353(14):1481–1488
27. Casiero D, Frishman WH. Cardiovascular complications of eating disorders. *Cardiol Rev.* 2006;14(5):227–231
28. Chial HJ, McAlpine DE, Camilleri M. Anorexia nervosa: manifestations and management for the gastroenterologist. *Am J Gastroenterol.* 2002;97(2):255–269
29. Kerem NC, Katzman DK. Brain structure and function in adolescents with anorexia nervosa. *Adolesc Med.* 2003;14(1):109–118
30. Golden NH, Jacobson MS, Schebendach J, Solanto MV, Hertz SM, Shenker IR. Resumption of menses in anorexia nervosa. *Arch Pediatr Adolesc Med.* 1997;151(1):16–21
31. Golden NH, Jacobson MS, Sterling WM, Hertz S. Treatment goal weight in adolescents with anorexia nervosa: use of BMI percentiles. *Int J Eat Disord.* 2008;41(4):301–306
32. Misra M, Aggarwal A, Miller KK, et al. Effects of anorexia nervosa on clinical, hematological, biochemical, and bone density parameters in community-dwelling adolescent girls. *Pediatrics.* 2004;114(6):1574–1583
33. Castro J, Toro J, Lazaro L, Pons F, Halperin I. Bone mineral density in male adolescents with anorexia nervosa. *J Am Acad Child Adolesc Psychiatry.* 2002;41(5):613–618
34. Rigotti NA, Neer RM, Skates SJ, Herzog DB, Nussbaum SR. The clinical course of osteoporosis in anorexia nervosa: a longitudinal study of cortical bone mass. *JAMA.* 1991;265(9):1133–1138
35. Lucas AR, Melton LJ 3rd, Crowson CS, O'Fallon WM. Long-term fracture risk among women with anorexia nervosa: a population-based cohort study. *Mayo Clin Proc.* 1999;74(10):972–977

36. Misra M, Klibanski A. Anorexia nervosa and osteoporosis. *Rev Endocr Metab Disord.* 2006; 7(1–2):91–99
37. Konstantynowicz J, Kadziela-Olech H, Kaczmarski M, et al. Depression in anorexia nervosa: a risk factor for osteoporosis. *J Clin Endocrinol Metab.* 2005;90(9):5382–5385
38. Mika C, Holtkamp K, Heer M, Günther RW, Herpertz-Dahlmann B. A 2-year prospective study of bone metabolism and bone mineral density in adolescents with anorexia nervosa. *J Neural Transm.* 2007;114(12):1611–1618
39. Zipfel S, Seibel MJ, Lowe B, Beumont PJ, Kasperk C, Herzog DW. Osteoporosis in eating disorders: a follow-up study of patients with anorexia and bulimia nervosa. *J Clin Endocrinol Metab.* 2001;86(11):5227–5233
40. Golden NH, Iglesias EA, Jacobson MS, et al. Alendronate for the treatment of osteopenia in anorexia nervosa: a randomized, double-blind, placebo-controlled trial. *J Clin Endocrinol Metab.* 2005;90(6):3179–3185
41. Miller KK, Grieco KA, Mulder J, et al. Effects of risedronate on bone density in anorexia nervosa. *J Clin Endocrinol Metab.* 2004;89(8):3903–3906
42. Grinspoon S, Thomas L, Miller K, Herzog D, Klibanski A. Effects of recombinant human IGF-1 and oral contraceptive administration on bone density in anorexia nervosa. *J Clin Endocrinol Metab.* 2002;87(6):2883–2891
43. Mühlau M, Gaser C, Ilg R, et al. Gray matter decrease of the anterior cingulate cortex in anorexia nervosa. *Am J Psychiatry.* 2007;164(12):1850–1857
44. Rome E, Ammerman S, Rosen DS, et al. Children and adolescents with eating disorders: the State of the Art. *Pediatrics.* 2003;111(1). Available at: www.pediatrics.org/cgi/content/full/111/1/e98
45. Le Grange D, Binford R, Loeb KL. Manualized family-based treatment for anorexia nervosa: a case series. *J Am Acad Child Adolesc Psychiatry.* 2005;44(1):41–46
46. Lock J, Couturier J, Agras WS. Comparison of long-term outcomes in adolescents with anorexia nervosa treated with family therapy. *J Am Acad Child Adolesc Psychiatry.* 2006;45(6):666–672
47. Dunican KC, DelDotto D. The role of olanzapine in the treatment of anorexia nervosa. *Ann Pharmacother.* 2007;41(1):111–115
48. Mondraty N, Birmingham CL, Touyz S, Sundakov V, Chapman L, Beumont P. Randomized controlled trial of olanzapine in the treatment of cognitions in anorexia nervosa. *Australas Psychiatry.* 2005;13(1):72–75
49. Claudino AM, Hay P, Lima MS, Bacaltchuk J, Schmidt U, Treasure J. Antidepressants for anorexia nervosa. *Cochrane Database Syst Rev.* 2006;(1):CD004365
50. Kaye W, Nagata T, Weltzin TE, et al. Double-blind placebo-controlled administration of fluoxetine in restricting- and restricting-purging-type anorexia nervosa. *Biol Psychiatry.* 2001; 49(7):644–652
51. Walsh BT, Kaplan AS, Attia E, et al. Fluoxetine after weight restoration in anorexia nervosa: a randomized clinical trial. *JAMA.* 2006;295(22):2605–2612
52. Birmingham CL, Gritzner S. How does zinc supplementation benefit anorexia nervosa? *Eat Weight Disord.* 2006;11(4):e109–e111
53. Fichter MM, Quadflieg N, Hedlund S. Twelve-year course and outcome predictors of anorexia nervosa. *Int J Eat Disord.* 2006;39(2):87–100
54. Herzog DB, Greenwood DN, Dorer DJ, et al. Mortality in eating disorders: a descriptive study. *Int J Eat Disord.* 2000;28(1):20–26
55. Lindblad F, Lindberg L, Hjern A. Improved survival in adolescent patients with anorexia nervosa: a comparison of two Swedish national cohorts of female patients. *Am J Psychiatry.* 2006;163(8):1433–1435
56. Schneider M. Bulimia nervosa and binge-eating disorder in adolescents. *Adolesc Med.* 2003; 14(1):119–131
57. Austin SB, Ziyadeh NJ, Vohra S, et al. Irregular menses linked to vomiting in a non-clinical sample: findings from the national eating disorders screening program in high schools. *J Adolesc Health.* 2008;42(5):450–457

58. Bacaltchuk J, Hay P, Mari JJ. Antidepressant versus placebo for the treatment of bulimia nervosa: a systematic review. *Aust N Z J Psychiatry*. 2000;34(2):310–317
59. Herzog D, Dorer DJ, Keel PK, et al. Recovery and relapse in anorexia and bulimia nervosa: a 7.5-year follow-up study. *J Am Acad Child Adolesc Psychiatry*. 1999;38(7):829–837
60. Pope HG, Laloned JK, Pindyck LJ, et al. Binge eating disorder: a stable syndrome. *Am J Psychiatry*. 2006;163(12):2181–2183
61. Fairburn CG, Cooper Z, Doll HA, Norman P, O'Connor M. The natural course of bulimia nervosa and binge eating disorder in young women. *Arch Gen Psychiatry*. 2000;57(7):659–665
62. McElroy SL, Hudson JI, Malhotra S, Welge JA, Nelson EB, Keck PE Jr. Citalopram in the treatment of binge-eating disorder: A placebo-controlled trial. *J Clin Psychiatry*. 2003;64(7): 807–813

Adolesc Med 19 (2008) 573–591

Bone Metabolism During Adolescence: The Known, the Unknown, and the Controversial

Zeev Harel, MD*

Division of Adolescent Medicine/Hasbro Children's Hospital/Rhode Island Hospital, 593 Eddy Street, Providence, RI 02903, USA

Department of Pediatrics, Warren Alpert Medical School of Brown University, 97 Waterman Street, Providence, RI 02912, USA

Bone formation and bone resorption are continuous processes throughout life. During adolescence, bone formation prevails over resorption, resulting in accumulation of 40% of peak bone mass. The amount of skeletal mass acquired during adolescence is one of the most important factors in determining the risk of osteoporosis and fractures later in life.[1] It is clear that to prevent osteoporosis, efforts should be made to ascertain that adolescents attain 100% of their potential peak bone mass.

In adolescents, bone modeling (construction) and remodeling (reconstruction) modify the external size and contours of bone and its internal architecture and lead to cortical and trabecular bone thickening. Both processes are performed by the same effector cells, osteoblasts and osteoclasts, but differ in the way these cells are arranged. During modeling, periosteal osteoblasts deposit new bone on an extended surface area and over an extended period of time without being interrupted by osteoclasts. During remodeling, osteoblasts and osteoclasts are linked ("coupled") tightly in time and space. The purpose of modeling and remodeling during growth is to improve bone quality and establish the skeleton's peak bone strength. The strength of bone is determined by its material composition and structure. Bone is composed of type I collagen stiffened by crystals of calcium hydroxyapatite. To allow flexibility, human bone is only ~60% mineralized. The composition and degree of collagen cross-linking also influence bone strength.[2]

The accretion of bone mass in adolescents involves the interaction of multiple calcitrophic hormones such as growth hormone (GH), insulin-like growth factor 1 (IGF-1), and gonadal hormones.[3] In addition to genetic and ethnic/racial factors

*Corresponding author.
E-mail address: zharel@lifespan.org (Z. Harel).

 ISSN 1934-4287

Table 1
Factors that affect bone-mass accretion

Nonmodifiable	Modifiable
Genetics	Nutrition
Age, gynecological age	Weight-bearing physical activity
Race and ethnicity	Smoking
History of pregnancy	Alcohol use
A chronic disease	Hormonal status

that affect this process, environmental factors such as dietary habits and physical activity (Table 1) may influence the accretion of bone mass during adolescence.[3]

Imaging techniques such as dual-energy radiograph absorptiometry (DEXA) have been used to assess bone-mineral content (BMC) and bone-mineral density (BMD) in children and adolescents.[4] In addition, biochemical markers of bone turnover have been used to evaluate bone formation and bone resorption in this age group.[5]

MEASUREMENT OF BONE MASS

Imaging Techniques

Dual-Energy Radiograph Absorptiometry

DEXA is widely accepted as the preferred method for assessing bone mass in children and adolescents because of its speed, precision, availability, and modest radiation exposure.[6] BMC (grams) of the entire body and BMD (grams per centimeter squared) of the spine and hip are obtained. However, DEXA is limited, because it calculates a two-dimensional projected area and not a volumetric BMD. As a result, DEXA may overestimate true bone mass in larger individuals and underestimate bone mass in smaller individuals, although the growth process is attenuated in the postmenarchal years in girls, it can still lead to a much greater change in bone volume than in bone area. Therefore, several investigators have derived models to estimate volumetric bone density to reduce the influence of bone size on DEXA measurements.[7,8] Standardization conversion equations have also been developed to account for the different DEXA scanners (Hologic Inc [Waltham, MA] or Lunar [Madison, WI]) used in some multiple-center studies.[9,10] The use of gender- and ethnic-specific normative standards has been recommended when interpreting bone densitometry data of adolescents.[8,11,12] The World Health Organization osteoporosis criteria that use *t* scores (comparing patient data to a reference population of young adults) should not be applied to adolescents because of the age discrepancy.[13] The *z* score is a measure that reports patient data as the SD compared with a reference population of the same age and is more useful when interpreting adolescent DEXA reports.

A z score lower than −2 has been used to define "low bone density for chronological age" in adolescents. Bone-density measurement should be considered for adolescents with an underlying chronic condition that predisposes to a low BMD and for adolescents with risk factors for low BMD or with a strong family history of osteoporosis. When following patients longitudinally, an attempt should be made to use the same densitometer and reference data.[14]

Axial Quantitative Computed Tomography

Axial quantitative computed tomography (QCT) circumvents the measurement artifact associated with DEXA by measuring volumetric BMD directly. However, QCT is not widely available and requires considerably higher radiation exposure than DEXA.[6] Peripheral QCT (pQCT) requires less radiation (similar to DEXA radiation) and has the ability to differentiate cortical bone from trabecular bone. Parameters such as cortical density, total cross-sectional bone area, cortical bone area, and cortical thickness can be assessed by using pQCT.[15,16] As it becomes more readily available, pQCT could be used to assess volumetric BMD in the adolescent population.

Quantitative Ultrasound

Quantitative ultrasound (QUS) is an attractive method for evaluating adolescent bone mass, because it is portable and inexpensive and requires no ionizing radiation.[6] However, this technique is less precise,[6] and pediatric reference data are limited.[17]

Markers of Bone Turnover

Sensitive indicators for bone formation include blood osteocalcin and bone-specific alkaline phosphatase (BAP). Osteocalcin is the major noncollagenous protein of bone matrix. Osteocalcin is synthesized by osteoblasts in the bone, partly incorporated into the bone matrix, and partly delivered to the circulatory system. Bone-derived alkaline phosphatase (BAP) is an enzyme localized to the membrane of osteoblasts, and it is released into the circulation.

Urinary *N*-telopeptide (uNTX), the amino telopeptide cross-linking domain of type I collagen, and urinary pyridinoline and deoxypyridinoline, the nondeductible crosslinks between the telopeptide regions of the collagen molecules, are good indicators of bone resorption.[5]

Markers of bone formation (serum BAP and osteocalcin) and of bone resorption (uNTX) are typically measured by enzyme immunoassays in most laboratories. Because of the diurnal variability of uNTX, it is recommended to obtain a urine sample at the same time during the day (typically second void).

Studies have shown marked increases in bone-turnover markers throughout the growth spurt in adolescents. These increases last until the time of peak height velocity.[18–20] After menarche in girls, there is a decline in bone-turnover markers, but bone accretion in the postmenarchal years may continue in the face of this slowdown in bone turnover.[21]

BONE ACCRETION IN FEMALE ADOLESCENTS

Although longitudinal growth is most rapid during early pubertal stages in girls, bone-mineral accrual is greatest around the time of menarche.[22] Peak velocity of bone-mass accumulation has been reported to be ~0.7 years after the peak in longitudinal growth velocity.[23] Menarche is a milestone for both longitudinal growth and bone-mass accretion in adolescent girls. Although there is a decrease in the rate of longitudinal growth immediately after menarche, intensive bone accrual continues for several years after this physiologic milestone.[24]

This postmenarcheal increase in bone accretion is probably caused by the high levels of estrogen, GH, and IGF-1 during these later stages of pubertal development in girls. However, toward the end of puberty, the high levels of estradiol inhibit chondrocyte proliferation and reduce bone turnover despite the presence of high levels of GH and IGF-1.[5,22] This inhibition of chondrocyte proliferation and bone turnover ultimately results in attenuation of the bone-accretion process in girls' late adolescence years.[3,5,25]

On average, young women attain 92% of their total body BMC by the age of 18 and 99% by age 26.[26] However, the attainment age of peak bone mass in young women is site specific; peak bone mass seems to be attained in the femoral neck by the age of 16,[24] whereas in the lumbar spine, bone mass continues to increase throughout the third decade of life.[27]

The time in life in which spine peak bone mass in women is attained is the subject of considerable controversy, with estimates for the axial skeleton ranging from soon after the completion of sexual and skeletal maturity at the end of the second decade, to the fifth decade of life. Most reports, but not all, have indicated that bone mass does not significantly increase after the third decade. These discrepancies may be attributed, at least in part, to differences in the technique and methodology used in the various studies. For example, Wren et al[28] have shown that bone acquisition in the lumbar spine measured by computed tomography reaches its peak by sexual and skeletal maturity, whereas bone values measured by DEXA continue to increase after puberty and cessation of longitudinal growth. The conflicting results between computed tomography and DEXA are likely a reflection of the influence of soft tissues around the spine and/or the inclusion of the posterior elements of the vertebrae in DEXA measurements.[28]

BONE ACCRETION IN MALE ADOLESCENTS

BMC accretion accelerates in boys ~2 years later than in girls, reflecting the later onset of puberty in boys. The highest rate of BMC accumulation in boys is at late puberty.[20,25] Although there are no differences in BMC between prepubertal boys and girls, boys have a greater increase in BMC during puberty, resulting in greater values of skeletal mass.[11] The greater bone mass in males is partly a result of their greater bone size. Although earlier reports suggested that peak bone mass in boys occurs between 17 and 20 years of age, a more recent report indicated that peak bone mass in boys is attained within the third decade of life.[29]

FACTORS THAT AFFECT BONE ACCRETION IN ADOLESCENTS

Factors That Cannot Be Modified

Genetics

The genetic contribution to BMD is well established from both twin and family studies. Duncan et al[30] reported a total heritability range of 61% to 67% at the lumbar spine and 44% to 67% at the femoral neck. Although there has been progress in identifying some genetic variants, most of the genes and genetic variants that regulate bone mass and susceptibility to osteoporosis remain undiscovered.[31] A family history of osteoporosis is an important risk factor for low BMD, particularly in women.[32] However, this is sometimes difficult to assess in adolescents, given that the adolescents' mothers are too young to have experienced osteoporosis, and that adolescents might not know the medical histories of their grandmothers.

Age

The influence of age on BMD in adolescents is related to the effects of puberty on BMD, particularly during the early pubertal stages. In general, BMD during adolescence is more a function of pubertal stage than of chronological age. Because the age of onset and the progression of puberty are highly variable, several authors have included Tanner stages in presentation of normative BMD data for adolescents.[11,33]

In girls, there is a wide individual variation in the age of menarche (onset of the first menstrual period). Menarche occurs during Tanner stage 3 in 25% of girls, Tanner stage 4 in 60% of girls, and Tanner stage 5 in 15% of girls. Because of these variations, gynecologic age (time since menarche) has been used in assessing BMD during the postmenarchal years in adolescent girls. In a recent study of postmenarchal adolescents, chronological age was significantly associated solely with BMD values of the lumbar spine, whereas gynecologic age was significantly associated with the BMD values of both the lumbar spine and the total hip.[21]

Race

Multiple studies have found that black adolescent girls have significantly higher BMD values compared with those of their nonblack counterparts.[34,35] In a recent study, after adjusting for chronological age, gynecologic age, and BMI, the BMD of black participants was still significantly higher than the BMD of nonblack participants at the total hip ($P < .05$) and the femoral neck ($P < .05$) but not at the lumbar spine.[21] In addition to possible effects of several anthropomorphic factors such as greater BMI and muscle mass, some studies have suggested that the greater accumulation of bone mass in black girls is a result of more-efficient renal calcium retention[36,37] and skeletal resistance to the bone-resorption effect of parathyroid hormone.[38] More studies are needed to elucidate the mechanisms behind this observed difference.

History of Pregnancy

The negative impact of pregnancy on the BMD of adolescent girls is not well established, but it seems to be greater than that found in older women. Bone loss may be more significant in adolescent mothers, because in this age group the fetus' demands for calcium compete with the ongoing needs of the adolescent for bone-mineral accrual. Sowers et al[38] have shown that adolescent mothers lose more BMD during pregnancy than older mothers (5.5% vs 1.9%, respectively).

Moreover, lactation during the first 5 months after delivery has been shown to further decrease BMD.[39] Although the BMD of most adult women returns to preconception values,[39,40] it is unclear whether BMD losses during pregnancy and lactation in adolescents are completely reversible. In a recent study of adolescents, previous history of pregnancy was significantly associated with a lower BMD at the lumbar spine ($P < .0001$) and total hip ($P < .01$) when compared with the BMD of adolescents who had never been pregnant.[21] It remains to be determined in long-term prospective studies whether the pregnancy- and lactation-induced bone loss in adolescent mothers is completely reversible.

Chronic Disease

In addition to bone diseases such as osteogenesis imperfecta, many other conditions may impair bone accretion and place adolescents at risk for poor skeletal health (Table 2). Many of these illnesses also require use of medications that have deleterious skeletal effects (Table 2).

Factors That Can Be Modified

Weight/BMI

Several reports have shown that weight and BMI have an effect on BMD.[35,41,42] These reports have led a few authors to include weight in their normative BMD

Table 2
Chronic medical conditions and medications that can impair bone-mineral accrual

Chronic Medical Conditions	Endocrinopathies	Medications
Prolonged immobilization	Cushing syndrome (hypercortisolism)	Anticonvulsants
Anorexia nervosa	GH deficiency	Glucocorticoids
Inflammatory bowel disease	Hyperthyroidism	Cyclosporine A
Celiac disease	Hypothyroidism	Gonadotropin-releasing hormone agonists
Cystic fibrosis	Hyperparathyroidism	Heparin
Cerebral palsy and other neuromuscular conditions	Hyperprolactinemia	Lithium
Chronic renal failure	Hypogonadism/sex hormone deficiency	DMPA
Status post cranial irradiation (particularly pituitary)		Chemotherapeutic agents (such as methotrexate)
Diabetes mellitus		
Epilepsy		
HIV infection		
Malignancies		
Status post organ transplantation		
Rheumatologic diseases		
Sickle cell disease		
Thalassemia		
Turner syndrome		
Asthma		

value analysis.[35,41] The positive correlation of higher weight/BMI and BMD is commonly believed to be a result of the impact of greater weight bearing on the BMD of overweight females. Increased loading of long bones produces the greatest mechanical stresses on the subperiosteal surface and stimulates bone formation by subperiosteal expansion.[42] Hormonal influences, such as increased conversion of androstenedione to estrogen and increased circulating leptin concentrations, also play a role and contribute to the increased skeletal mass observed with obesity.[43]

Nutritional Factors

Calcium Approximately one third of the BMC consists of calcium.[44] In addition to providing the structural strength, bone calcium also serves as a reservoir that can be tapped to maintain extracellular calcium concentration.[45] The growth of the skeleton requires a positive calcium balance, with relatively high calcium retention needed for adequate bone calcium accretion during childhood and adolescence.[46] Jackman et al examined the relation between calcium retention and calcium intake in adolescent girls and found an increase in retention with increase in calcium intake.[46] The Institute of Medicine, with its dietary reference intakes, recommend a calcium intake of 1300 mg/day for adolescents, with a tolerable upper intake limit of 2500 mg/day.[47]

The amount of calcium deposited in a well-prepared osteoid matrix during childhood and adolescence may determine the risk of osteoporosis and fractures in adulthood.[48,49] Although peak bone mass has a large genetic component, there is evidence that it can be enhanced by increased calcium consumption.[50] Studies have shown that adequate milk consumption is associated with a greater BMD in teenagers and young adults,[51,52] and that calcium supplementation leads to an increase in BMD in children and adolescents.[53–56] Examining whether there is a threshold effect of calcium on bone mass, Matkovic and Heaney[57] analyzed data from 124 studies that involved children and young adults and reported a threshold effect of daily calcium intake of 1480 mg for 9- to 17-year-old children.

At this stage of increased need for calcium, the majority of adolescents consume significantly less than the recommended daily intake.[58] Knowledge that adequate calcium intake during adolescence is critical for prevention of osteoporosis was associated with higher consumption of calcium, and adolescents who were aware of the daily requirement for calcium tended to consume more of this essential mineral.[58] Thus, it is clear that adolescent health care providers, nurses, dietitians, and health teachers have to provide information about the health benefits of calcium. In particular, those who provide health care to adolescents have to emphasize the important role of calcium in peak bone-mass accretion during adolescence. With adolescents it is important to be specific. Concrete information about calcium sources and amounts should be provided. Adolescents should be recommended to drink 1 cup of milk in the morning and 1 cup of milk at bedtime. Adolescents should also be informed about nondairy sources of calcium, such as fruit juices and cereals enriched with calcium, which have been increasingly available in recent years. Because dietary habits of the family and peers, as well as advertising media, may affect adolescents' dietary habits, these factors should also be included in every calcium educational program for adolescents.

It remains controversial whether to recommend calcium supplementation for improving BMD in healthy adolescents. Although studies have shown increases in BMD with calcium supplementation,[53–56] these increases may not be maintained. A recent meta-analysis of randomized, controlled trials in children aged 3 to 18 years found a small effect of calcium supplementation on total BMC and upper-limb BMD but no effect on femoral-neck or lumbar-spine BMD.[59] The effect persisted after the end of supplementation only at the upper limb. The authors concluded that although it is possible that the small increase in BMD from calcium supplementation could reduce the risk of upper-limb fractures, the public health benefit of this is likely to be small.[59] Thus, these results do not support the use of calcium supplementation in healthy adolescents as a public health intervention. However, conclusions cannot be extrapolated to adolescents with medical conditions that affect bone metabolism.

Protein An adequate intake of protein is essential for the synthesis of bone matrix. In particular, protein is necessary for the production of IGF-1, which is an essential bone growth factor. Although excessive dietary protein from foods with high potential renal acid load may adversely affect bone and lead to increased calcium excretion,[60] it is believed that excess protein will not harm the skeleton as long as calcium intake is adequate.[61] An ideal diet for adolescents should include 20% protein, which constitutes ~1 g of protein per kg of body weight.

Vitamin D Vitamin D increases intestinal absorption of calcium, and phosphate, and is an essential factor in the mineralization of the skeleton. Vitamin D is obtained either from dietary sources or from cutaneous synthesis through a process initiated by ultraviolet radiation on the skin. The body's vitamin D stores can be assessed by measuring the serum concentration of 25-hydroxyvitamin D (25[OH]D). When the serum 25(OH)D concentration decreases, parathyroid hormone concentrations increase, which leads to increased osteoclast activity and bone resorption. Although there has been an intense debate as to which serum 25(OH)D concentrations are optimal for the acquisition and maintenance of bone mass,[62–64] it is believed that serum 25(OH)D levels of 80 nmol/L are needed for optimal calcium-absorption efficiency and optimal suppression of serum parathyroid hormone concentrations.[65]

Vitamin D deficiency has been reported among children, particularly during the dark seasons of the year.[63] In a study of healthy US teenagers, 24.1% were found to have vitamin D deficiency (serum 25[OH]D concentration <37.5 nmol/L), with a higher prevalence of vitamin D deficiency observed in black adolescents and during winter.[66] In another study by Harness and Cromer,[67] 17% of the girls were found to be vitamin D deficient (serum 25[OH]D concentration <27.5 nmol/L). Pubertal girls with hypovitaminosis D seem to be at risk of not reaching the maximum peak bone mass, particularly at the lumbar spine.[68]

The reference intake of vitamin D for children and adolescents is 200 IU/day.[47,69] However, to achieve serum 25(OH)D concentrations of 80 nmol/L in female adolescents aged 12 to 19 years, there is a need to consume an additional 863 IU/day of vitamin D.[59] To avoid hypervitaminosis D, which is associated with serum 25(OH)D levels in excess of 400 nmol/L, an upper level of safe intake of vitamin D was set at 2000 IU/day for all ages.[47,65]

Magnesium Approximately 60% of the body's magnesium is found in bone. Magnesium, which plays an important role in adenosine triphosphate metabolism and is a cofactor for many enzymes, is essential for both bone-matrix and bone-mineral metabolism.[70] Inadequate dietary magnesium intake has been reported in adolescents and young adults.[71] Efforts should be made to raise adolescents' intake of magnesium to the recommended intake of 360 mg/day for girls (ages 14–18 years) and 410 mg/day for boys (ages 14–18 years). Magnesium sources include dairy products, nuts, whole grains, and green leafy vegetables.

Phosphorus Approximately 85% of the body's phosphorus is in bone. Recommended daily intake for adolescents is 1250 mg/day,[47] and most adolescents and young adults meet this requirement.[71] The main food sources are the protein food groups of meat and milk. Fruits and vegetables contain only small amounts of phosphorus. A meal plan that provides adequate amounts of calcium and protein also provides an adequate amount of phosphorus.

Vitamin K Vitamin K mediates the carboxylation of glutamyl residues on several bone proteins, notably osteocalcin. Carboxylation of these bone proteins is essential for their biological activity and for their affinity for calcium.[72,73] Optimal carboxylation of bone proteins requires a higher vitamin K intake than the recommended daily intake (0.5–1.0 μg/kg body weight) needed for carboxylation of blood coagulation factors.[73] In one study, supplementation with vitamin K (1–10 mg/day) increased markers for bone formation, decreased markers for bone resorption, and reduced urinary calcium loss.[74] Dietary sources of vitamin K include green vegetables such as spinach, kale, and broccoli, which are rich in vitamin K_1 (phylloquinone), and cheese and liver, which are rich in vitamin K_2 (menaquinones). At the present time, data are insufficient to recommend vitamin K supplements for adolescents.

Dietary Phytoestrogens Phytoestrogens are naturally occurring plant compounds that have estrogenic and/or antiestrogenic activity.[75,76] Tentative evidence suggests that phytoestrogens may have a positive effect on bone density similar to the effects of a related pharmaceutical compound (ipriflavone).[75] Although phytoestrogens are ubiquitous in many foods including beans, sprouts, cabbage, spinach, and grains, the 2 main phytoestrogens (lignans and isoflavones) are found in particularly high concentrations in flaxseeds and soybeans, respectively.[75] Current data about phytoestrogens are not sufficient to recommend particular dietary phytoestrogens for adolescents.

Other Dietary Factors Consumption of vegetables has been shown to increase bone mass.[77] A decrease in bone resorption as well as a decrease in urinary secretion of calcium may explain this beneficial effect, although the active compound in vegetables leading to this remains to be identified.

By contrast, high consumption of carbonated beverages may lead to a reduction in BMD during adolescence.[78] In addition to milk displacement from the diet, the acid load of carbonated soft drinks may lead to an increase in urinary excretion of calcium.

Nutrient Interactions Although consumption of a high-calcium diet has not interfered with iron status,[79] zinc retention,[80] or magnesium kinetics,[81] there is evidence to suggest that some dietary factors may inhibit calcium absorption or increase calcium excretion. Oxalic acid (found in spinach, beans, sweet potatoes, and rhubarb) and phytic acid (the storage form of phosphorus in seeds) are known inhibitors of calcium absorption. Adolescents who consume these foods should be encouraged to increase consumption of calcium-rich foods to compensate for possible lower calcium absorption. High consumption of sodium chloride and protein increases urinary calcium excretion. In adolescent girls, every additional gram of salt consumed leads to an extra 26 mg of calcium excreted in the urine,[82] whereas an additional gram of protein consumed leads to an extra 1 mg of calcium excreted in the urine. Adolescents should be informed about these interactions and be advised to limit their dietary salt intake to <2400 mg/day and their dietary protein intake to 1 g/kg per day. More studies about nutrient-nutrient interactions in adolescents, as well as studies about interactions of nutrients with other parameters such as exercise and hormonal changes during adolescence, are warranted.

Physical Activity

Moderate amounts of exercise have been shown to have a positive impact on bone.[83] One consistent finding is that moderate physical activity of a weight-bearing nature, such as running or jumping, generally has a more positive impact on bone than non–weight-bearing activities such as swimming.[84] Nickols-Richardson et al[85] examined BMD in young female gymnasts (aged 8–13 years) over 12 months compared with that in height- and weight-matched controls. Despite lower body fat among the gymnasts, larger increases in BMD were observed in this group when compared with the control group. There seems to be a threshold of intensity of physical activity over which a negative impact on bone occurs, particularly when the exercise is anaerobic or is performed by very thin, amenorrheic participants. The negative relationship between high levels of exercise and BMD is not restricted to women. Bilanin et al[86] found significantly decreased BMD in male long-distance runners (mean distance: 92 ± 6.3 km/wk) when compared with that in male nonrunners. A common explanation is relatively low circulating levels of sex hormones commonly observed in very thin athletes with intensive training schedules.[87] A second theory is hypercortisolism from chronic physical stress.[88] A third theory posits that B-endorphins, produced by intensive exercise, suppress hypothalamic production of gonadotropin-releasing hormone with resultant low levels of estrogen.[89] Finally, the loss of calcium in sweat may contribute to low BMD in athletes who participate in strenuous exercise. Klesges et al[90] examined collegiate male basketball players practicing outside in a Southern state during the summer. Acute losses in BMD were observed in the players, and these BMD changes were correlated with levels of calcium in sweat.

Cigarette Smoking and Alcohol Consumption

There is evidence to suggest that cigarette smoking is associated with lower peak BMD levels during adulthood, particularly in those who started smoking cigarettes at an early age.[91,92] Although a direct toxic effect of nicotine on bone cells has been suggested, the exact mechanism by which smoking affects bone metabolism remains to be elucidated. The association between smoking and BMD during adolescence may be gender dependent. Although smoking was associated with lower BMD and reduced cortical thickness in young (aged 18–20) men,[93] a study of adolescent girls did not show a relationship between cigarette smoking and BMD.[21] Similarly, although excessive alcohol consumption has been shown to suppress bone metabolism,[94] alcohol-use history showed no correlation with the BMD of female adolescents.[21] However, investigators in the study[21] did not collect information on quantity, frequency, or duration of cigarette smoking and alcohol use; thus, it is possible that the girls who smoked cigarettes or drank alcohol did so at a very low level that would not affect BMD.

Calcitrophic Hormones

The accretion of bone mass in adolescents involves the interaction of multiple calcitrophic hormones such as GH and gonadal hormones, together with growth factors such as IGF-1 and IGF-2.[3] Puberty is triggered by increased pulsatile secretion of gonadotropin-releasing hormone by the hypothalamus, leading to increases in serum gonadotropin levels and, thus, to increases in secretion of gonadal sex hormones. The increase in serum estrogen enhances pulsatile GH secretion in both genders, and this increase, in turn, increases circulating, and possible osteoblast, IGF-1 concentrations.

There is evidence that the calcitrophic hormones active in the bone-remodeling process exert a major part of their effects through the IGF regulatory system.[95,96] IGF-1 enhances chondrocyte proliferation and differentiation in the growth plate and stimulates osteoblast proliferation and differentiation and collagen synthesis.[95,96]

Sex steroids also seem to increase bone mass during skeletal maturation independent of the effects of circulating levels of GH and IGF-1. The 25% greater bone mass in postpubertal boys over postpubertal girls is likely caused mainly by the pubertal increase in serum testosterone, because increases in GH secretion and IGF-1 production are similar or even greater in girls than in boys. However, estrogen contributes substantially to volumetric BMD in both genders. During puberty, estrogen promotes accrual of bone mass on the cortical endosteal surface and in trabecular bone. At the cellular level, estrogen affects the generation, life span, and functional activity of both osteoclasts and osteoblasts. Estrogen decreases osteoclast formation and activity, and by increasing apoptosis, it decreases osteoclasts' life span.[97] In addition, estrogen increases intestinal calcium absorption and increases renal calcium conservation by enhancing tubular calcium resorption.[98]

As with estrogen, the major action of testosterone at the tissue level is to reduce bone resorption. However, much of this action is indirect via aromatization of testosterone to estrogen. Testosterone may differ from estrogen by acting at different stages of osteoblast differentiation, and testosterone and estrogen may affect osteoblasts differently at various skeletal locations.[98]

PROGESTERONE AND THE BONE

Although estrogen plays an important role in growth and maturation of bone in adolescents and in protecting against excessive bone resorption in adults, the effect of progesterone on the bone is less clear. In women with hypogonadism, there is evidence that progesterone acts as a bone-trophic hormone[99] and prevents bone loss.[100,101] Progestins, including medroxyprogesterone acetate, have been shown to have positive effects on bone metabolism, manifested by the reduction of urinary ratios of calcium and hydroxyproline to creatinine, as well as the reduction of other indices of bone resorption. In addition, progestins may increase intestinal absorption of calcium and may have a positive effect on calcitonin. However, in healthy women using a progestin-only contraceptive such as depo-medroxyprogesterone acetate (DMPA), possible osteopenia is a concern because of the induced partial estrogen deficiency.

DMPA AND THE BONE IN ADOLESCENTS

Longitudinal studies of adolescent girls on DMPA showed a decrease of 1.8% to 3.5% in BMD of the lumbar spine over 12 months of use, compared with increases of 1.2% to 2.9% in the control group.[102–104] Another longitudinal study reported a mean decrease of 2.2% in the femoral-neck BMD of girls using DMPA over 12 months, compared with a mean increase of 2.3% in the control group.[105] A recent prospective study of adolescents showed significant losses of BMD at the spine and hip while on DMPA, with a rapid recovery of BMD, particularly at the spine and whole body, after discontinuation of the method.[106] However, the design of that study made it impossible to determine what the adolescents' BMD would have been had they never used DMPA.

The exact mechanism that leads to the reduction in BMD in adolescents on DMPA is as yet unknown. Ott et al[107] reported an increase in *N*-telopeptide excretion, a bone-resorption marker, in DMPA users, suggesting an accelerated bone turnover with bone resorption exceeding bone formation in users of DMPA. This increased bone turnover was consistent with findings observed in hypogonadism conditions, although measurements of hormones involved in bone resorption, such as estrogen and parathyroid hormone, were not obtained in that study. Conversely, Rome et al[108] reported a decrease in urinary deoxypyridinoline (a bone-resorption marker) excretion and a decrease in serum BAP (a bone-formation marker) in adolescents using DMPA, suggesting lower bone turnover. This last study raised the possibility that, in addition to relative estrogen deficiency,[109] other factors might be involved in the reduction of BMD in adolescents on DMPA.

Based on these studies, on November 17, 2004, the US Food and Drug Administration issued a "black-box warning" for DMPA, stating that prolonged use of the method may result in significant loss of BMD, that the loss is greater the longer the drug is administered, and that BMD loss may not be completely reversible after discontinuation of the drug.[110] In a 2006 position paper of the Society for Adolescent Medicine, Cromer et al[111] provided a list of clinical guidelines for continuation of DMPA use in the adolescent age group.

CONCLUSIONS

Throughout the past several years there has been considerable progress in identifying and understanding the factors that affect bone metabolism in adolescents. Although genetic predisposition, age, race, and ethnicity cannot be modified, factors such as nutrition, physical activity, and lifestyle choices can be changed. Promoting a healthy lifestyle, regular weight-bearing physical activity, and a healthy diet with adequate calcium and vitamin D intake may prove to be the best way to optimize bone accretion in this age group.

REFERENCES

1. Johnston CC, Slemenda CW. Peak bone mass, bone loss and risk of fracture. *Osteoporos Int.* 1994;4(suppl 1):S43–S45
2. Seeman E, Delmas PD. Bone quality: the material and structural basis of bone strength and fragility. *N Engl J Med.* 2006;354(21):2250–2261
3. Davies JH, Evans BA, Gregory JW. Bone mass acquisition in healthy children. *Arch Dis Child.* 2005;90(4):373–378
4. Glastre C, Braillon P, David L, et al. Measurement of bone mineral content of the lumbar spine by dual energy x-ray absorptiometry in normal children: correlations with growth parameters. *J Clin Endocrinol Metab.* 1990;70(5):1330–1333
5. Blumsohn A, Hannon RA, Wrate R, et al. Biochemical markers of bone turnover in girls during puberty. *Clin Endocrinol (Oxf).* 1994;40(5):663–670
6. Genant HK, Engelke K, Fuerst T, et al. Noninvasive assessment of bone mineral and structure: state of the art. *J Bone Miner Res.* 1996;11(6):707–730
7. Lu PW, Cowell CT, Lloyd-Jones SA, Briody JN, Howman-Giles R. Volumetric bone mineral density in normal subjects, aged 5–27 years. *J Clin Endocrinol Metab.* 1996;81(4):1586–1590
8. Bachrach LK, Hastie T, Wang MC, Narasimhan B, Marcus R. Bone mineral acquisition in healthy Asian, Hispanic, black, and Caucasian youth: a longitudinal study. *J Clin Endocrinol Metab.* 1999;84(12):4702–4712
9. Hanson J. Standardization of femur BMD. *J Bone Miner Res.* 1997;12(8):1316–1317
10. Hui SL, Gao S, Zhou XH, et al. Universal standardization of bone density measurements: a method with optimal properties for calibration among several instruments. *J Bone Miner Res.* 1997;12(9):1463–1470
11. Faulkner RA, Bailey DA, Drinkwater DT, McKay HA, Arnold C, Wilkinson AA. Bone densitometry in Canadian children 8–17 years of age. *Calcif Tissue Int.* 1996;59(5):344–351
12. Binkley TL, Specker BL, Wittig TA. Centile curves for bone densitometry measurements in healthy males and females ages 5–22 yr. *J Clin Densitom.* 2002;5(4):343–353
13. Khan AA, Bachrach L, Brown JP, et al. Standards and guidelines for performing central dual-energy x-ray absorptiometry in premenopausal women, men and children. *J Clin Densitom.* 2004;7(1):51–64
14. Lewiecki EM, Watts NB, McClung MR, et al. Official positions of the Internal Society for Clinical Densitometry. *J Clin Endocrinol Metab.* 2004;89(8):3651–3655
15. Neu CM, Manz F, Rauch F, Merkel A, Schoenau E. Bone densities and bone size at the distal radius in healthy children and adolescents: a study using peripheral quantitative computed tomography. *Bone.* 2001;28(2):227–232

16. Leonard MB, Shults J, Elliott DM, Stallings VA, Zemel BS. Interpretation of whole body dual energy x-ray absorptiometry measures in children: comparison with peripheral quantitative computed tomography. *Bone*. 2004;34(6):1044–1052
17. Mughal MZ, Ward K, Qayyum N, Langton CM. Assessment of bone status using the contact ultrasound bone analyzer. *Arch Dis Child*. 1997;76(6):535–536
18. Mora S, Prinster C, Proverbio MC, et al. Urinary markers of bone turnover in healthy children and adolescents: age-related changes and effect of puberty. *Calcif Tissue Int*. 1998;63(5):369–374
19. Mora S, Pitukcheewanont P, Kaufman FR, Nelson JC, Gilsanz V. Biochemical markers of bone turnover and the volume and the density of bone in children at different stages of sexual development. *J Bone Miner Res*. 1999;14(10):1664–1671
20. Van Coeverden SCCM, Netelenbos JC, de Ridder CM, Roos JC, Popp-Snijders C, Delemarre-van de Waal HA. Bone metabolism markers and bone mass in healthy pubertal boys and girls. *Clin Endocrinol (Oxf)*. 2002;57(1):107–116
21. Harel Z, Gold M, Cromer B, et al. Bone mineral density in postmenarchal adolescent girls in the United States: associated biopsychosocial variables and bone turnover markers. *J Adolesc Health*. 2007;40(1):44–53
22. Cadogan J, Blumsohn A, Barker ME, Eatell R. A longitudinal study of bone gain in pubertal girls: anthropometric and biochemical correlates. *J Bone Miner Res*. 1998;13(10):1602–1612
23. Bailey DA. The Saskatchewan Pediatric Bone Mineral Accrual Study: bone mineral acquisition during the growing years. *Int J Sports Med*. 1997;18(suppl 3):S191–S194
24. Theintz G, Buchs B, Rizzoli R, et al. Longitudinal monitoring of bone mass accumulation in healthy adolescents: evidence for marked reduction after 16 years of age at the levels of lumbar spine and femoral neck in female subjects. *J Clin Endocrinol Metab*. 1992;75(4):1060–1065
25. Bonjour JP, Theintz G, Buchs B, Slosman D, Rizzoli R. Critical years and stages of puberty for spinal and femoral bone mass accumulation during adolescence. *J Clin Endocrinol Metab*. 1991;73(3):555–563
26. Teegarden D, Proulx WR, Martin BR, et al. Peak bone mass in young women. *J Bone Miner Res*. 1995;10(5):711–715
27. Recker RR, Davies KM, Hinders SM, Heaney RP, Stegman MR, Kimmel DB. Bone gain in young adult women. *JAMA*. 1992;268(17):2403–2408
28. Wren TA, Kim PS, Janika A, Sanches M, Gilsanz V. Timing of peak bone mass: discrepancies between CT and DXA. *J Clin Endocrinol Metab*. 2007;92(3):938–941
29. Høiberg M, Nielsen TL, Wraae K, Abrahamsen B, Hagen C, Andersen M, Brixen K. Population-based reference values for bone mineral density in young men. *Osteoporos Int*. 2007; 18(11):1507–1514
30. Duncan EL, Cardon LR, Sinsheimer JS, Wass JA, Brown MA. Site and gender specificity of inheritance of bone mineral density. *J Bone Miner Res*. 2003;18(8):1531–1538
31. Ralston SH, de Crombrugghe B. Genetic regulation of bone mass and susceptibility to osteoporosis. *Genes Dev*. 2006;20(18):2492–2506
32. Bainbridge KE, Sowers M, Lin X, Harlow SD. Risk factors for low bone mineral density and the 6-year rate of bone loss among premenopausal and perimenopausal women. *Osteoporos Int*. 2004;15(6):439–446
33. Mølgaard C, Thomsen BL, Michaelsen KF. Influence of weight, age and puberty on bone size and bone mineral content in healthy children and adolescents. *Acta Paediatr*. 1998;87(5):494–499
34. Gilsanz V, Roe TF, Mora S, Costin G, Goodman WG. Changes in vertebral bone density in black girls and white girls during childhood and puberty. *N Engl J Med*. 1991;325(23):1597–1600
35. Cromer BA, Binkovitz L, Ziegler J, Harvey R, Debanne SM. Reference values for bone mineral density in 12 to 18 year old girls categorized by weight, race, and age. *Pediatr Radiol*. 2004;34(10):787–792
36. Bell NH, Greene A, Epstein S, Oexmann MJ, Shaw S, Shary J. Evidence for alteration of the vitamin D-endocrine system in blacks. *J Clin Invest*. 1985;76(2):470–473

37. Meier DE, Luckey MM, Wallenstein S, Clemens TL, Orwoll ES, Waslien CI. Calcium, vitamin D, and parathyroid hormone status in young white and black women: association with racial differences in bone mass. *J Clin Endocrinol Metab.* 1991;72(3):703–710
38. Sowers MF, School T, Harris L, Jannausch M. Bone loss in adolescent and adult pregnant women. *Obstet Gynecol.* 2000;96(2):189–193
39. Karlsson C, Obrant KJ, Karlsson M. Pregnancy and lactation confer reversible bone loss in humans. *Osteoporos Int.* 2001;12(10):828–834
40. Pearson D, Kaur M, San P, Lawson N, Baker P, Hosking D. Recovery of pregnancy mediated bone loss during lactation. *Bone.* 2004;34(3):570–578
41. Southard RN, Morris JD, Mahan JD, Hayes JR, Torch MA, Sommer A, Zipf WB. Bone mass in healthy children: measurement with quantitative DXA. *Radiology.* 1991;179(3):735–738
42. Leonard MB, Shults J, Wilson BA, Tershakovec AM, Zemel BS. Obesity during childhood and adolescence augments bone mass and bone dimensions. *Am J Clin Nutr.* 2004;80(2):514–523
43. Klein KO, Larmore KA, de Lancey E, Brown JM, Considine RV, Hassink SG. Effect of obesity on estradiol level, and its relationship to leptin, bone maturation, and bone mineral density in children. *J Clin Endocrinol Metab.* 1998;83(10):3469–3475
44. Mølgaard C, Thomsen BL, Michaelsen KF. Whole body bone mineral accretion in healthy children and adolescents. *Arch Dis Child.* 1999;81(1):10–15
45. Power ML, Heaney RP, Kalkwarf HJ, et al. The role of calcium in health and disease. *Am J Obstet Gynecol.* 1999;181(6):1560–1569
46. Jackman LA, Millane SS, Martin BR, et al. Calcium retention in relation to calcium intake and postmenarchal age in adolescent females. *Am J Clin Nutr.* 1997;66(2):327–333
47. Institute of Medicine, Standing Committee on the Scientific Evaluation of Dietary Reference Intakes, Food and Nutrition Board. *Dietary Reference Intakes for Calcium, Phosphorus, Magnesium, Vitamin D, and Fluoride.* Washington, DC: National Academy Press; 1997
48. Matković V, Kostial K, Simonović I, Buzina R, Brodarec A, Nordin BE. Bone status and fracture rates in two regions of Yugoslavia. *Am J Clin Nutr.* 1979;32(3):540–549
49. Sandler RB, Slemanda CW, LaPorte RE, et al. Postmenopausal bone density and milk consumption in childhood and adolescence. *Am J Clin Nutr.* 1985;42(2):270–274
50. Matkovic V, Fontana D, Tominac C, Goel P, Chesnut CH. Factors that influence peak bone mass formation: a study of calcium balance and the inheritance of bone mass in adolescent females. *Am J Clin Nutr.* 1990;52(5):878–888
51. Teegarden D, Lyle RM, Proulx WR, Johnston CC, Weaver CM. Previous milk consumption is associated with greater bone density in young women. *Am J Clin Nutr.* 1999;69(5):1014–1017
52. Merrilees MJ, Smart EJ, Gilchrist NL, et al. Effects of diary food supplements on bone mineral density in teenage girls. *Eur J Nutr.* 2000;39(6):256–262
53. Johnston CC, Miller JZ, Slemenda CW, et al. Calcium supplementation and increases in bone mineral density in children. *N Engl J Med.* 1992;327(2):82–87
54. Lloyd T, Martel JK, Rollings N, et al. The effect of calcium supplementation and Tanner stage on bone density, content and area in teenage women. *Osteoporos Int.* 1996;6(4):276–283
55. Stear SJ, Prentice A, Jones SC, Cole TJ. Effect of a calcium and exercise intervention on the bone mineral status of 16–18-y-old adolescent girls. *Am J Clin Nutr.* 2003;77(4):985–992
56. Prentice A, Ginty F, Stear SJ, Jones SC, Laskey MA, Cole TJ. Calcium supplementation increases stature and bone mineral mass of 16- to 18-year-old boys. *J Clin Endocrinol Metab.* 2005;90(6):3153–3161
57. Matkovic V, Heaney RP. Calcium balance during human growth: evidence for threshold behavior. *Am J Clin Nutr.* 1992;55(5):992–996
58. Harel Z, Riggs S, Vaz R, White L, Menzies G. Adolescents and calcium: what they do and do not know and how much they consume. *J Adolesc Health.* 1998;22(3):225–228
59. Winzenberg T, Shaw K, Fryer J, Jones G. Effects of calcium supplementation on bone density in healthy children: meta-analysis of randomised controlled trials. *BMJ.* 2006;333(7572):775–780
60. Barzel US, Massey LK. Excess dietary protein can adversely affect bone. *J Nutr.* 1998;128(6):1051–1053

61. Heaney RP. Excess dietary protein may not adversely affect bone. *J Nutr*. 1998;128(6):1054–1057
62. Hollis BW. Assessment of vitamin D nutritional and hormonal status: what to measure and how to do it. *Calcif Tissue Int*. 1996;58(1):4–5
63. Docio S, Riancho JA, Pérez A, Olmos JM, Amado JA, González-Macías J. Seasonal deficiency of vitamin D in children: a potential target for osteoporosis-preventing strategies? *J Bone Miner Res*. 1998;13(4):544–548
64. Malabanan A, Veronikis IE, Holick MF. Redefining vitamin D insufficiency. *Lancet*. 1998; 351(9105):805–806
65. Weaver CM, Fleet JC. Vitamin D requirements: current and future. *Am J Clin Nutr*. 2004;80(6 suppl):1735S–1739S
66. Gordon CM, DePeter KC, Feldman HA, Grace E, Emans SJ. Prevalence of vitamin D deficiency among healthy adolescents. *Arch Pediatr Adolesc Med*. 2004;158(6):531–537
67. Harkness LS, Cromer BA. Vitamin D deficiency in adolescent females. *J Adolesc Health*. 2005;37(1):75
68. Lehtonen-Veromaa MKM, Mottonen TT, Nuotio IO, Irjala KM, Leino AE, Viikari JS. Vitamin D and attainment of peak bone mass among peripubertal Finnish girls: a 3-y prospective study. *Am J Clin Nutr*. 2002;76(6):1446–1453
69. Gartner LM, Greer FR; American Academy of Pediatrics, Section on Breastfeeding and Committee on Nutrition. Prevention of rickets and vitamin D deficiency: new guidelines for vitamin D intake. *Pediatrics*. 2003;111(4 pt 1):908–910
70. Sojka JE, Weaver CM. Magnesium supplementation and osteoporosis. *Nutr Rev*. 1995;53(3): 71–74
71. Zive MM, Nicklas TA, Busch EC, Myers L, Berenson GS. Marginal vitamin and mineral intakes of young adults: the Bogalusa Heart Study. *J Adolesc Health*. 1996;19(1):39–47
72. Vermeer C, Gijsbers BL, Crăcium AM, Groenen-van Dooren MM, Knapen MH. Effects of vitamin K on bone mass and bone metabolism. *J Nutr*. 1996;126(4 suppl):1187S–1191S
73. Vermeer C, Knapen MH, Schurgers LJ. Vitamin K and metabolic bone disease. *J Clin Pathol*. 1998;51(6):424–426
74. Knapen MHJ, Jie KSG, Hamulyak K, Vermeer C. Vitamin K-induced changes in markers for osteoblast activity and urinary calcium loss. *Calcif Tissue Int*. 1993;53(2):81–85
75. Tham DM, Gardner CD, Haskell WL. Clinical review 97: potential health benefits of dietary phytoestrogens—a review of the clinical, epidemiological, and mechanistic evidence. *J Clin Endocrinol Metab*. 1998;83(7):2223–2235
76. Setchell KD, Cassidy A. Dietary isoflavones: biological effects and relevance to human health. *J Nutr*. 1999;129(3):758S–767S
77. Mühlbauer RC, Li F. Effect of vegetables on bone metabolism. *Nature*. 1999;401(6751):343–344
78. McGartland C, Robson PJ, Murray L, et al. Carbonated soft drink consumption and bone mineral density in adolescence: the Northern Ireland Young Hearts project. *J Bone Miner Res*. 2003;18(9):1563–1569
79. Ilich-Ernst JZ, McKenna AA, Badenhop NE, et al. Iron status, menarche, and calcium supplementation in adolescent girls. *Am J Clin Nutr*. 1998;68(4):880–887
80. McKenna AA, Ilich JZ, Andon MB, Wang C, Matkovic V. Zinc balance in adolescent females consuming a low- or high-calcium diet. *Am J Clin Nutr*. 1997;65(5):1460–1464
81. Sojka J, Wastney M, Abrams S, et al. Magnesium kinetics in adolescent girls determined using stable isotopes: effect of high and low calcium intake. *Am J Physiol*. 1997;273(2 pt 2):R710–R715
82. Matkovic V, Ilich JZ, Andon MB, et al. Urinary calcium, sodium, and bone mass of young females. *Am J Clin Nutr*. 1995;62(2):417–425
83. Bradney M, Pearce G, Naughton G, et al. Moderate exercise during growth in prepubertal boys: changes in bone mass, size, volumetric density, and bone strength: a controlled prospective study. *J Bone Miner Res*. 1998;13(12):1814–1821

84. Taaffe D, Harter-Snow C, Connolly D, Robinson TL, Brown MD, Marcus R. Differential effects of swimming versus weight-bearing activity on bone mineral status of eumenorrheic athletes. *J Bone Miner Res.* 1995;10(4):586–593
85. Nickols-Richardson SM, O'Connor PJ, Shapses SA, Lewis RD. Longitudinal bone mineral density changes in female child artistic gymnasts. *J Bone Miner Res.* 1999;14(6):994–1002
86. Bilanin JE, Blanchard MS, Russek-Cohen E. Lower vertebral bone density in male long-distance runner. *Med Sci Sports Exerc.* 1989;21(1):66–70
87. Wheeler GD, Wall SR, Belcastro AN, Cumming DC. Reduced serum testosterone and prolactin levels in male distance runners. *JAMA.* 1984;252(4):514–516
88. Luger A, Deuster P, Kyle S, et al. Acute hypothalamic-pituitary-adrenal responses to the stress of treadmill exercise: physiologic adaptations to physical training. *N Engl J Med.* 1987;316(21): 1309–1315
89. De Crée C. Endogenous opioid peptides in the control of the normal menstrual cycle and their possible role in athletic menstrual irregularities. *Obstet Gynecol Surv.* 1989;44(10):720–732
90. Klesges RC, Ward KD, Shelton ML, et al. Changes in bone mineral content in male athletes: mechanisms of action and intervention effects. *JAMA.* 1996;276(3):226–230
91. Law MR, Hackshaw AK. A meta-analysis of cigarette smoking, bone mineral density and risk of hip fracture: recognition of a major effect. *BMJ.* 1997;315(7112):841–846
92. Elgán C, Samsioe G, Dykes AK. Influence of smoking and oral contraceptives on bone mineral density and bone remodeling in young women: a 2-year study. *Contraception.* 2003;67(6):439–447
93. Lorentzon M, Mellström D, Haug E, Ohlsson C. Smoking is associated with lower bone mineral density and reduced cortical thickness in young men. *J Clin Endocrinol Metab.* 2007;92(2): 497–503
94. Clark MK, Sowers MF, Dekordi F, Nichols S. Bone mineral density and fractures among alcohol-dependent women in treatment and in recovery. *Osteoporos Int.* 2003;14(5):396–403
95. Ljunghall S, Lindh E, Johansson AG. Endocrine interactions of insulin-like growth factor I on bone. *Acta Paediatr Supp*l. 1994;399:178–179
96. Rosen CJ, Donahue LR, Hunter SJ. Insulin-like growth factors and bone: the osteoporosis connection. *Proc Soc Exp Biol Med.* 1994;206(2):83–102
97. Hughes DE, Dai A, Tiffee JC, Li HH, Mundy GR, Boyce BF. Estrogen promotes apoptosis of murine osteoclasts mediated by TGF-B. *Nat Med.* 1996;2(10):1132–1136
98. Riggs BL, Khosla S, Melton LJ. Sex steroids and the construction and conservation of the adult skeleton. *Endocr Rev.* 2002;23(3):279–302
99. Prior JC. Progesterone as a bone-trophic hormone. *Endocr Rev.* 1990;11(2):386–398
100. Gallagher JC, Kable WT, Goldgar D. Effect of progestin therapy on cortical and trabecular bone: comparison with estrogen. *Am J Med.* 1991;90(2):171–178
101. Prior JC, Vigna YM, Barr SI, Rexworthy C, Lentle BC. Cyclic medroxyprogesterone treatment increases bone density. *Am J Med.* 1994;96(6):521–530
102. Cromer BA, Blair JM, Mahan JD, Zibners L, Naumovski Z. A prospective comparison of bone density in adolescent girls receiving depot medroxyprogesterone acetate (Depo Provera), levonorgestrel (Norplant), or oral contraceptives. *J Pediatr.* 1996;129(5):671–676
103. Busen NH, Britt RB, Rianon N. Bone mineral density in a cohort of adolescent women using depot medroxyprogesterone acetate for one to two years. *J Adolesc Health.* 2003;32(4):257–259
104. Lara-Torre E, Edwards CP, Perlman S, Hertweck SP. Bone mineral density in adolescent females using depot medroxyprogesterone acetate. *J Pediatr Adolesc Gynecol.* 2004;17(1): 17–21
105. Cromer BA, Stager M, Bonny A, et al. Depot medroxyprogesterone acetate, oral contraceptives and bone mineral density in a cohort of adolescent girls. *J Adolesc Health.* 2004;35(6):434–441
106. Scholes D, LaCroix AZ, Ichikawa LE, Barlow WE, Ott SM. Change in bone mineral density among adolescent women using and discontinuing depot medroxyprogesterone acetate contraception. *Arch Pediatr Adolesc Med.* 2005;159(2):139–144

107. Ott SM, Scholes D, LaCroix AZ, Ichikawa LE, Yoshida CK, Barlow WE. Effects of contraceptive use on bone biochemical markers in young women. *J Clin Endocrinol Metab.* 2001; 86(1):179–185

108. Rome E, Ziegler J, Secic M, et al. Bone biochemical markers in adolescent girls using either depot medroxyprogesterone acetate or an oral contraceptive. *J Pediatr Adolesc Gynecol.* 2004;17(6):373–377

109. Clark MK, Sowers M, Levy BT, Tenhundfeld P. Magnitude and variability of sequential estradiol and progesterone concentrations in women using depot medroxyprogesterone acetate for contraception. *Fertil Steril.* 2001;75(5):871–877

110. Food and Drug Administration. Physician information [Depo-Provera]. Available at: www.fda.gov/medwatch/SAFETY/2004/DepoProvera_Label.pdf. Accessed January 27, 2005

111. Cromer B, Scholes D, Berenson A, et al. Depot medroxyprogesterone acetate and bone mineral density in adolescents:the black box warning—a position paper of the Society for Adolescent Medicine. *J Adolesc Health.* 2006;39(2):296–301

Adolesc Med 19 (2008) 592–596

A

B